LABORATORY MANAGEMENT

Principles and Processes

Third Edition

DENISE M. HARMENING, PH.D., MT(ASCP), CLS(NCA)

*Director of the Online Master of Science Program
in Clinical Laboratory Management*

*Adjunct Professor, Department of Medical Laboratory Science
Rush University
Chicago, Illinois*

D.H. Publishing & Consulting, Inc. WE CREATE SOLUTIONS
St. Petersburg, Florida 33711

Distributed by D.H. Publishing & Consulting, Inc.
www.DHBOOKPUBLISHING.com

Library of Congress Control Number: 2011912075

Publisher: *D.H. Publishing & Consulting, Inc.*

Director of Production and Manufacturing: *Jesse A. Javens*

Production Editor: *Denise M. Harmening*

Cover Design: *Jesse A. Javens*

Editorial Assistant: *Anastasiya O. Sepikova*

Composition: *Bookmasters*

Printing and Binding: *Bookmasters*

Distribution Publishers: *D.H. Publishing & Consulting, Inc.*, 32 Jefferson Court South, St. Petersburg, FL, www.dhbookpublishing.com

 D.H. Publishing & Consulting, Inc.
St. Petersburg, Florida 33711

ISBN: 978-0-943903-12-5

Contents

SECTION I   *Principles of Laboratory Management*

SECTION IV   *Operations*

SECTION V   *Strategies for Career Success*

Dedication

This book is dedicated to my family especially, my husband, who has always supported all of my work and who has encouraged me to fulfill my potential . . . .

And

To all laboratory personnel—past, present, and future—who have touched and will continue to touch the lives of so many students and patients . . . . I also dedicate this book to you in the hope of inspiring an unquenchable thirst for knowledge.

Preface

Currently, there is a great demand for laboratory managers, with a national vacancy rate of 18.6%. The rapidly changing laboratory environment is constantly responding to diverging trends in healthcare. This mandates the requirement for effective management. Laboratory managers will need to create new solutions to today's problems. This book is designed to give a problem-based approach to teaching the principles of laboratory management. The focus is to present underlying managerial concepts and then assist the learner in the successful application of theoretical models to real-life situations. Each chapter begins with an illustrative case to present a management problem followed by thought-provoking questions to stimulate the learners' critical thinking skills. In addition, each chapter contains an outline and educational objectives that can be used in teaching. Internet and website references permit the learner to acquire advanced and current information in each of the major topic areas. Problem-based learning activities are listed at the end of each chapter to serve as a guide for instruction and reinforcement of the content presented. Twenty chapters are divided into five major areas of management: Principles of Laboratory Management, Human Resource Management, Financial Management, Operations, and Strategies for Career Success. Unique to this book are chapters on Quality Management in the Laboratory, Education and Training, the Cost of Quality, Ethical Issues in Laboratory Management, and a chapter on Career Planning. Summary charts of important items to know for each chapter and a glossary of key terms facilitate the learning process.

The Author and contributors of *Laboratory Management: Principles and Processes, Third Edition* present detailed management and educational information along with real-life problem-based learning activities designed to engage learners by assuming managerial roles. Learners are encouraged to use these problem-based activities not only to review knowledge presented in this text, but also to gain further knowledge related to the management and educational aspects of laboratory science. I would like to acknowledge and thank my husband, Jesse A. Javens, for his contribution, dedication and support of this book. I would also like to thank Anastasiya O. Sepikova, who served as the project manager and dedicated many hours of devotion to making this third edition a reality.

Denise M. Harmening, Ph.D., MT(ASCP), CLS(NCA)

Contributors

Matthew M. Anderson, MS
Manager of Business Affairs
College of Health Sciences
Rush University
Chicago, Illinois

Lani Barovick, MS
Associate VP of Human Resource
Services
Office of Administration and Finance
Baltimore University of Maryland
Baltimore, Maryland

Lucia M. Berte, MA, MT(ASCP)SBB,
DLM; CQA(ASQ)CMQ/OE
Laboratories Made Better! P.C.
Broomfield, Colorado

Elaine M. Brett, MS, MT(ASCP)
Performance Development Consultant
EMB Associates
Bowie, Maryland

Sandra S. Brown, MBA, MT(ASCP)
Laboratory Manager
Maryland Heights, Missouri

Marie A. Cato, MBA, MT(ASCP)
Vice President of Operations, Wisconsin
Aurora Consolidated Laboratories, Inc.
West Allis, Wisconsin

George M. Chuzi, ESQ
Law Offices
Kalijarvi, Chuzi & Newman, P.C.
Washington, D.C.

Joseph J. Collins, MS, CPA
Washington Township, New Jersey

Susan L. Conforti, EdD, MT(ASCP)SBB
Medical Laboratory Technology
Farmingdale State College
Farmingdale, New York

Jill Dennis, MEd, MLS
Chair of Math and Science
CLS Program Director
Associate Dean of Academic Operations
Thomas University
Thomasville, Georgia

Jeanne M. Donnelly, MBA, RHIA
Assistant Professor, Department of
Health Information Management
Saint Louis University
Saint Louis, Missouri

Sharon S. Ehrmeyer, PhD, MT(ASCP)
Director, Clinical Laboratory Science/
Medical Technology Program
Professor, Department of Pathology
and Laboratory Medicine
University of Wisconsin Medical School
Madison, Wisconsin

Vicki S. Freeman, PhD, MLS^{CM}
(ASCP)SC
Chair and Professor, Department of
Clinical Laboratory Sciences
School of Allied Health Services
University of Texas Medical Branch
Galveston, Texas

Heather J. Hall, MBA, MT(ASCP), CG(ASCP)^{CM}
Instructor, Medical Laboratory Sciences Department of Chemistry and Biochemistry
South Dakota State University
Brookings, South Dakota

Janet S. Hall, MS, CC(NRCC)
Associate Administrator
Laboratories of Pathology
Outreach Referral and Business Services
University of Maryland Medical Center
Baltimore, Maryland

Denise M. Harmening, PhD, MT(ASCP), CLS(NCA)
Director, Online MS Program in Clinical Laboratory Management
Adjunct Professor, Department Medical Laboratory Science
Rush University
Chicago, Illinois

Jan R. Heier, DBA, CPA
Professor, Department of Accounting and Finance,
Auburn University Montgomery
Montgomery, Alabama

Ellen Hope Kearns, PhD, SH(ASCP), MASCP
President, HOPE for Healthcare Professionals International
Huntington Beach, California

Michael E. Kurtz, MS, MBA
Laboratory Administration/Marketing Manager, Clinical Laboratories
Saint Louis University Hospital
Saint Louis, Missouri

Paul Labbe, NMT, MCLT
V.P. Operations
CompuNet Clinical Laboratories
Dayton, Ohio

Randall S. Lambrecht, PhD, MT(ASCP), CLS(NCA)
Vice President, Research and Academic Relations, Aurora Health Care,
Aurora Sinai Medical Center
Milwaukee, Wisconsin

Irina Lutinger, MPH, H(ASCP), DLM
Senior Administrator-Director of Laboratories
New York University Medical Center
New York, New York

Kelly L. McLeay, RN, MSN
MSICU/NSU Nurse Manager
Morton Plant Hospital
Clearwater, Florida

David W. Matear, PhD, DDPH, MSc
President
Solumedix Management Consultancy, LLC
Al Ain, United Arab Emirates

Christine Pitocco, MS, MT(ASCP)BB
Clinical Assistant Professor
Clinical Laboratory Science Program
School of Health Technology and Management,
Stony Brook University
Stony Brook, New York

Dale C. Scutro, BS, MT(AMT)
Laboratory Manager,
Morton Plant Hospital,
Clearwater, Florida

Jane R. Semler, MS, MT(ASCP)
Assistant Professor, Medical Technology
Department of Allied Health Sciences
Austin Peay State University
Clarksville, Tennessee

Anastasiya O. Sepikova, BA
Project Manager and Editorial Assistant
D.H. Publishing & Consulting, Inc.
Saint Petersburg, Florida

Adil E. Shamoo, PhD, CIP
President and CEO
Human Research Technologies
Editor-in-Chief,
Accountability in Research
Baltimore, Maryland

Amber G. Tuten, MEd, MLS(ASCP)^{CM},
DLM(ASCP)^{CM}
CLS Program Director
Assistant Professor of CLS
and Chemistry
Thomas University
Thomasville, Georgia

Christine V. Walters, MAS, JD,
SPHR
Independent Consultant
Glyndon, Maryland

Joseph J. Wawrzynski, Jr., MBA, MT
(ASCP)BB, DLM^{CM}, CQA(ASQ)CQIA
Administrative Director
Clinical Laboratory Services
Methodist Division
Thomas Jefferson University Hospital
Philadelphia, Pennsylvania

Principles of Laboratory Management

In order for laboratory managers to be effective on the job, they must not only be technically competent in their specific area(s) of laboratory medicine but also familiar with the nontechnical side of management. This "other side" includes all of the topics addressed in this text. For ease of learning, these topics are combined into five sections as noted in the table of contents and the introduction of each section.

Section I introduces the learner to quality management in the laboratory, the global concept of organizational structure followed by specific discussions of leadership, management functions, and managerial problem solving, decision making, and process improvement. As one might imagine, some of the issues discussed in this section are appropriately brought out in more than one chapter where they best apply.

Section I Contents:

1

CHAPTER 1

Quality Management in the Medical Laboratory

Lucia M. Berte, MA, MT(ASCP)SBB, DLM; CQA(ASQ)CMQ/OE

OBJECTIVES

Following successful completion of this chapter, the learner will be able to:

1. Explain the relationship between the three levels of quality.
2. Describe the difference between compliance and quality management.
3. Describe the framework of a quality management system for the medical laboratory.
4. List 12 quality management system (QMS) essentials and the laboratory operations to which they are applied.
5. Use a flowchart to describe a process.
6. State the role of validation in introducing a new process.
7. Name at least five laboratory process controls.
8. Describe the difference between a form and a record.
9. Explain the importance of document control for procedures.

3

10. State the difference between remedial and corrective action.
11. Describe the role of auditing in a QMS.
12. Identify at least six sources of input for helping processes improve.
13. Define the activities in a problem-solving process.

KEY TERMS

Accreditation Standards
Analytic Activity
Compliance
Continual Improvement
Corrective Action
Document Control
Flowchart
Information Management
Internal Audit
Management Review
Nonconformance
Opportunities for Improvement
Path of Workflow
Postanalytic Activity
Preanalytic Activity

Procedure
Process
Process Control
Proficiency Testing (PT)
Quality
Quality Assurance (QA)
Quality Control (QC)
Quality Indicators
Quality Management (QM)
Quality Management System (QMS)
Quality System Essentials (QSEs)
Records
Regulatory Requirements
Remedial Action
Validation

Case Study   Fundamentals of Quality Management

You've become the manager of a community hospital laboratory shortly after the previous manager was terminated because of deficiencies in laboratory accreditation assessments and no documented plan for quality. Upon review of previous accreditation assessment reports, you discover several instances of deficiencies repeated from cycle to cycle despite the laboratory's documented responses of "corrective actions." Your review of the laboratory's administrative manual reveals no logical organization and a lot of missing information that, if present, would have alleviated many of the deficiencies. You've been asked to ensure significant improvement on the laboratory's next accreditation assessment 18 months away.

Issues and Questions to Consider:

1. *What is the laboratory's path of workflow?*
2. *What are the levels of laboratory quality?*
3. *How are compliance and quality management different?*
4. *What are the generic quality management fundamentals for any laboratory?*
5. *What is the link between laboratory quality management and patient safety?*
6. *How can a laboratory administrative manual be organized to promote quality management?*

INTRODUCTION

Several dictionaries define **quality** as "the degree to which a product or service meets requirements." Laboratories need to provide quality to their customers in many forms, most importantly the following:

- Safe, comfortable phlebotomy experiences provided to all patients.
- Properly collected and labeled specimens provided for testing.
- Timely, accurate test results and reports provided to physicians and other health care personnel.
- Informative and helpful consultations and answers to questions.

To best meet **regulatory** and **accreditation** requirements, the laboratory needs to bring a quality philosophy into all its activities. The best quality philosophy that provides a high degree of assurance of meeting regulatory, accreditation, and customer requirements includes these three perspectives:

- Quality, safety, and effectiveness are built into a product.
- Quality cannot be inspected or tested into a product.
- Each step in the process must be controlled to meet quality standards.[1]

THE LABORATORY'S PATH OF WORKFLOW

The laboratory's **path of workflow** is the core business in transforming a test order into the results report. The path of workflow is a sequence of processes that begins with the input of the clinician's ordering of a test through the activities of sample collection, sample transport, sample receiving and accessioning, testing, review, report preparation, and report delivery and ends with the output of accurate test results and interpretations back to the clinician. It's important to recognize that the laboratory does not perform or control some of these processes. For example, test ordering is usually done by health care professionals authorized to order laboratory testing. Also, the laboratory does not collect all samples to be tested or examined; surgeons remove tissues and organs during surgery; gynecologists collect samples for Pap smears; and nurses collect non-blood samples such as wound swabs and urine specimens, as well as blood samples from patients' central infusion lines. Whether or not the laboratory has control over or performs activities in the path of workflow, these activities still need to be performed correctly every time to ensure accurate results in a timely manner for patient care. Figure 1-1 depicts the sequence of activities in the laboratory's path of workflow. This sequence has been shown to be true for any size, scope, or specialty laboratory, anywhere in the world.[3]

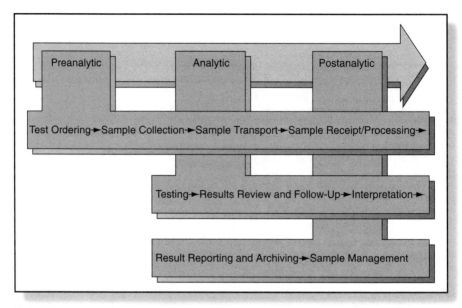

FIGURE 1-1. Laboratory Path of Workflow

QUALITY AS A TARGET

The method previously mentioned for bringing the quality philosophy into the laboratory's workflow is to understand and develop the aspects of quality, which are **quality control (QC), quality assurance (QA),** and **quality management system (QMS).** When these quality aspects are properly implemented and the facility's management and staff are actively involved in monitoring and maintaining the QMS, true quality management has been achieved. Figure 1-2 demonstrates these aspects of quality and their internationally accepted definitions.[2]

Quality Control (QC)

It is useful to think of laboratory quality as a target—such as those used for archery or shooting practice. Quality control is the innermost circle of the target because the target for each and every laboratory test is accurate results. Quality control (QC) provides a high degree of confidence that testing and examination results are accurate for the batch of samples being tested or examined at that time. QC is method control; samples with known expected results are tested before or along with patient samples. When the expected QC results are obtained it can be said that all the patient samples' unknown results obtained within defined QC time periods (e.g., each sample, batch, shift, daily, weekly, etc.) are likely to be accurate. However, QC neither implies nor verifies that those accurate results necessarily belong to the patient whose name is on the sample! All the QC ever performed in the past or into the future will *never* prevent a patient misidentification or a

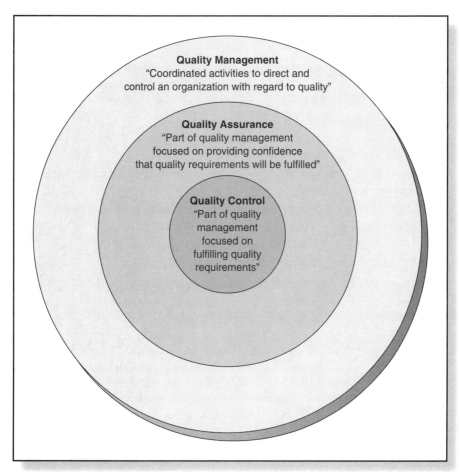

FIGURE 1-2. **Levels of Quality**

sample switch. In the laboratory's **preanalytic, analytic, and postanalytic activities**, QC hits only the target's center—the analytic methods.

Requirements for the type and frequency of QC are specified in regulations, **accreditation standards**, manufacturers' operator manuals, package inserts, and by state and local authorities. Regular performance of QC reveals when a method, piece of equipment, or procedure is not working as expected.

Quality Assurance (QA)

Quality assurance (QA) is the next outer ring of the target. QA is a set of planned actions to provide confidence that processes other than testing that influence the quality of the laboratory's results and reports are working as expected, individually and collectively.[2] QA answers the question, "How does the laboratory know it is delivering a high quality service to its customers?" This is a very different question from whether laboratory test results are accurate. In QA, the laboratory measures its contributions to patient care by answering questions such as these:

- From how many patients did a phlebotomist attempt to collect a blood sample only to find that the patient was not wearing proper identification?
- How many samples are not acceptable upon receipt into the laboratory and from which locations do they come?
- How well does the collection time of the sample reflect the administration time of a therapeutic drug?
- How timely are laboratory results compared with physician, nurse, and patient needs?
- How many times did the laboratory have to notify clinicians about corrections to released results found to be erroneous?
- How do the laboratory's results compare with those of other laboratories for the same analytic method or instrument?
- How well do final interpretations correspond to frozen section diagnoses?
- How well do interpretations from fine needle aspiration biopsies correlate with interpretations from the tissue biopsy?

These questions—and many more that could and should be asked—measure the effects of activities in the laboratory's preanalytic, analytic, and postanalytic processes well beyond method control. QA looks beyond the performance of just the test method or piece of equipment to assess how well the laboratory's entire workflow is functioning. This is particularly important in processes that cross over functional or departmental lines. Therefore, QA is bigger than QC and covers all the preanalytic, analytic, and postanalytic processes. Table 1-1 lists common QC and QA activities practiced by most laboratories.

Quality Management System (QMS)

A quality management system (QMS) is the outermost ring of the target, which encompasses all the management activities needed to ensure that the laboratory's workflow proceeds smoothly to provide laboratory services to customers and patients. All the management activities described in this entire textbook—such as meeting design and safety requirements for the laboratory's physical facilities; staff training and competence assessment; equipment management; procuring, storing and managing reagents and supplies; and creating, approving, revising and controlling the laboratory's documents and records—support the laboratory's ability to meet regulatory and accreditation requirements and fulfill the need for accurate results in a timely manner. A model for a generic quality management system that meets all the requirements of U.S. laboratory regulatory and accreditation organizations has been published by the Clinical and Laboratory Standards Institute (CLSI) in a guideline that describes how to use 12 **Quality System Essentials (QSEs)** as a means to organize all the policies, processes, and procedures that any laboratory needs to meet those requirements.[3]

TABLE 1-1. **Common Laboratory QC Activities and QA Indicators**

QC Activities	QA Indicators
Test Methods	• Number and source of improper test requests
• Testing of reagents, stains, and kits with samples of known values (e.g., reactive vs. nonreactive; abnormal vs. normal values; growth vs. no growth, etc.)	• Number of test requests with incomplete or incorrect information
• Point-of-Care testing instruments	• Number and location of patients without proper identification at time of specimen collection or transfusion
• Automated testing systems	
Laboratory Equipment	• Number of, source of, and reasons for unacceptable specimens
• Refrigerators	• Number of and reasons for incomplete testing (e.g., analyzer failures, method problems, technical problems)
• Freezers	
• Heating instruments	
• Incubators, all types	• Number of and reasons for invalid test results (e.g., QC failures, calibration failure, etc.)
• Water baths	
• Thawing devices	
• pH meters	• Number of and reasons for turnaround time failures
• Weighing scales	
• Centrifuges, all types	• Number of times that incorrect results were reported and had to be called back and corrected (i.e., reporting error)
• Cell washers	
• Blood irradiators	
• Blood warmers	• Number of and reasons for re-sent reports
• Shipping containers	

A QMS includes both QC and QA, as well as the management activities described above—and more—necessary to make your laboratory's best contribution to patient care.

Organizations that license and accredit medical laboratories have established their quality requirements to be more comprehensive and more coordinated than either QC or QA alone. A QMS provides a framework for building quality principles and practices into *all* laboratory operations, starting with test ordering and proceeding through delivery of test reports.

Figure 1-3 demonstrates that the QMS essentials are the foundational building blocks that support the laboratory's preanalytic, analytic, and postanalytic workflow for all types, sizes, specialties, and scopes of laboratories.

COMPLIANCE WITH REQUIREMENTS VERSUS QUALITY MANAGEMENT

Compliance with federal regulations and accreditation standards for medical laboratories is required by the following organizations:

- Centers for Medicare and Medicaid Services (CMS)[4]
- Occupational Safety and Health Administration (OSHA)[5]

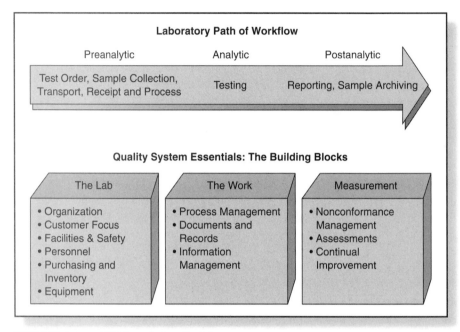

FIGURE 1-3.   QMS Foundation Model

- Food and Drug Administration (FDA)[6,7]
- The Joint Commission (TJC)[8,9]
- College of American Pathologists (CAP)[10]
- Commission on Laboratory Assessment (COLA)[11]
- American Association of Blood Banks (AABB)[12]

Laboratories need to comply with all applicable requirements to maintain licensure and accreditation. Compliance inspections (also called surveys or assessments) measure the state of the laboratory's program with respect to the applicable requirements at a single point in time and are usually conducted every 1 to 2 years. Through observation and detection of errors, deficiencies, and deviations, the inspections evaluate how effectively the laboratory meets the requirements. Although this process may seem logical, compliance programs alone are inadequate to find and prioritize a laboratory's problems. Compliance simply requires the correction of identified deviations and deficiencies and usually leaves the laboratory with the false sense that it has solved its problems and has been brought into compliance. However, subsequent inspections often reveal the same deviations and deficiencies, because the laboratory's current QC and QA programs neither identify nor correct fundamental quality problems. Remember that quality cannot be inspected into a process because regulatory and accreditation inspections only find deviations and deficiencies *after* they occurred. Laboratories need to design work processes in a way that *prevents* deficiencies and errors from occurring in the first place. A philosophy of prevention provides for the best economic use of the laboratory's limited resources and also helps ensure that activities are performed correctly the first time.

Whereas participation in compliance inspections is a periodic activity, **quality management (QM)** is actively and continuously practiced by the laboratory's medical and administrative leaders, managers, and staff throughout all laboratory operations all the time. This is an important distinction because with QM, the laboratory is always ready for an inspection through validating that processes work as intended before implementation; monitoring process performance; knowing where the problems are; continuously determining root causes of problems and removing them; and documenting the actions taken. In QM organizations, quality is everyone's job all the time. For QM organizations, quality is not something done in addition to one's job or in preparation for an inspection—it's *built into* the job! Laboratory professionals are well advised to adopt this statement as a personal philosophy to make their best professional contributions to patient care and safety.

QUALITY MANAGEMENT SYSTEM (QMS) ESSENTIALS

The QMS essentials are in a logical order that be explained as follows for any new or changed laboratory test or service. The laboratory *Organization* develops its mission, vision, values, goals, and objectives around the tests and services it plans to offer and whether those services are for physicians, nurses, and patients, such as in a hospital or physician office laboratory setting, or to other laboratories, as in a referral laboratory setting. The laboratory should have a *Customer Focus* by determining the needs and expectations of its various customers and designing its processes and procedures to meet those needs as well as meet all applicable regulatory and accreditation requirements. The laboratory needs to have adequate physical *Facilities* to support the testing and services offered and ensure that all applicable *Safety* requirements are met. The laboratory determines the qualifications needed for each job and hires qualified *Personnel* who are trained and maintain competence in their assigned work processes and procedures. Equipment, reagents, and materials need to be *Purchased* and adequate stores maintained in *Inventory*. The laboratory needs an *Equipment Management* plan that meets manufacturer's, regulatory, and accreditation requirements. Before any work can commence, the laboratory needs to design, document, and validate preanalytic, analytic, and postanalytic *Processes* with appropriate *Management* and control to ensure their correct performance. *Documents* provide instructions for work processes and procedures; performing the procedures generates *Records* of work performance. Patient *Information* is *Managed* in a way to ensure confidentiality, information integrity, and appropriate information access. The process of capturing particulars of *Nonconformances* is *Managed* to identify recurring process problems that can affect patient safety, laboratory credibility, and the operating budget. Internal and external *Assessments* measure and monitor the laboratory's performance to identify opportunities for improvement. The facility should constantly strive for **Continual Improvement**.

The discussion of each Quality System Essential (QSE) in the following sections summarizes key regulatory and accreditation requirements for that QSE; however, the requirements described are not all-inclusive. Laboratories need to maintain the communication resources that will alert them to current, new, and changed requirements.

Organization

The type and size of the laboratory determine the configuration of the laboratory's QMS. In hospitals, laboratory systems, and large referral laboratories there is usually an organization-wide quality function or department that prioritizes and coordinates quality projects, approves resources, and receives reports and information from all departments. The laboratory needs to participate in laboratory-wide quality initiatives, organizational quality-related activities, and the organization's continual improvement program. The laboratory should state in writing its policies, goals, and objectives for each of the QMS essentials and relate them to the bigger organization's quality goals.

The organization of the laboratory needs to be described—usually depicted in an organization chart—showing:

- relationships among laboratory personnel by job title;
- the laboratory's link to the hospital or parent organization; and
- how the laboratory links to the organization's quality function.

The laboratory may choose to have a quality council represented by management and staff from the various laboratory sections that provides quality-related input to the laboratory's top management. The council develops the laboratory's QMS policies, goals, and objectives to support laboratory and larger organization initiatives; develops the processes for QMS implementation; recommends resources needed for support; recommends identified improvement projects for prioritization by management; and supports cross-functional process improvements. There may also be a quality steering committee composed of senior managers and department staff who operationalize the quality objectives and strategies and implement process improvements.

Customer Focus

Although the laboratory toils on behalf of patients, the real customer is the entity or person that receives and must be satisfied with a product or service. For laboratories, the customers are the physicians and nurses, who want accurate timely results for the laboratory tests and examinations they order, and patients, who want a safe and comfortable phlebotomy experience. For all types of laboratories, internal customers are the laboratory employees themselves. For example, the staff who perform testing and examinations are the direct customers of the staff who receive and accession samples into the laboratory's information system.

Having a customer focus means understanding the customer's expectations and designing the laboratory's workflow to meet those expectations. In the examples given above, the laboratory needs to design laboratory processes to provide accurate results in a timely manner to physicians and nurses; provide a timely, safe, and comfortable phlebotomy experience for patients; and deliver to the testing staff acceptable samples that have accurate patient identification and accession numbers. In addition to fulfilling customer expectations, the processes and procedures must also meet regulatory and accreditation requirements.

Facilities and Safety

The laboratory's allocated space should be designed to provide for efficient workflow and effective ergonomics. All regulatory, accreditation, and larger organization requirements for current and planned space need to be met. Sample collection areas need to consider accommodations for disabled patients, comfort, privacy, and safety, in addition to optimizing collection conditions. Effective separation is needed between adjacent laboratory sections when there are incompatibilities or the chance of cross-contamination. Examples include a quiet, interruption-free workspace for cytology screening, a contamination-free area for molecular testing, and temperature control for computer systems.

In hospitals, the TJC mandates an environmental control program that addresses all significant environmental issues for facility management and maintenance such as temperature control, electrical safety, fire protection, and so forth.[8] The CMS and TJC require that hospital laboratories have training programs for all laboratory personnel on emergency preparedness, chemical hygiene, and infection control.[4,9] In addition, any blood bank that performs irradiation of blood components must also have a radiation safety program and document appropriate radiation training.[12]

Personnel

Quality begins and ends with people. However, a quality problem is seldom an individual employee's fault. Rather, quality problems are almost always due to faulty work processes. All the quality policies, goals, and objectives ever written do not ensure accurate laboratory test results in a timely manner unless laboratory staff know how their job fits into the organization, are trained to perform their respective work processes and procedures, and demonstrate ongoing competence by doing it right the first time, every time. Laboratory management needs to work with the organization's human resources departments to define qualifications for all laboratory jobs and to write job descriptions that include educational qualifications, experience, and federal, state, and local licensing requirements, where applicable, so that qualified persons can be hired. Table 1-2 shows the major types of training that personnel need to receive once they are hired. This training extends significantly beyond just the task specifics of a

TABLE 1-2.   Training for New Employees

Orientation	*Safety Training*
• Organization	• Emergency preparedness
• Department	• Accident reporting
• Section	• Chemical hygiene program
	• Hazardous waste disposal program
Quality Training	• Infection control (including
• Quality Management System	universal precautions, bioterrorism)
• Team skills	• Radiation safety, where applicable
• Problem-solving skills	
	Work Processes and Procedures Training
Computer Training	
• Facility information system (e.g., parent organization or hospital)	• Work processes performed on the job
• Department information system (e.g., laboratory)	• Procedures performed
• Personal computers	• New work processes and procedures
• e-mail	• Revised work processes and procedures
• scheduling	
• on-line documentation	*Compliance Training*
	• Medicare necessity requirements
	• Fraud and abuse reporting
	• Concerns about quality and safety

particular job. After the assessment of initial competence after training is concluded, periodic evaluation and documentation of the continuing competence of personnel to perform their assigned job functions and tasks is also required. Competence assessment challenges can include direct observation of job task performance, review of records, and written, verbal, or practical tests.

Purchasing and Inventory

In hospital-based laboratories, contract and purchasing issues are usually handled by the hospital's purchasing department. Laboratory personnel may or may not have control over the specific vendors with which the organization has agreements to purchase reagents and kits for testing, equipment and automated test systems, other important supplies and materials, and blood components. Therefore, the laboratory may need to work with the larger organization's specified processes for selecting vendors of equipment, supplies, and services, and for entering into and amending agreements. At a minimum, all laboratories need to have a process by which incoming supplies are inspected; the performance of those supplies (e.g., reagents and test kits) verified where required; and the supplies and reagents stored according to manufacturer's directions. Due to the very high cost of storing inventory, the laboratory also needs to have effective processes for managing inventories of reagents, supplies, and blood components.

Equipment

The laboratory needs to have a process for installing new equipment and ensuring its proper functioning before use in daily operations. Schedules for calibration and preventive maintenance are required, with frequencies determined by regulations, accreditation requirements, manufacturers' written instructions, usage, testing volume, and equipment reliability. In addition to temperature-controlled equipment (e.g., refrigerators, freezers, incubators), instruments such as automated analyzers, readers, pipettors, and washers—as well as general purpose equipment such as centrifuges and microscopes—also need to be installed and functioning properly before routine use. Defective equipment and instruments must be identified and repaired when necessary. Laboratory records of all installation, calibration, maintenance, use, troubleshooting, service, and repair activities are required to be maintained for the life of the equipment's use and for specified times after decommission.

Process Management

A **process** can be defined as a set of interrelated resources and activities that transforms inputs into outputs. **Process control** is a set of activities that ensures that a given work process will keep operating in a state that is continuously able to meet process goals without compromising the process itself. *Total process control* is the evaluation of the performance of a process, comparison of actual performance to a goal, and action taken on any significant difference. Process control is a means to build quality, safety, and effectiveness into the product or service from the beginning. Table 1-3 lists the important elements of controlling the laboratory's many and varied processes, both technical and non-technical.

The CMS has published its requirements for process control as the current *Clinical Laboratory Improvement Act (CLIA)* amendments that are cited in the Code of Federal Regulations.[4] The CLIA requirements specify that facilities design their processes and procedures to ensure that laboratory results are produced to meet the quality standards appropriate for their intended use. Figure 1-4 is a sequential flow of the elements of total process control.

Process Flowcharting

The best tool for understanding a process is to flowchart it. Flowcharting graphically represents the sequence of activities in a process and shows how the inputs are converted into outputs. Such charts help people develop a common understanding

TABLE 1-3.   Important Elements of Process Control

- Understand and document (e.g., flowchart) the sequence of activities in a process
- Develop and write procedures for the individual process activities
- Validate the entire process to ensure that it works as expected before actual use (to include all equipments, reagents, instruments, documents, and staff)
- Measure process parameters to see that they stay in control
- Understand when and why the process has variations
- Take action to remove unwanted variation

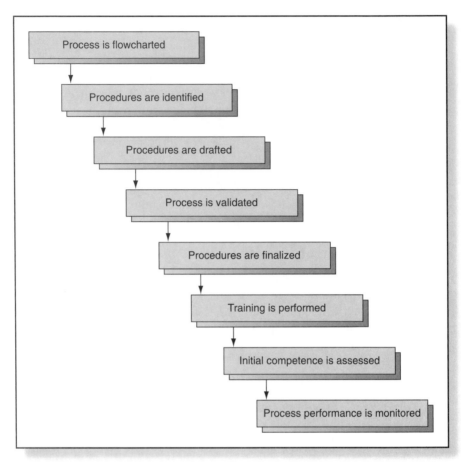

FIGURE 1-4.   TPC Diagram

of a process. Mapping a laboratory's current work processes reveals bottlenecks, missing actions, decision points, dead ends, and choices that can lead to errors, delays, and unnecessary work. Mapping a new process facilitates understanding of where resources will be needed for successful accomplishment. Flowcharting can be done on paper or with commercially available software programs. Figure 1-5 is a generic flowchart for the activities in setting up and performing testing on an automated analyzer. It illustrates different decision points and actions.

Laboratory Procedures

A work process involves one or more persons who perform a defined sequence of activities over a period of time. A process flowchart describes "who does what and when" in a visual manner and provides a big picture of "how it happens." The boxes in the flowchart represent activities performed by one person; these activities need instructions that answer the question, "How do I do this activity?"

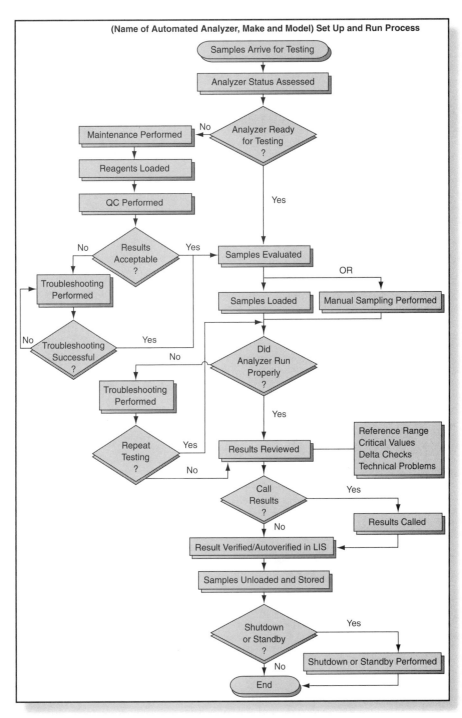

FIGURE 1-5. **Analyzer Set Up Flowchart**

Procedures provide instructions for each activity in the larger process. For example, the process to collect a blood sample involves the defined sequence of greeting the patient; verifying the patient's identity; assessing the patient's condition and vascular access; washing one's hands; assembling the appropriate collection materials for this collection; collecting the sample by venipuncture or capillary puncture; labeling the sample; and preparing the sample for transport to the laboratory. The process activities need to be performed in this sequence to ensure the correct end result—for example, one is *never* to label the samples before identifying the patient! In this process, there needs to be specific written procedures for each of the activities described above. Although some laboratories may combine all this information into one very long document (often called an "SOP"), it benefits both the laboratory and the reader to graphically depict the activities in their correct sequence in a process flowchart and write separate instructions for each activity.

Validation

To ensure that new processes will work as intended, they are required to be validated before being put into use. **Validation** challenges all activities in a new process to provide a high degree of assurance that the process will work as intended in the live environment. For example, when a new blood test for a tumor marker is offered, the entirety of the new testing process—from test order through report delivery—must be validated in each laboratory that will perform the new test. The new test method—with its associated instrument/s, test kits, computer functions, and procedures—must be verified as meeting the manufacturer's functional specifications and the laboratory's intended use. Validating the new testing process ensures that it will perform as expected with that laboratory's workflow, instrumentation, personnel, written procedures, and information systems. The culmination of this validation effort is a defined process and set of new procedures on which all personnel who will collect samples, process samples, and perform the new test need to be trained. Training needs to be documented and personnel competence in the new process and procedures needs to be verified before the new test is implemented in the live environment.

Process Controls

It is essential to monitor a process to ensure that it is performing as required, to correct process problems before they affect output, and to improve processes to meet changing needs and technology. Routine process controls include:

- QC of test methods and reagents;
- reviews of work and QC records; and
- capture of nonconformances when the process did not perform as expected.

These routine process controls monitor whether a process is functioning as needed. **Proficiency testing (PT)** is another example of a process control. In proficiency testing, one laboratory's methods and procedures are compared with those of other laboratories for the ability to get the same results on a set of samples whose values are known only to the PT provider. Regulations require that all laboratories participate in proficiency testing for specified diagnostic laboratory tests.

Other process controls include automated and manual steps to prevent the occurrence of errors. One common process control performed by a laboratory's computerized information system (LIS) is the comparison of a patient's current results to previous results stored in the system (delta checking) to detect any significant differences. The differences may be due to the patient's condition or could also signal a possible sample switch such that the current results do not actually belong to that patient. Another common process control is the manual review of results by a different person who may detect errors or inconsistencies before results are released.

Documents and Records

Documents are approved information contained in a written or electronic format. *Documents* define the QMS for external inspectors and internal staff. Examples of documents include written policies, process flowcharts, procedures/ instructions, forms, manufacturers' package inserts, computer software, instrument operator manuals, and copies of regulations and standards. **Records** capture the results or outcomes of performing procedures and testing in written forms or electronic media such as manual worksheets, instrument printouts, tags, or labels. Both documents and records must be controlled to provide evidence that regulations and standards are being met.

Document Control

A structured **document control** system links a laboratory's policies to respective processes and procedures and ensures that only the latest approved versions of documents are available for use. A typical document control system is structured as a pyramid, as shown in Figure 1-6.

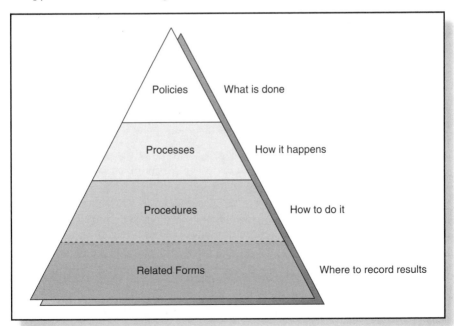

FIGURE 1-6.   **Document Pyramid**

The following example best illustrates how a laboratory should link its policies, processes, and procedures. A laboratory should have a written policy stating that it maintains a process and relevant procedures for correcting erroneous entries or results on paper records or in the computer. A second document (such as a process flowchart) describes the sequence of activities in identifying the need for a correction; obtaining any necessary approvals for the change; making the correction in the computer, on paper, or both; and notifying all appropriate parties of the correction. Third-level procedure documents instruct staff members how to record the need for a correction, how to obtain any necessary approvals for making the change, how to properly record a change to an entry on a paper record, how to properly record a change to an entry in a computer record, and how to notify appropriate parties of the change and document the notification. The process and procedures should be written in a way that ensures that all regulatory and accreditation requirements are met. The records of the actions taken throughout the process provide a tracking mechanism to provide evidence that the requirements were met.

There needs to be a system to control identification, approval, revision, and archiving of a laboratory's policies, process descriptions, procedures, and related forms. The document control system includes: instructions for creating documents in approved formats, assigning document identification and version designation, approving new and revised documents, preparing a master document list, and maintaining document history files. This "change control" process usually requires the completion and routing of a form that contains information about the reason for a new document or changes to an existing one. Other important change information includes when the change was requested; who wants the change; what other documents, if any, are affected by this change; and dates for approval, training, and in-use. A master copy of the new approved version is added to the master document history file, which contains copies of all previous versions of that same document. The hard copies in this master file capture the original signatures and provide a paper backup when electronic files cannot be accessed. The master document list is updated with the new version number. When a revised version of a document is ready to be released, the distribution process needs to be controlled to ensure that copies of the obsolete document (e.g., procedures in a working manual) are replaced with the new version and the obsolete copies destroyed. Laboratory staff should not keep and refer to copies of procedures and forms stashed in lockers, drawers, and personal files. Use of unapproved outdated documents could lead to errors or omissions that could cause harm to patients.

Records Management

Forms are specially designed documents—either paper or electronic—on which are recorded the results or outcomes of performing a given procedure. Forms are also controlled documents. The document system should link the form to its respective procedure. Instructions for completion of forms, when needed, can be conveniently placed on the front or back side of the form. When entries are made into a blank form (either paper or a computer screen), the form becomes a record. Regulations and accreditation requirements mandate the review of records by supervisory personnel and specify the type of records and length of time they need to be stored for possible future reference. State, local, and facility requirements for record retention periods may also apply. Records need to be stored in a manner that allows for access by authorized persons and prevents damage or inadvertent destruction.

Information Management

Whereas documents and records provide information about what to do, how to do it, and what happened when it was done, this quality system essential on information management includes the activities of using, manipulating, and transferring the patient information, test results, and reports in the laboratory's paper and/ or electronic information systems. For example, maintaining the confidentiality of privileged patient information is mandated by government regulations; the laboratory's information handling processes need to ensure that confidentiality is preserved. The laboratory also needs to verify that the integrity of any data or information sent inside or outside the facility is maintained, whether the medium used is paper-based or electronic. For example, the facility needs to verify that the processes for faxing, e-mailing, or sending information across instrument and computer interfaces maintains the original information without adulteration.

Nonconformance Management

Each laboratory needs to have a process for detecting, reporting, evaluating, and correcting deviations and nonconformances in its procedures, products, or services. "Nonconformance management" is one name for such a process. Other commonly used names include occurrence, incident, or variation management. Table 1-4 provides some definitions of terms used to further classify laboratory nonconformances.

Nonconformance Reporting

Information about events involving the laboratory that deviate from accepted policy, process, or procedure needs to be captured and acted upon. Hospitals usually have an organization-wide risk management program in place, but mostly this program captures information about events involving patients and visitors that could result in financial loss. An internal laboratory nonconformance management system captures and analyzes information about nonconformances that occurred across the entire laboratory workflow whether or not a patient was involved.

All employees need to participate in nonconformance reporting. However, it is essential that nonconformance reporting not be perceived by the staff as a tool for finger-pointing or disciplinary action. Instead, all staff needs to understand that nonconformances present information about laboratory processes that do not work as they should and, thus, knowledge of these problems provides opportunities for improvement. Nonconformances may be identified either by staff in the course of routine activities or by supervisors during review of records. Complaints received in the laboratory are also considered nonconformances. The

TABLE 1-4.   Common Classifications of Various Types of Nonconformances

Nonconformance Type	Definition
Accident	Nonconformance generally not attributable to a person's mistake, such as a power outage or an aged instrument's malfunction
Adverse reaction	Complications that occurred to a patient during or after the sample collection process or to a recipient of transfused blood components
Complaint	Expression of dissatisfaction from internal customers (employees) or external customers (physicians, nurses, patients)
Discrepancy	Difference or inconsistency in the outcomes of a process, procedure, or test results
Error	Nonconformance attributable to a human or system problem, such as a problem from failure to follow established procedure or a part of a process that did not work as expected

laboratory needs to capture information about all nonconformances, including those identified before test results were released. In the reporting process, employees describe the "who," "where," and "when" and then briefly describe what happened and what they did at the time to remediate the problem. A standard report form can be used to capture information on all occurrences. The elements of such a form are shown in Table 1-5.

Investigation and Corrective Action
Supervisors and quality function personnel record the nonconformances in a spreadsheet or database so that the resolution process can be tracked. The nonconformances are reviewed, investigated, and could be further classified as to severity of impact to patients and/or whether the nonconformance was discovered before or after test results were released.

The immediate action taken by the person discovering the nonconformance is known as **remedial action** and is the initial quick-fix solution. Remedial actions most often do not address the real cause of the problem, which can be determined only through investigation. Therefore, investigation of complaints or errors provides an opportunity to identify factors that contributed to the problem. Process improvement tools (discussed later in this chapter) are used to identify the contributing factors and to determine the best way to remove them through implementing corrective action.

Most **corrective action** involves making changes in the process. All employees performing that process must then be informed of the change and retrained when necessary. Sometimes the corrective action involves only retraining specific individuals who may not have been adequately trained initially or who have been taking unapproved personal deviations from the established process and/or procedures.

TABLE 1-5. Elements of a Nonconformance Management Report Form

Nonconformance data	• Site of nonconformance (hospital, laboratory, other) • Date and time nonconformance discovered • Person initiating the report • Date and time of initiating the report • Problem identified by (physician, nurse, laboratory, other)
Problem data	• Before testing (preanalytic): sample collection, labeling, transport, data entry, or identification problems or errors • During testing (analytic): delay in testing, incomplete test run due to method or instrument problem, invalid test run (QC or calibration failure) • After testing (postanalytic): critical result not communicated, patient report sent to incorrect location, corrected report, archived sample not found • Other: other equipment problem, computer problem, safety problem, supplies problem, complaint, patient injury
Corrected report information	• Error identified by • Identity of original person entering the result • Identity of person making correction • Explanation of how error was discovered • Copy of pre-error and post-error laboratory report
Remedial (immediate) action taken	• Description of immediate action taken • Identity of person providing immediate action • Date and time of immediate action
Supervisor/Manager investigation and comment	• How/why did this happen? • What changes have been made to prevent recurrence?
Quality function review	• Date and time of entry into database • Identity of person entering into database • Is report completed appropriately? • Has this problem been noted before? If yes, any trends or patterns? • Is a root cause analysis needed? • Is this nonconformance reportable to the FDA?

The **nonconformance** reporting process needs to be clearly defined so that information is tracked and acted upon and feedback is provided. The person responsible for the laboratory's quality function (often called the QA officer or quality manager) reviews all nonconformance reports, assigns each an accession number, and forwards the report to the laboratory areas that will be involved in the investigation. After the investigation, the completed report is returned to the quality officer, who reviews it for completeness and appropriateness of remedial and corrective action. Medical device-related deaths, injuries, and adverse events (e.g., due to problems and failures with laboratory equipment and diagnostic tests) need to be reported to the FDA.[13]

In a good nonconformance management program, the nonconformances are also mapped to the specific involved process(es) in the laboratory's path of workflow. This information is trended to determine which processes have the most problems. The trending information provides significant support for defending when a process needs to be changed. Laboratory staff must make a conscious decision not just to respond to nonconformances with remedial actions but to use nonconformance information to take corrective action to remove the underlying root cause(s) of the problem and to make improvements that truly contribute to the safety and efficacy of the laboratory's services.

Assessments—Internal and External

Internal Assessments

The laboratory needs to have an internal assessment process in place to continuously monitor the effectiveness of its QMS. See Figure 1-3 for a review of the QSEs supporting the laboratory's path of workflow. Both the quality essentials and the laboratory's technical operations need to be assessed. Compliance inspection and other checklists [9–12] can be used; however, they assess the adequacy of only the listed items. The **quality indicators** monitored in the laboratory's QA program are also helpful but do not usually cover all important aspects of the laboratory's path of workflow.

Each laboratory should review all its processes and ask the question, "What can we monitor on a scheduled basis to ensure that this process is working as needed?" Quantitative indicators can then be derived for which the numerator is the number of times the process did or did not work and the denominator is the total number of times the process was performed. Common laboratory examples include the number of specimens received that were not acceptable for testing, the reasons samples were unacceptable and the locations from which they arrived, and the frequency with which the laboratory met its established turnaround times for various testing. Because the laboratory's main service is the provision of test results and reports, a most important indicator that directly affects patient safety is the number of times the laboratory sent out an erroneous result or report that had to be corrected. See Table 1-1 for additional examples of quality indicators.

The best internal assessment tool is the **internal audit** conducted by laboratory staff themselves. Unlike externally delivered compliance inspections, internal audits assess a specific laboratory process and determine, by review of documents and records, conducting interviews, and observing staff in action whether the laboratory is following its own processes and procedures as well as meeting applicable requirements. In a retrospective records audit, for example, a laboratory staff member (auditor) could randomly select a specimen accession number and track through each activity involved in how the specimen was received, accessioned, tested, and results reported. The training and competence assessment records of each laboratory employee involved from collection through results release are reviewed, as are the temperature records for the storage refrigerator(s), the QC records of reagent testing, and the maintenance and calibration records for centrifuges and other instruments used in testing on that specimen. The performance on the proficiency testing most recent to the specimen's receipt is also reviewed. Copies of procedures and forms used at the workstations for all testing and QC are examined to determine whether they are the most current version, according to the master list. A sampling of records is reviewed for inclusion of all required information, interpretations, any necessary follow-up action, and any required supervisory reviews.

When prospective audits are conducted, the auditor watches the staff performing activities in the selected process. The auditor may ask questions of staff members such as, "Were you trained to perform this procedure and, if so, when?" or "Where in the procedure are the instructions for what you just did?" or "Why are you doing [that action]?"

Audits should be conducted by laboratory staff who have been trained to perform audits and identify system problems. Auditors should not audit the laboratory processes and procedures they are responsible for or perform due to the conflict of interest. However, in a small laboratory, there may be insufficient personnel to have a separate quality function, and the supervisor and/or senior personnel may have to perform some auditing activities of staff work and vice versa.

The auditor presents his or her findings to the appropriate management and operations staff at a closing meeting. The auditor may request corrective action for each finding. A process should be in place for the evaluation and review of the audit by management staff to ensure that corrective actions were implemented. Follow-up audits may be necessary to ensure that the corrective action was successful in removing the cause(s) of the findings. Laboratory accrediting organizations usually want to look at summaries of laboratory audit findings and the corrective actions taken.

External Assessments

There are two types of external assessments. Proficiency testing (PT) is a means to demonstrate that the laboratory's testing processes provide results comparable to those of other laboratories with the same instruments and methods. In PT, the laboratory receives samples for testing from a designated PT provider and performs the testing using its routine processes, procedures, and staff. Results are compared to those of the PT provider and the other laboratories and the laboratory gets a report of its performance. Successful performance on PT challenges is a requirement for laboratory licensure and accreditation.[4]

The second type of external assessment is the inspection/assessment/ survey performed by regulatory and accreditation organizations for the purposes of obtaining and maintaining the laboratory's license or accreditation. External assessments are periodically conducted by the CMS, the FDA (for hospital blood banks with blood collection facilities), the TJC, the CAP, and the AABB to determine the laboratory's compliance with the respective requirements.[4-12]

Continual Improvement

Identifying Opportunities for Improvement

Opportunities for improvement can be identified from at least six main sources:

- the nonconformance trending process pointing to laboratory processes that are not functioning as well as intended;
- customer feedback such as complaints, solicited feedback, or suggestions from external customers whom the laboratory serves, as well as feedback from internal customers (employees);
- information derived from monitoring quality indicators of laboratory operations, particularly when it is compared with that of peer groups in other organizations;
- internal audit feedback, whereby objective evidence collected by the auditor should support the laboratory's understanding of why corrective action is needed and should be taken;
- feedback from periodic external compliance inspections (however, if the laboratory is already seriously involved in the previous four activities, there should be little new information learned of which it is not already aware), and
- reports from other departments in the hospital's organization-wide quality function, such as nursing or emergency department problems in dealing with the laboratory.

Summaries and data from the above sources should periodically be put into a report (often called the "quality report") that is sent to the laboratory's management team for review.

Management Review

The laboratory's management team should carefully review the quality report and set priorities for the problems that need the most immediate attention. Problems can be prioritized by considering all of the issues in Table 1-6. The importance of the problems will be unique to each laboratory's situation and not necessarily represented by the order in which they are presented in Table 1-6.

Using Teams

Many organizations have successfully used teams to solve problems or to design process improvements. Names such as "process improvement teams," "quality

TABLE 1-6.   Ways to Prioritize Improvement Projects

- How the problems affect patient safety
- Which problems are making the most customers the most unhappy
- How the problems affect the laboratory's licensure or accreditation
- How much the problems are adversely affecting the laboratory's operating budget

action teams," "continuous improvement teams," and "corrective action teams" have all been used to refer to groups of people representing different parts of a given process who have been brought together to identify and implement ways to remove the cause(s) of the problem and thereby improve the process. Teams need good team skills to perform their assignments successfully. Members of teams, including laboratory pathologists, scientists, and management staff, should receive team-building and problem-resolution training to ensure the most effective outcome for the time and resources expended.[14] Common processes that teams should focus on to improve, and those issues teams should not address are listed in Table 1-7.

Problem Resolution

Many approaches to the problem-solving process have been published. All the published problem-solving approaches contain essentially the same activities, as shown in Table 1-8.

Table 1-9 depicts one common approach to managing the problem-solving process that includes these main activities:[15]

- Developing a customer-oriented action plan
- Putting the plan into action
- Measuring and monitoring to determine effectiveness of the action
- Determining what to do based on the measurements

TABLE 1-7. Process Improvement Teams Should Focus on Opportunities to Improve Work Processes

Teams Should Improve Processes That Affect:	Teams Should Not Work on These Issues:
Quality of product	Problems governed by or directly related to union contracts
Quality and reliability of service to internal and external customers	Grievances and grievance procedures
Efficiency and accuracy of job performance	Seniority
Waste reduction, scrap, rework, and operating costs	Job classifications
Equipment performance, up-time, and reliability	Job assignments
Interdepartmental and intradepartmental communications	Pay rates or benefits
Improved process controls	
Safety, hygiene, and work environment	
Processes, procedures, training, and competence	
Learning new skills, upgrading knowledge of the business, developing personal capabilities, team process	

Adapted from Scholtes PR, Joiner BL, Streibel BJ: *The Team Handbook*, ed 3. Goal-QPC, Salem, MA, 2003. [14]

TABLE 1-8.   Phases of the Problem Resolution Process

- Problem identification
- Prioritization
- Problem selection
- Analysis
- Data collection
- Identifying possible solutions
- Choice of solution
- Implementation of chosen solution
- Monitoring
- Evaluation of effectiveness of chosen solution
- Sustaining the gains

TABLE 1-9.   A Common Quality Improvement Process

Plan-Do-Check-Act (PDCA)

Plan

A mission-consistent, customer-oriented action plan.

- Identify opportunities for improvement from data and information
- Prioritize improvement activities
- Develop an action plan for the selected activity by either
  - Initiating a new process, or
  - Improving an existing process
- Identify
  - Customer's needs
  - Participants
  - Timeframes
  - Outcome measurements
  - Success criteria

Do

Put the plan into action.

- Implement the action plan
  - Do a pilot project first
  - Broaden only after success
- Collect performance data

Check

Has the planned and implemented change created intended improvement?

- Analyze collected data
- Compare performance data to established success targets and original performance data to determine if improvement was achieved
- Identify any unexpected peripheral benefits
- Identify unanticipated problems in other areas

TABLE 1-9.   A Common Quality Improvement Process (*Continued*)

Act

Decide what to do next.

- Determine if customer's needs were met
- Take action based on the results
  - Success
    - Revise the process for further improvements (optional);
    - Assess again to determine if improvement is maintained, and
    - If a pilot project, standardize to the larger group
  - Lack of success—re-do the action plan and repeat

A formalized problem resolution process is just one piece of continual improvement. The same Plan-Do-Check-Act cycle can be applied to every process in the entire laboratory, whether problematic or not, to effect continual improvement.

SUMMARY

Today, working in a QMS environment is needed to achieve the standards of excellence necessary for surviving the changes facing the nation's health care industry and providing the level of patient safety that our patients both expect and deserve. Purchasers of health-care services want evidence that health-care providers such as hospitals and laboratories are involved in organization-wide quality improvement programs that increase patient safety. Only those organizations demonstrating measurable quality improvements are approved for agreements to provide products and services. The cultural change needed to create a QMS takes time, and laboratories that have not started need to begin immediately to keep pace. Consumers of laboratory services accept no less than total quality. Laboratories that provide less will not survive.

SUMMARY CHART:
Important Points to Remember

➤ Quality, safety, and effectiveness cannot be inspected into the laboratory's services; they must be *built into* those services.

➤ The laboratory's path of workflow contains preanalytic, analytic, and postanalytic processes that need to be performed correctly each and every time.

➤ Laboratory quality can be depicted as a series of concentric circles with QC at the center, QA as the middle ring, and a QMS encompassing the whole.

➤ Quality control (QC) provides control only of test methods by testing prepared samples with known expected results before or along with patient samples.

➤ Quality assurance (QA) measures the performance of laboratory processes, not tests.

➤ A quality management system (QMS) is the means to organize all the management activities that support the laboratory's preanalytic, analytic, and postanalytic processes in a way that meets applicable requirements.

➤ Compliance with federal regulations and accreditation requirements is mandated by the CMS, TJC, CAP, and AABB.

➤ Compliance inspections measure the state of the laboratory's program with respect to the applicable requirements at a single point in time and are usually conducted every 1 to 2 years.

➤ A laboratory quality management system contains 12 QMS essentials that can be organized as the building blocks of quality.

➤ The laboratory should have a description of reporting relationships among laboratory staff as well as the laboratory's relationship to any parent organization and its quality function.

➤ The laboratory needs to identify the expectations of its external and internal customers and design its workflow to meet those expectations.

➤ The laboratory needs to meet all applicable regulatory and accreditation requirements for facility design and safety.

➤ The competence of staff in performing their assigned job tasks needs to be assessed initially after training and periodically thereafter.

➤ Incoming laboratory supplies and reagents need to be inspected on receipt, tested where applicable, and stored according to manufacturer's directions.

➤ An equipment management plan includes schedules for and records of equipment calibration and maintenance and records of servicing and any repairs.

➤ Process control is a set of activities that ensures that a given work process will keep operating in a state that is continuously able to meet process goals without compromising the process itself.

➤ Flowcharting graphically represents the sequence of activities in a process and shows where instructions are needed.

➤ Process validation challenges all activities in a new process before implementation to provide a high degree of assurance that the process will work as intended.

➤ Routine QC procedures, review of records, and capture of nonconformances when the process did not perform as expected are routine process control measures that monitor whether a process is functioning as needed.

➤ Laboratory documents include policies, process descriptions, and procedures that tell staff what to do and how to do it.

➤ Information management is the set of processes that ensures the confidentiality and integrity of patient information and test results.

➤ Nonconformance management is a name for processes that detect, report, evaluate, and correct events in laboratory operations that do not meet the laboratory's or other requirements.

➤ An internal audit reviews a specific laboratory process and determines by examination of documents, records, interviews, and observations whether the process meets applicable requirements and follows the laboratory's policies, processes, and procedures.

➤ The laboratory should prepare a quality report, identify opportunities for improvement, prioritize improvement projects, and take action to resolve the quality problems they represent.

SUGGESTED PROBLEM-BASED LEARNING ACTIVITIES

Chapter 1: Quality Management in the Medical Laboratory

Instructions: Use Internet resources, books, articles, colleagues, etc. to present solutions to the problems listed below. There is no one correct solution to any problem.

Note to Instructor: Students may be divided into groups and given the problem-based learning activity to discuss and solve. Once the group has reached consensus on a solution, the group may present it to other students in the class, thus providing all students with information about potential solutions.

Problem #1

Use the information in this chapter to organize a table of contents for your laboratory's revised administrative manual. Indicate which information could go into which section. Identify at least four non-path-of-workflow procedures in the administrative manual that staff members perform.

Problem #2

Discuss and document the sequence of activities for participating in your laboratory's proficiency testing program; that is, the entire program, not simply performing testing. Think generically—what the activities are, rather than the details of each activity. Identify which laboratory positions (i.e., job titles) perform each activity in the sequence.

Problem #3

Your laboratory is receiving complaints from the emergency department that the turnaround time (TAT) for STAT testing is too slow. Describe how you would use continual improvement tools to solve this problem. Identify the persons involved and the activities you would undertake.

REFERENCES

1. Food and Drug Administration, Center for Biologics Evaluation and Research: *Guideline on General Principles of Process Validation.* Food and Drug Administration, Rockville, MD, 1987. Reprinted May 1993, accessed 2010.

2. International Organization for Standardization: *ISO 9000: 2005 Quality management systems—Fundamentals and vocabulary.* International Organization for Standardization, Geneva, 2005.

3. [In press] Clinical and Laboratory Standards Institute: *Quality Management System: A Model for Laboratory Services,* Approved Guideline, GP26-A4. Wayne, PA, 2010.

4. Centers for Medicare and Medicaid Services: *Code of Federal Regulations, Title 42, Parts 430 to end.* U.S. Government Printing Office, Washington, DC, revised annually.

5. Occupational Safety and Health Administration (OSHA): *Code of Federal Regulations, Title 21, Part 1910.* U.S. Government Printing Office, Washington, DC, revised annually.

6. Food and Drug Administration, Department of Health and Human Services: *Code of Federal Regulations, Title 21, Parts 200–299.* U.S. Government Printing Office, Washington, DC, revised annually.

7. Food and Drug Administration, Department of Health and Human Services: *Code of Federal Regulations, Title 21, Parts 600–799.* U.S. Government Printing Office, Washington, DC, revised annually.

8. The Joint Commission: *Comprehensive Accreditation Manual for Hospitals.* Oakbrook Terrace, IL, 2010.

9. The Joint Commission: *Comprehensive Accreditation Manual for Laboratories and Point-of-Care Testing.* Oakbrook Terrace, IL, 2010.

10. College of American Pathologists: *Inspection Checklists for Laboratory Accreditation.* Northfield, IL, 2009.

11. COLA: *Accreditation Program Criteria.* Columbia, MD, 2007.

12. American Association of Blood Banks: *Standards for Blood Banks and Transfusion Services,* ed 26. Bethesda, MD, 2009.

13. Food and Drug Administration, Department of Health and Human Services: *Code of Federal Regulations, Title 21, Part 803.* U.S. Government Printing Office, Washington, DC, revised annually.

14. Scholtes PR, Joiner BL, Streibel BJ: *The Team Handbook,* ed 3. GOAL/QPC, Salem, MA, 2003.

15. McCloskey LA, Collet DN: *TQM: A Primer Guide to Total Quality Management.* GOAL/QPC, Methuen, MA, 1993.

BIBLIOGRAPHY

Berte LM: Laboratory Quality Management: A Roadmap. In: Friedberg RC, Weiss RL, eds. *Clinics in Laboratory Medicine* 2007: 27(4); 771–790.

Berte LM: *Transfusion Service Manual of SOPs, Training Guides and Competence Assessment Tools,* ed 2. American Association of Blood Banks, Bethesda, MD, 2007.

Clinical and Laboratory Standards Institute: *Laboratory Documents: Development and Control,* Approved Guideline, GP2A-5. Wayne, PA, 2006.

Clinical and Laboratory Standards Institute: *Training and Competence Assessment,* Approved Guideline, GP21-A3. Wayne, PA, 2009.

Tague NR: *The Quality Toolbox,* ed 2. ASQC Press, Milwaukee, WI, 2005.

INTERNET RESOURCES

American Association of Blood Banks (AABB)
http://www.aabb.org

American Society for Quality (ASQ)
http://www.asq.org

American Society for Quality (ASQ)—Knowledge Center
http://www.asq.org/knowledge-center/

Centers for Medicare and Medicaid Services (CMS)
http://www.cms.gov/

Clinical and Laboratory Standards Institute (CLSI)
http://www.clsi.org

COLA: LabUniversity Online Learning Courses
http://www.cola.org/labu.html

College of American Pathologists (CAP)
http://www.cap.org/

International Organization for Standardization (ISO)
http://www.iso.org/iso/home.html

Occupational Safety and Health Administration (OSHA)
http://www.osha.gov/

The Joint Commission (TJC)
http://www.jointcommission.org/

U.S. Food and Drug Administration (FDA)
http://www.fda.gov/

CHAPTER 2

Organizational Structure: A Look at Concepts and Models

Heather J. Hall, MBA, MT(ASCP), CG(ASCP)^{CM}
Elaine M. Brett, MS, MT(ASCP)

CHAPTER OUTLINE

OBJECTIVES

Following successful completion of this chapter, the learner will be able to:

1. Describe some of the historical influences on organizational structures.
2. Define mechanistic and organic models of organizations.
3. Evaluate organizational needs using the open system.
4. Evaluate current organizational structures' ability to meet customer/patient needs and environmental influences.
5. Propose new structures based on customer/patient needs and environmental forces.
6. Identify and describe the impact of five organizational trends.

KEY TERMS

Browser-Server Model
Closed System
Congruence Model
Functional Structure
Matrix Organizations
Mechanistic Structure
Network Structures

Open System
Organic Structure
Organizational Structure
Process-Based Structure
Self-Contained Unit Structure
Systems

Case Study   Organizational Structure

Use your own laboratory or one with which you are familiar in the following situation. You have been asked to participate in a strategic planning exercise representing the laboratory for a multisite health system. Your hospital has had a traditional approach to managing the organization. The health system desires to take a "fresh look" at all aspects of the organization.

Issues and Questions to Consider:

1. Describe the current structure of the health system, the hospital, and the laboratory.
2. Looking at the laboratory as an open system, list some things external to the laboratory that will influence its operation and structure.
3. What are some factors internal to the laboratory that you will need to consider in making any changes to the system?
4. Consider the organizational structures described in this chapter. Visualize your laboratory in each of these structures. Prepare a rough sketch of your laboratory using each of the following structures:
   a. Functional
   b. Self-Contained Units
   c. Matrix
   d. Process-Based
   e. Network
5. Which organizational structure works best for your system and why?

INTRODUCTION

An organization is a collection of people working together under a defined structure for the purpose of achieving predetermined outcomes through the use of financial, human, and material resources. There are a number of approaches to the structure and management of organizations. *Structure* is defined by Merriam-Webster as "something arranged in a definite pattern of organization". [1] Selection of the management organizational structure will depend on factors such as size, content, complexity, and distribution of work in the laboratory.

As laboratories move into the new century, they must redefine and explore the possibilities of our organizations. We live in a world of communities and organizations. These are **systems** made up of individuals who share a common purpose and perform tasks in service of that purpose. Success of any organization is a function of the capabilities of the individuals rather than the way in which they are organized. Talented personnel will perform well in most organizational structures and much better in a good organization. The structures of these organizational systems are both a creation and a creator of our behavior. Organizations provide vision and focus, they consist of technical and social components, they provide boundaries and creative freedom, and they are open to the changing environment yet contain their own culture within.

Organizations serve the following functions:

- Provide society with products and services.
- Offer employment and economic exchange for members.
- Give a framework for a social system (i.e., organizations are social habitats for people).

Albert Einstein said, "We cannot solve the problems we have created with the same thinking that created them." Organizations, like individuals, must learn from past successes and failures and look for creative ways to find solutions for the future. Organizations perform best where information flows rapidly. Information must flow both internally and externally to permit accurate decisions to be made. The clinical laboratory is no different from any other system in this regard.

The clinical laboratory is typically an organization within an organization. It functions as part of the larger health system and provides specific services that are vital to the overall mission of providing patient care. The laboratory may also function across health systems, providing specialized services and "centers of excellence." Understanding basic concepts of organizational structure and function can give insight into how we act and react in our own systems. Optimizing the technical and social aspects of the organization can enhance and maximize performance and outcomes. In almost any laboratory, you will find an organizational chart that can help you understand the levels of authority and lines of communication. By convention, the organizational chart with boxes and lines describes a structural plan. This chapter provides information about the background of **organizational structures**. It describes a broader concept of the organization as a complex system and its design as an "architecture" that includes work and social components in addition to formal structure. It examines organizations through several different lenses: historical, system models, and design/structure. In addition, it describes 21st Century organizational trends.

Fundamentally, a look at organizations should help answer the question, "How do we divide up the work?" To adequately function in the complex healthcare environment, it is important for the medical laboratory scientist to understand the structure and politics of their organization. Such an appreciation can foster better communication, better understanding of system decisions, and help in career advancement opportunities.

HISTORICAL PERSPECTIVE

The structures of organizations in the West are really "recent" inventions. The most familiar structures developed as the 19th Century shifted from a basically agrarian society to an industrial society. The effect, as we shall see, was to provide a dedicated workforce that required a top-down flow of information and instructions.

The concepts were based on a bureaucratic approach derived from military organizations. The cultural changes that unfolded as a result of our moving into the Information Age in the last quarter of the 20th Century, require that our organizations take on new and different forms. Unfortunately, many of the modern day organizations—including those in healthcare—are still using a 19th Century model!

In the early part of the 1900s, the stage was set for modern organizations. As the Industrial Age took hold, the need for managing large numbers of people in complex activities required an efficient way to organize people. Max Weber, a German sociologist, introduced the concept of bureaucracy or *rational-legal* system. The structure and processes required a strong hierarchy of authority, extensive division of labor for optimum functional performance, impersonal rules and rigid procedures that account for nearly every contingency, and decision making based on rules and tactics developed to guarantee consistent and effective pursuit of organizational goals. The model presents the image and characteristics of a "well-oiled" machine working particularly well in businesses involving routine tasks that can be specified in writing and that do not change quickly or frequently.

Near the turn of the 20th Century, Frederick Taylor introduced the discipline of scientific management as a means to organize work. In the introduction to his book, *The Principles of Scientific Management,* he states, "In the past the man has been first; in the future the system must be first."[2] Taylor dealt with the problem of how to get more productivity out of workers, and used time and motion studies to break jobs into smaller repetitive tasks and find the best way to do a job. He introduced several principles including the following:

- Specialization—the creation of specialist jobs and "thinking departments"[2]
- "Piecework" pay-systems designed to increase motivation and reduce "slacking-off" by workers[2]

Taylor advocated a strong division of labor between management (thinking) and worker (doing). It was the manager's job to understand the task and plan a method of executing it, and then coerce the worker to do it, by motivating the worker with pay.[2]

The essence of Weber and Taylor and other classic theorists was to organize working groups in a rational manner, a noble effort for their times. These were days of assembly lines and unskilled immigrant labor. These approaches had many desirable features in terms of motivation, efficiency, and use of expertise. However, the pure application of the theories was challenged in the studies of the effects of social factors on morale and productivity in the decades that followed. The beginnings of a "human relations movement" came out of studies from the Hawthorne plant of the Western Electric Company in the late 1920s and early 1930s. In short, these studies, which influenced the organization of the workforce through the 1960s, suggested that informal social structures had much to do with the way an organization runs. Feelings and attitudes about the work, the environment, and the supervisor all contributed to performance. "Just doing their job" left workers feeling alienated and dispirited.

Formal organization provides the direction and the stability of the infrastructure. The informal organization has well-developed social structures, histories, and culture. Informal groups have a powerful influence on productivity, sometimes more so than economic incentives. Human relations approach advocated paying greater attention to workers' needs, training in interpersonal skills for supervisors, and generally "humanizing" the workplace.

The inclusion of the human element in organizations continued. In the 1950s and 1960s, the development and application of behavioral and social sciences in combination with advancements in industrial and information technology created new questions about the work environment. Global competition and demands for greater efficiency and productivity prompted efforts to redesign existing processes.

One influencing approach was sociotechnical systems theory, which was based on the premise that an organization is a combination of people (social aspect) and technology (technical aspect) and is open to its environment. Both parts must work together to accomplish tasks and produce both physical products or services and social/psychological outcomes. The social and technical parts are jointly optimized in contrast with traditional methods that first design the technical component and then "fit" the people to it. Implementation of sociotechnical systems is highly participative, involving all relevant stakeholders and promoting employee involvement at all levels in the work design. The formation of self-managing work groups, training of group members in multiple skills and delegation of the work creates process changes that influence the productivity and efficiency of the organizations. Sharing of information, knowledge, and learning is characteristic of this approach. In the context of clinical laboratory, this means organizing a department by considering the instrumentation and technology *and* by focusing on people issues, communication, and social interactions.

In 1961, after observing trends in many organizations, Burns and Stalker described a range of organization management structures that they referred to as mechanistic to organic structures.[3] A **mechanistic structure** may be appropriate in an environment of slow change and relative stability. The organization is highly structured with direction and communication from the top-down and relies on authority-obedience relationships. In the extreme, there is centralized decision making, strict division of labor, and insistence on loyalty and conformity to policy and procedures. At the opposite end is the **organic structure**, which is preferred in an environment of high change. This system features decentralized decision making and a fluid design, which facilitates flexibility and adaptation, and encourages a wide sharing of responsibility.

In the 1980s and 1990s, different types of process improvements influenced organizational structures in business and healthcare. French and Bell summarized the variety of interventions that have affected structural changes in organizations over the past several decades.[3] Table 2-1 provides basic definitions of some of these approaches as well as some of the consequences to the organization. Many of these approaches foster a team concept for the work, regarding both the technical and social aspects of the organization. The changes represent a more results-focused application of processes and a collaborative sharing of information.

It appears that the structure of organizations is evolving. The traditional top-down mechanistic model that exists in many organizations will give way to an organic or network model where employees on the front line drive critical decisions to serve customer/client needs. The organization of the future will take on open system characteristics discussed in the next section.

ORGANIZATIONAL MANAGEMENT: A SYSTEMS APPROACH

Systems contained within larger structures help to categorize the large amount of information managed by the organizational structure. In contrast to the mechanistic and organic systems presented earlier, this section will provide comparisons of the closed, open and congruence systems. The nature of current and evolving expectations placed on the Clinical Laboratory lend to a larger discussion on the open system.

Using a simple abstract model, such as a biologic organism, organizational systems can be thought of as interdependent, interconnected elements that constitute an identifiable whole. Biologic systems are generally thought of as open systems that function as input-throughput-output/outcome mechanisms. As shown in Figure 2-1, systems exhibit activities that take input from the environment, do "something" to the input through transformation or conversion, and export a changed product back into the environment. In a single cell organism, the system is completely dependent on the flow of energy and matter. Beginning with the intake of food, water, and air, to the elimination of energy, waste, and by-products,

TABLE 2-1. **A Summary of Structural Interventions and Their Consequences on the Organization**

Intervention	Objective	Consequence
Self-Managed Teams	Provide teams with a grouping of tasks that make up a major unit of the total work to be performed.	Flattening the organization, improved productivity; reconceptualizing roles of managers as coordinators and coaches.
Work Redesign Theory	Motivation and performance can be enhanced by redesigning jobs.	Redistribution of tasks; greater individual accountability.
MBO—Management by Objectives	Assumes the need for systematic (quantifiable) goal setting linking the goals of superiors to subordinates.	May range from autocratic, unilateral mechanisms to enforce compliance to collaborative process with increased focus on organizational objectives.
Quality Circles	A form of group problem solving with primary focus on enhancing product quality.	Formation of cross-functional and multifunctional teams; greater employee participation; more creative integration.
Quality of Work Life	Restructuring of several dimensions of the organization to solve a problem and introduce sustained change.	Increase in employee participation in decision-making work teams.
Total Quality Management	A combination of approaches including quality circles, statistical quality control, self-managed teams. Focus is on customer needs and continuous improvement process.	Increase in employee participation and teamwork. Higher productivity. Supports participative management.
Reengineering	Focuses on redesigning business processes.	Top-down program. Combining, eliminating, restructuring activities to affect efficiency and productivity.

the components of the system are organized to handle the flow of energy, and they possess the capacity to change and adapt. In *Leadership and the New Science,* Dr. Margaret Wheatley expands on the metaphor:

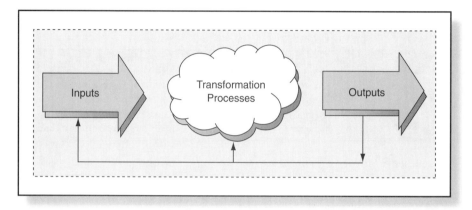

FIGURE 2-1.   Simple Open System Configuration

"Our concept of organizations is moving away from the mechanistic creations that flourished in the age of bureaucracy. We now speak in earnest of more fluid, organic structures, of boundaryless and seamless organizations. We are beginning to recognize organizations as whole systems, construing them as 'learning organizations' or 'organic' and noticing that people exhibit self organizing capacity."[4]

If we look at our organizations as **open systems**, we can start to see the interactions and influences of one part of the system with others and evaluate the needs of the organization. It can help us understand why some organizations perform well and why others may experience conflict. The clinical laboratory is an excellent example of the open system model. The laboratory receives input including specimens, test requests, and supplies from many sources. The laboratory staff, instruments, and processes "transform" the inputs to provide test results and information for patients and clinicians.

Open systems share the following characteristics:

1. There is an implied purpose or goal that is the reason for the system's existence. The primary mission or task of a system determines its distinct nature. The clinical laboratory, for example, may be dedicated to the output or production of timely and meaningful delivery of test results. This purpose will be a "guiding light" that helps all members accept direction and focus.

2. The external environment drives significant change. The requirements of the environment will direct and define the purpose. The environment consists of external elements and forces that affect an organization's ability to establish and reach its objectives. If the environment no longer requires the output of the system, the system will no longer have purpose and may cease to exist. Consider the medical need for laboratory testing and the influence of new technologies. There is a constant change in the demand for the kind of testing and the delivery of testing. An example is the influence of point-of-care

testing. The external environment (patients, clinicians) demand testing closer to the patient where immediate results could be obtained and decisions regarding treatment made. The available technology made this testing possible, streamlining the diagnostic process. These external influences have driven significant change on the laboratory organization and delivery of test results.

3. Systems have clearly defined boundaries. Physical structure, technology, or the type of work, give the system uniqueness and label its purpose and function. The individual parts or members within the system interact and work together toward a common purpose. An open system, however, is permeable to its environment and exchanges information and resources with the environment. The members of the Clinical Laboratory are recognized by the boundaries of the department or system and will act synergistically within the boundaries to provide quality test results. The laboratory boundary, however, must be open to the needs, processes, and contributions of the health system and the community that is served. For example, the differing work groups of Hematology and Immunohematology may communicate with each other within the boundaries of the laboratory to anticipate patient/clinician needs based on test results and current or prior treatments. In an open system, this communication between the work groups can be carried outside of the boundaries of the laboratory, and suggestions can be made or questions can be asked of the clinician to better reach the overall organizational goal of increased patient care.

4. Like biological systems, organizations seek to maintain a state of stability or equilibrium. Part of the plan of a successful organization is to maintain harmony with the potentially disruptive forces of the environment. The more complex and turbulent those forces are, the bigger the challenges and demands on the system. The paradox is that to achieve stability and equilibrium, a system must constantly change. It is a challenge and a frustration to leaders and managers to find the most agreeable ways to maintain order in the workplace, while at the same time, making continuous adjustments to meet the demands of the external environment. In modern organizations, leaders must acknowledge that there may be multiple paths and multiple adjustments to reach a particular outcome or goal. This becomes quite evident by observing many different laboratory organizations. All laboratories have similar purpose: generating quality results. Yet each laboratory is unique in the way it accomplishes the tasks to meet the needs of its particular community.

5. As a system grows and becomes more complex, it forms differentiated, specialized components or subsystems including work teams, sections, or departments. The subsystems seek to be unique and different and eventually evolve into a hierarchy. In the hospital laboratory, specialization takes place on several levels. Even though the laboratory has its unique purpose in receiving specimens and delivering data, it functions as a subsystem in the larger hospital organization.

The laboratory, in turn, is differentiated into sections, such as blood bank, virology, or molecular diagnostics that function as self-contained sub-sections, which meet special needs and technical requirements.

6. Feedback is important to the alignment and performance of the system. Positive feedback will inform whether the purpose and goals are aligned with the environmental needs, and whether the targets are appropriate. Adjustments in the system can be made to serve the purpose. Negative feedback monitors whether the system is on course with the purpose and goals, and prompts corrective action. For the laboratory, interdepartmental meetings and communications are important feedback mechanisms that can help monitor performance, provide information, and prompt necessary changes.

Despite their behavior as open systems, many laboratory organizations remain in a relatively closed system framework. Table 2-2 compares certain organizational elements and behaviors in Open and Closed Systems. The **closed system**, being less considerate of external forces, is internally focused. The closed system uses mechanistic structures as previously described. Top-down authority and reliance on policy and procedures are typical. As mentioned, in a relatively stable, slow changing environment, the closed, mechanistic approach may be appropriate. It is a challenge for the laboratory manager to recognize inconsistencies, and be able to implement changes that improve the organization.

One way of approaching the changes is to look more closely at what must happen within an open system to support a state of equilibrium. The **congruence model** described by David Nadler shows a little more detail of the elements of an organization as an open system and some of the dynamics involved. The model

TABLE 2-2.   A Comparison of Open and Closed Organizational Systems

	Relatively Closed System	Relatively Open System
Leadership Style	Independent Superior-Subordinate basis	Collaborative Collegial basis
Decision Making	Hierarchically determined	At the level where the problem and the information reside
Authority and Responsibility	Located together Single accountability	May be separate with multiple accountability
Conflict	Eliminate or suppress	Manage
Performance Appraisal	Hierarchical or external	Self-review
Distribution of Work	Allocate jobs to people	Negotiate work among groups
Thinking Mode	Euclidean Sequential and logical	Multiple frames of reference
Power Base	Hierarchy or status	Control over uncertainty
Managing Arena	Within the system	At the system boundary

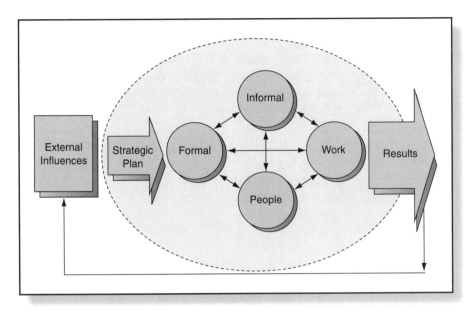

FIGURE 2-2. **A Congruence Model Showing the Organization as an Open System**

Adapted from Nadler, DA & Nadler, MB: *Champions of Change,* p. 41, 1998. [5]

can be used to analyze environmental relationships of an organization and assess the internal interdependence and alignment of its parts. In the model, the elements of the transformation process or, more appropriately, the operating organization are the major components that transform the inputs to the outputs through the implementation of a strategy. In Figure 2-2, the following components are represented and their interrelationships are shown as arrows:

- Work—the tasks performed to provide the products or services
- People—including skills, knowledge, and workforce expectations
- Formal Organization—formal structures, policies, and procedures for performing the work
- Informal Organization—culture and informal rules and understanding about how the system works

Table 2-3 provides examples of how some elements of the clinical laboratory might be represented in the congruence model.

Constituents of the system must be considered and must be congruent with each other to obtain maximum efficiency in transforming strategies to performance. The lack of fit between any of the components of the operating organization— between formal and informal structures, people and work requirements—will compromise the system and can produce huge problems including operational inefficiencies, tension among personnel, morale problems, miscommunication,

TABLE 2-3.   Application of Elements of the Clinical Laboratory to the Congruence Model

Inputs	Operating Organization	Outputs
Environmental Influences • Patient needs • Healthcare regulations • Health system requirements • Sample delivery • Competitors • Unions	*Formal Organization* • Structure • Policies • Procedures • Regulatory compliance	*System Information* • Test results • Diagnostic information • Consultation
Resources • Financial • Information • People • Supplies • Technology	*People* • Individual skills and knowledge • Needs and preferences • Expectations	*Department Contribution* • Financial performance • Patient response
Organization's History • Vision and mission • Values and norms • Location	*Work* • Test performance • Process flow • Automation/ Instrumentation • Point of care	*Individual* • Academic contribution • Teaching/learning • Personal growth and recognition
	Informal Organization • Informal working arrangements • Behavior of leaders • Patterns of relationships • Culture and climate • Communication patterns	

and overall dysfunction. Table 2-4 poses questions that may test how well your organization demonstrates "goodness of fit" between the four components of the operating organization. This assessment may help us understand how well the laboratory system is functioning and identify inconsistencies.

TABLE 2-4. **Assessment of "Goodness of Fit" Among the Four Components of the Operating Organization Based on the Congruence Model**

Fit	Issue	Questions
People—Formal Organization	Individual needs are met by the organization. Individuals are clear on organizational expectations and individual system goals are aligned.	Are goals communicated clearly? Are individuals aligned with the mission of the laboratory, or the health system? Are people working for or against the system? Are reward systems adequate?
People—Work	Individual needs are met by the work. Individuals are prepared with skills and knowledge for the work.	Is the work fulfilling? Is there enough creative freedom to do the job? Are people adequately trained? Are the right people in the job?
People—Informal Organization	Individual needs are met by the informal organization. The informal organization makes use of individual resources.	Do leadership behaviors promote the values and mission? Is the culture and climate conducive to achieving desired performance? Can individuals express themselves in a safe environment?
Work—Formal Organization	Organizational arrangements support the task. The organization motivates behavior that is consistent with expected performance.	Does the organization structure support the departmental task? Is the work being done consistent with the mission and values of the organization? Are work expectations being met? Are the right resources in place to successfully meet the goals? Are job descriptions appropriate?
Work—Informal Organization	The informal organization helps or hinders the performance of the work.	Does the culture support the execution of the tasks?
Formal—Informal Organization	The elements of the informal organization are consistent with the formal organization.	Are interdepartmental and intradepartmental communications supported? Are the goals and rewards of the informal organization consistent with the formal organization? Is alignment evident?

ORGANIZATION DESIGN: A STRUCTURAL PERSPECTIVE

Focus on regulatory policies and quality initiatives, along with advances in technology, have resulted in most laboratories being technically high-quality and demonstrating acceptable clinical competency. Changes in organizational design can further affect efficiencies, productivity, cost-containment, and personnel needs. Whereas system models help categorize the many aspects of the system, structural models show function and linkage of how groups in the organization relate to each other.

Five factors influence the design and structure of the organization:

- Organizational goals and strategic direction.
- Technologic capabilities, including information technology.
- Size (the laboratory subsystem and the larger health system).
- Environment (especially client/patient needs).
- Leadership style, member behaviors, and organization culture.

Five structural models illustrate the range from mechanistic to organic networks. These models include functional, self-contained units, matrix, process-based, and network structures. Although these models are not exclusive, they illustrate some basic advantages and disadvantages of recognizable approaches. Understanding the design helps us understand how the work is divided and how work efforts are coordinated. In reality, a clinical laboratory may be a hybrid of several of the structural models.

The **functional structure** is hierarchical and, in the extreme, rigidly bureaucratic. In this structure, specialized units report in an upward chain of command, and there is clear understanding of responsibility and authority. As with the closed system model, these organizations can function best in a stable, controlled environment where the organization is small to medium in size and departments are engaged in repetitive, efficient, routine tasks. The disadvantages of the functional structure are that communication among groups can be compromised with departments acting as silos and focused on only their areas of responsibility. There is a possibility that coordination between departments may become competitive and unresponsive. Functional laboratory organizations may have both a medical/technical and an administrative reporting scheme structure at the top of the organization. Specialized units such as Chemistry, Hematology, Microbiology, and others may be represented as sections or departments with a hierarchy of supervision and management, as shown in Figure 2-3A.

In the restructuring of clinical laboratories, efforts at consolidation and creating more cost-effective structures have resulted in a flattening of the hierarchical structure and elimination of some supervisory and management layers. Although there may be fewer steps in the decision-making process, the top-down control remains (Figure 2-3B).

The **self-contained unit structure** is organized around a common basis. This may be a discipline, a location, a customer group, or a technology. Each unit contains all relevant skills and processes to successfully operate. The grouping of

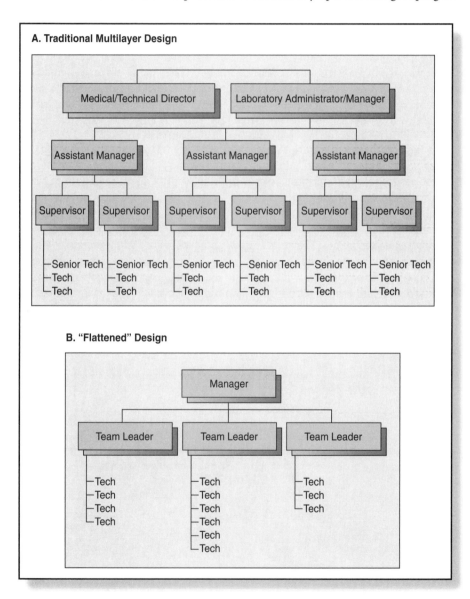

FIGURE 2-3. Functional Laboratory Organizational Chart

disciplines in the laboratory (e.g., Chemistry, Hematology, Microbiology) in large health system environments with their own functional expertise and supervisory structure are examples of self-contained units. In addition, satellite laboratories or service specialty areas responsible for their own outcomes may be self-contained "pods" providing their own special skills and services. Figure 2-4 represents one approach to a self-contained unit or team approach, where members of each unit are grouped by function around centralized support and management services. Team approaches work well if resources are coordinated toward a common goal. Good communication plans and sharing of information maximize efficiency. A disadvantage to this structure is duplication of resources and expertise, requiring a larger facility and more employees; possible lack of work for specialty areas; and feelings of isolation from other specialty areas of the laboratory. Advantages are the ability for each unit to function efficiently, as all resources are included in each unit, and the ability to meet changing conditions quickly.

Matrix organizations take advantage of skills and function. Matrix designs allow departments or areas to simultaneously concentrate on specialized functions and on production. In the clinical laboratory, restructuring from a functional system with specialty disciplines such as Chemistry, Hematology, or Microbiology toward a production focus as a core or rapid response laboratory, may result in the matrixing of technical and production operations responsibilities as shown in Figure 2-5. Vertical lines represent responsibility for functional and operational issues; horizontal lines provide subject or discipline expertise; circles designate teams that are formed for optimal skills and performance. A matrix design works best when the demands of the environment are changing and uncertain, and where

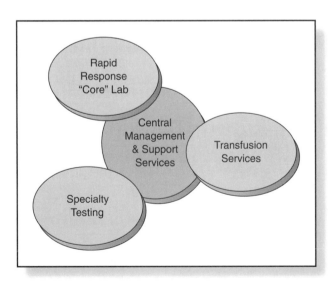

FIGURE 2-4.   **Example of a Self-Contained Unit Structure**

Note: Circles represent overlapping teams, each with specialized functions and tasks.

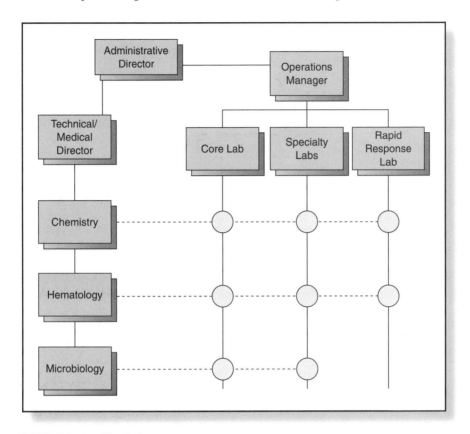

FIGURE 2-5.   Matrix Structure

Note: Solid lines indicate formal direct reporting; dashed lines indicate informal reporting. Circles represent functional departments or teams.

there is a high interdependency on technical expertise and specialization. This type of structure promotes skill diversification (cross-training) and efficiency in sharing human resources. The disadvantage of matrix structures is that roles and reporting structures can be confusing and ambiguous. An individual may report to more than one boss and may be asked to assume different roles depending on the team they are on. Employees may feel "pulled in many directions" until they completely understand the structure and access to resources. Success of Matrix structures relies on interpersonal and conflict management skills.

Process-based structures emphasize the lateral relationships in an organization and allow the organization to use resources for customer satisfaction. Figure 2-6 provides an outline of a process-based structure. The process-based structure focuses around the process driving the structure and the customer defining the performance. The goal of the clinical laboratory is to provide accurate and timely results to patients and their physicians. Specimen collection and

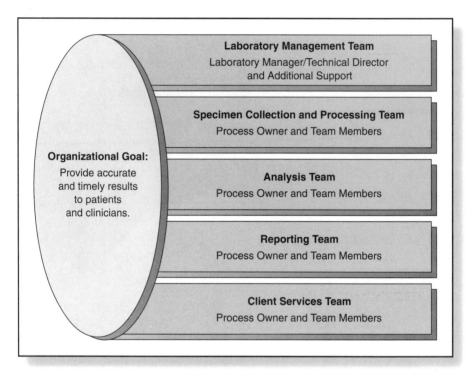

FIGURE 2-6.   Example of a Process-Based Structure

processing, analyzing and reporting are all processes required to reach this goal and can be the basis for the teams developed in this structure. The teams are the functional unit of this structure, are self-managed and responsible for all outcomes of the assigned process. Transitioning to this structure can be difficult from traditional hierarchical structures as the approach flattens the structure and can change the focus of the leadership to processes rather than departments. Additional obstacles to manage are drastic changes in mindset and duplication of resources that may be scarce.[6]

Network structures are evolving as information technology allows instantaneous access and distribution of data and information. For many years, organization structures emulated machine structures. References to "well-oiled" parts and "lean-machines" implied control of knowledge and resources. Networked organizations reflect information technology models with customer focus and information sharing. Network structures consist of specialized units, either internal or external to the organization, that are linked together by informal or formal agreements. Networks may take on a variety of forms because they run from the customer/patient back, not from the top down. They combine innovation and responsiveness of small entrepreneurial structures with the economies of scale of large organizations.

One concept is the human network organization patterned after a **browser-server model** as portrayed by Harry Dent in Figure 2-7.[7] On the front line, employees serve client needs and make critical decisions. Employees on the

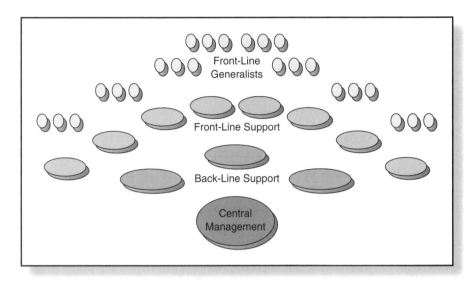

FIGURE 2-7.   **Human Network Organization**
Adapted from Dent, H: The *Roaring* 2000s. p.150, 1998. [7]

back lines, who specialize in a particular skill or knowledge base, support the front line. Unlike traditional organizations, network organizations have a center, not a top. The role of management is to coordinate, facilitate, and serve. In a laboratory setting, the front line may represent those activities that are closest to the patient such as point-of-care testing and client services. The next layer, front-line support, represents less urgent batched testing. Back-line support includes specialized technical areas that offer more complex and esoteric tests. The back line also serves as a resource for front line in technical or clinical matters. A central management provides necessary resources and serves as support of functions such as information systems, facilities, and personnel.

Another network model used in the clinical laboratory incorporates the need to consolidate services, reduce duplications, and expand revenue-generating services while delivering high-quality cost-effective results. Depending on the scope of the health system, the network may incorporate, point-of-care, internal (inpatient) operations, and external (outreach) functions. The network may also have alliances and partnerships with other systems or centers of excellence. Figure 2-8 shows a model of three levels of service from point-of-care to core laboratory in a large geographic region. In this network model hospitals or outreach laboratories (labeled H) handle immediate testing that requires quick turnaround. Batched tests typically with next-day turnaround are done in regional core laboratories. A central laboratory provides low-volume and esoteric testing and serves as a medical and technical resource. This networked system depends on strong collaborative leadership, an efficient information system, appropriate clinical instrumentation, and flexible staffing.

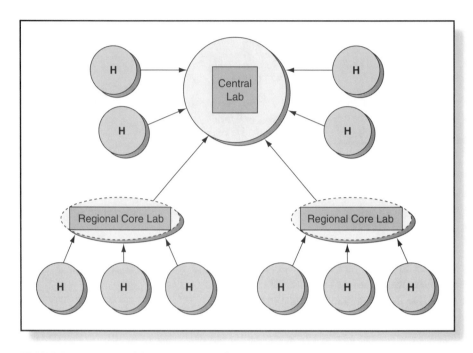

FIGURE 2-8.   A Health System Network
Adapted from Lu, S. et al.: *Clin Lab Manage Rev.*, p. 509, 1996.[8]

Network structures have emerged to respond to the dynamically changing environment that is growing more and more complex, interdependent and client driven. Our access to information is overwhelming and individual customers/patients demand personalized and immediate attention. The network structure is highly flexible and streamlines responses. However, the model requires radical change in how we view working relationships and leadership/management roles. Without that change, it is difficult to manage the equilateral interactions across organizations and to maintain commitment of members to the network.

21st CENTURY ORGANIZATIONAL TRENDS

In general, some trends in organizations will be prompted by the requirements for efficiency, speed, cost-effectiveness, and customer/patient focus.

1. Technology advancements continue to evolve providing faster, more comprehensive platforms that will become more and more accessible. Information handling, telecommunications, increasing point-of-care testing

availability and emerging noninvasive medical devices will have significant effects on the structure of laboratory systems. The balance of economies of scale through consolidated platforms along with the demand for patient-focused (customer) testing will create a healthy tension that will challenge the traditional clinical laboratory system and will necessitate new models for service delivery.

2. Diversity in both the workforce and the consumer population emerges as a key issue to organizational structure, culture, and management. Changing demographics resulting a workforce that is more heterogeneous sexually, ethnically, culturally, generationally, and individually are a source of both innovation and conflict. How an organization copes with different styles of interaction, communication, and appearance will challenge its structure.

3. Flexibility and organizational agility are necessary to respond to demands of patients and healthcare providers. Rigid structures that are bound by rules and regulations will give way to those that can quickly respond with innovative solutions. Structures that are flexible allow greater autonomy and encourage decision making at the point-of-care. Systems will emphasize lifetime employability by creating learning environments rather than lifetime employment through career tracks.

4. Flattening of organizations will result in fewer management levels and empowerment of employees to make decisions. The access to information through more robust technology means less need for the communication and control functions managers have traditionally held. In some ways the role of management is challenged with the "automation of management" by accessibility of information systems capable of storing and "sharing" organizational goals, plans, policies, and procedures. Aspects of the management role that can be programmed free up managers to be facilitators and coaches instead of "corporate cops." In addition, the expectation of employees to be self-directed and accountable reduces requirements for managers as caretakers. Adequate learning environments that promote leadership development and individual empowerment will need to be created.

5. Trends toward strategic alliances, partnerships, mergers, and industry information sharing contribute to a networked approach to organizational structures. Internal signs that organizations are trending toward networks include an increase in direct communications across unit and department boundaries, formation of cross-functional teams, and decentralization of services to meet customer/patient demands. The increased use of the Internet and health system *intranets* will complement the trend toward point-of-care and self-testing and broaden the network even more. Patients will take on the perspective of consumers of laboratory and other medical information and will expect faster, more efficient delivery of services.

SUMMARY

Laboratory professionals should be challenged to look for new and creative designs to the meet the needs of the environment, particularly customers and patients. There is no single structure and no "right way" to divide up the work. Each organization must evaluate their unique situation and anticipate the future trends. The leadership of the system must find and recognize the future and not be blinded by the day-to-day business at hand or paralyzed by past practices. We must ask the questions that help us understand the interdependencies of the components of the organization. We must look at the forces in our environment that will drive change and create new opportunities. We must look to align processes and the people in our organizations to carry out strategic plans that will guide us to the organization's goals and vision.

SUMMARY CHART:
Important Points to Remember

➤ The structure and systems used in organizations are influenced by several factors: size, content, complexity, distribution of work, organizational goals, technology, environment and organizational culture.

➤ The organizational structure is the way in which an organization divides its tasks and coordinates them for overall goal achievement. Commonly represented visually as an organization chart.

➤ Organizational systems can range from mechanistic to organic or closed to open to organize information and processes.

➤ A mechanistic structure is an organizational model consisting of a highly structured environment with communication from the top down and reliance on authority-obedience relationships; appropriate in environments of slow change and relative stability.

➤ An organic structure is an organizational model consisting of an environment that features decentralized decision making, and encourages adaptability and flexibility; appropriate in environments of change.

➤ Structures have changed from rigid rational-legal or mechanistic to more organic and open to provide quality service and product to customer and clients.

➤ Systems are designed to obtain inputs, transform the inputs and provide quality outputs or outcomes.

➤ Five common structures present in organizations include functional, self-contained, matrix, process based and network.

➤ Future systems and organizational structures will be driven by trends in technology, diversity of the populations, and flexibility of the organization to meet needs internally and externally, flattening of the structure to provide quicker and more accurate communication, and strategic alliances and partnerships in the field.

SUGGESTED PROBLEM-BASED LEARNING ACTIVITIES

Chapter 2: Organizational Structure: A Look at Concepts and Models

Instructions: Use Internet resources, books, articles, colleagues, etc., to present solutions to the problems listed below. There is no one correct solution to any problem.

Note to Instructor: Students in class may be divided into groups and given the problem-based learning activity to discuss and solve. Once the group has reached consensus as to a solution, the group will present it to the other students in the class. This activity will provide all students with information regarding solutions to the problem.

Problem #1

Design a traditional organizational chart for an institution and then re-structure the chart for a client-focused design. Discuss formal and informal structures related to the organizational chart. Discuss advantages, disadvantages, and potential problems related to the transition of the organization from the traditional chart to the client-focused design.

Problem #2

A new administration has taken charge in your institution and you (the laboratory manager) have been directed to form self-directed work groups to focus on each component of the mission of your department.

Problem #3

Your hospital administration has asked you to develop an organizational structure to facilitate productivity and cost-effectiveness.

Problem #4

The Center for Medicare and Medicaid services now requires all orders to be written and signed by a physician. Develop a laboratory structure that will maintain efficiency in providing results to the physician and maintain patient satisfaction.

REFERENCES

1. "Structure." Def. 2b. *Merriam-Webster Online Dictionary.* Retrieved 26 Dec 2010, from: http://www.merriam-webster.com/dictionary/structure

2. Taylor FW: *The Principles of Scientific Management.* Kessinger Publishing, Whitefish, MT, 2004.

3. French WL, Bell CH Jr: *Organization Development.* Prentice Hall, Upper Saddle River, NJ, 1999.

4. Wheatley MJ: *Leadership and the New Science.* Barrett-Koehler Publishers, San Francisco, CA, 1999.

5. Nadler DA, Nadler MB: *Champions of Change.* Jossey-Bass, San Francisco, CA, 1998.

6. Sims RR: *Managing Organizational Behavior.* Quorum Books, Westport, CT, 2002.

7. Dent HS Jr: *The Roaring 2000s.* Touchstone—Simon & Schuster, New York, NY, 1998.

8. Lu S, et al: Outreach, Consolidation, and Networking: Columbia's Approach to Successful Integration of Laboratory Services in California. *Clin Lab Manage Rev* 1996: 10(5); 507-517.

BIBLIOGRAPHY

Aldridge JW: Socio-Technical Systems. In: DiStefano A, Rudestam KE, Silverman RJ, eds. *Encyclopedia of Distributed Learning,* 2004.

Borgotti SP: 21st Century Organizational Trends. 2001. Accessed 27 Dec 2010, from: http://www.analytictech.com/mb021/trendsin.htm

Bradford DL, Burk WW: *Reinventing Organizational Development.* Pfeiffer, San Francisco, CA, 2005.

Farwell DC: Hospital Laboratory Consolidation. *Clin Lab Manage Rev* 1995: 9(5); 411-420.

Friedman BA: Integrating Laboratory Processes into Clinical Processes, Web-Based Laboratory Reporting, and the Emergence of the Virtual Clinical Laboratory. *Clin Lab Manage Rev,* 26(5):333–38, 1998.

Hoffman P: Socio-Technical Systems and Organizational Values. Jan 2007. Accessed 26 Dec 2010, from: http://www.expertarticles.com/article/Business/Networking/Socio-Technical-Systems-and-Organizational-Values.html

Holman D, et al: *The Essentials of the New Workplace: A Guide to the Human Impact of Modern Working Practices.* John Wiley & Sons, Indianapolis, IN, 2004.

Howells J: *The Management of Innovation.* Sage Publications USA, Thousand Oaks, CA, 2005.

Rothwell WJ, et al: *Practicing Organization Development: A Guide for Consultants.* Jossey-Bass/Pfeiffer, San Francisco, CA, 1995.

INTERNET RESOURCES

The Association for Quality and Participation (AQP)
http://www.aqp.org

Free Management Library
http://www.managementhelp.org

Reference for Business—Encyclopedia of Small Business
http://www.referenceforbusiness.com

Systems Thinking Press—A resource for publications on systems thinking and strategic management.
http://www.systemsthinkingpress.com

Tavistock Institute
http://www.tavinstitute.org

CHAPTER 3

Principles of Leadership: Past, Present, and Future

Ellen Hope Kearns, PhD, SH(ASCP), MASCP
David W. Matear, PhD, DDPH, Msc

CHAPTER OUTLINE

OBJECTIVES

Following successful completion of this chapter, the learner will be able to:

1. Define three work-related situations and describe appropriate effective versus ineffective leadership styles and behaviors.
2. Briefly explain Leadership Theories X, Y, and Z.
3. Describe Full Range Leadership Theory and its components.
4. Describe Transformational Leadership and its components.
5. Describe Global Transformational Leadership and related competencies.
6. Compare and contrast leadership versus management.
7. Briefly describe three key functions of a formal leader.
8. Assess one's own leadership qualities according to attributes presented.
9. Describe four competencies for effective leadership.
10. Explain the Blake-Mouton Managerial Grid.
11. Assess one's own leadership style according to leadership styles presented.

KEY TERMS

Behavioral Approach
Blake-Mouton Managerial Grid
Character
Coercive Power
Courage
Credibility
Cultural Intelligence
Dependency Theory
Emotional Intelligence
Expert Power
Global Transformational Leadership
Humility
Insight
Integrity
Keirsey Temperament Theory

Leadership
Legitimate Power
Passion
Positive Self-Esteem
Power
Reciprocal Approach
Referent Power
Reward Power
Sense of Humor
Situational Contingency Approach
Theory X-Theory Y
Theory Z
Trait Approach
Vision

Case Study — **Leadership Styles**

Congratulations! You have just been promoted to Laboratory Manager in a medium-sized community hospital after six years of working in the Chemistry laboratory. You are well respected by your peers and knowledgeable of laboratory practices. However, some of the staff have questioned why you received the promotion, since you have had very little formal management or supervisory training.

The administrator asks you to lead a task force to increase outreach business for the hospital. She tells you that you must increase market share in the next six months.

Issues and Questions to Consider:

1. *What management characteristics will you need to exhibit?*
2. *What leadership attributes will be needed to achieve success?*
3. *Name at least three things you will do first to get this project going.*
4. *Describe how you can use the leadership styles in Table 3-6 to maximize your effectiveness.*
5. *What are your strengths?*
6. *What traits or styles will you need to improve?*
7. *What do you anticipate are some leadership challenges that you will need to overcome?*

INTRODUCTION

The chronology and history of leadership research have revealed a variety of central themes. Table 3-1 lists the various themes of leadership research. The Southwest Educational Development Laboratory Report highlights some of the major works of leadership research published in the 1900s.

In this chapter, examples are cited of popular leadership theories, paradigms, and principles written by contemporary scholars who have inspired us and influenced our understanding of leadership. This chapter begins with a historical perspective on researchers' approaches to leadership and includes definitions of leadership and a section on leadership development. Whether you are reading this chapter because you are taking a required course, have recently accepted a new leadership role in the laboratory, or are already a leader, it is our hope that you will understand your leadership role better after utilizing this chapter.

TABLE 3-1.   Central Themes of Leadership Research

- Relationships between leadership styles and behaviors
- Leadership skills
- Leader and follower characteristics
- Personality traits of leaders
- Situational leadership
- Organizational leadership theories
- Leaders versus managers
- Visionary leadership
- Transformational leadership
- The role of leaders and leadership

WHAT WE MEAN BY LEADERSHIP

"Leadership is not domination, but the art of persuading people to work toward a common goal."

—Daniel Goleman on Emotional Intelligence[1]

Leadership is defined in many different ways; however, many definitions of leadership contain common elements. For example, Susan Komives and her colleagues suggest that leadership is viewed and valued differently by various cultures and disciplines.[2] A multidisciplinary approach to leadership fosters a shared understanding of similarities and differences in leadership principles and practices across disciplines and cultures.[2] Thurgood noted that leadership does not fit into any one experience, theory, or historical study[3]; rather, leadership is a cumulative effect of many factors. The education and development of a leader requires a broader perspective that emphasizes leadership as both a process (science) and an art (ineffable instinct) to be developed. In addition, Nahavandi suggests that cultures may have an impact on leadership approach.[4] For example, cultures with a strong tradition for prophetic salvation may be more accepting to charismatic or transformational leadership through emotional bonds and accepted social norms within such cultures. As a result, **Cultural Intelligence (CQ)** is now considered to be important in leadership of multicultural groups or in a global or international setting. Cultural intelligence is a person's ability to function effectively in situations characterized by cultural diversity.[5, 6, 7] Cultural intelligence provides an understanding about individuals' capabilities to be successful within multi-cultural situations, cross-cultural interactions, and perform in culturally diverse work groups.[8]

In health care services, Longest and his colleagues note that leadership is, "a process of one individual influencing another individual or group to achieve particular objectives."[9] Southwest Airlines' view of leadership is, "a dynamic relationship based on mutual influence and common purpose between leaders and collaborators in which both are moved to higher levels of motivation and moral development as they affect real, intended change."[10] It is interesting to note that Southwest Airlines uses the word "collaborator" instead of "follower," a more commonly used term in leadership discussions. In their view, "collaborator" better describes the individuals at Southwest Airlines because leadership is what Southwest leaders and their collaborators do together. John Snyder, an outstanding leader in clinical laboratory sciences and higher education administration, defines leadership as:

"The ability to persuade others to seek defined objectives enthusiastically. It is the human factor which binds a group together and motivates it toward goals. Management activities such as planning, organizing, and decision-making are dormant cocoons until the leader triggers the power of motivation in people and guides them toward goals."[11]

David Glenn, CEO of Pathology Services, P.C., states that "the most valuable part of my leadership is to inspire and empower the staff to become leaders in their own areas of responsibility." (Glenn, D. Personal Communication, 7 Jan 2010). Notice that these leadership definitions include groups, individuals, organizations, management tasks, goals and objectives, attitudes and behaviors. Please note that influence is a common element.

LEADERSHIP VERSUS MANAGEMENT

Leadership and management are often thought of as the same thing. However, like other authors, we contend that there is an important distinction between the two. The primary difference between the two concepts is addressed in Michael Maccoby's article, "Understanding the Difference Between Management and Leadership."[12] Maccoby suggests that managers are primarily administrators who are able to influence decisions and actions; whereas, leaders influence the opinions and attitudes of others to accomplish a mutually agreed-on task while advancing the group's integrity and moral purpose. Simply put, the leader is the central person who guides the group toward achieving a goal. In other words, leadership takes place any time one attempts to influence the behavior of a group; whether it is to accomplish one's own goals, or to accomplish those of the organization.

John Kotter, in *Leading Change*, makes the distinction of management versus leadership in the following way. He describes management as a set of processes (such as planning, budgeting, organizing, and problem solving) that can keep a complicated system of people and technology running smoothly.[13] Leadership, on the other hand, creates organizations or adapts them to significant changes in circumstance.

Leadership defines the future and establishes direction, aligns the people and processes with a vision, and inspires the organization to make it happen. Zalesnick views managers and leaders as different types of people. In his view, "managers and leaders differ in attitudes toward goals, conceptions of work, behavior toward risk taking, relations with others, and their sense of self."[14] Further, Zalesnick suggests that different personality traits exist between leaders and managers. Leadership traits will be discussed under the heading, "Attributes of Effective Leadership."

If this were a perfect world, all managers would be effective leaders that people would want to follow. However, based on feedback from our colleagues, managers can be ineffective and even resemble "the boss" portrayed in the poem entitled "The Leader," written by an unknown author, which appears below:

The boss drives group members, the leader coaches them.
The boss depends upon authority; the leader on good will.
The boss inspires fear; the leader inspires enthusiasm.
The boss says, "I"; the leader says, "We."
The boss assigns the task, the leader sets the pace.
The boss says, "Get there on time"; the leader gets there ahead of time.
The boss fixes the blame for the breakdown; the leader fixes the breakdown.
The boss knows how it is done; the leader shows how.
The boss makes work drudgery; the leader makes it a game.
The boss says, "Go"; the leader says, "Let's go."

According to Kevin Cashman, "Leadership is authentic self-expression that creates value . . . It involves awakening our inner identity, purpose and vision so that our lives are dedicated to a conscious, intentional manner of living."[15] Gardner and Stough suggest that the understanding of emotions is particularly important to leadership effectiveness.[16] Gill's integrative leadership model is supported by Goleman, Boyatzis, and McKee's primal leadership theory (PLT), which suggests that a leader's primal task is to manage emotions in a way that creates an environment that promotes confidence and collaborative work.[17, 18] Taking this further, Wood, Coppola, and Satterwhite identify key transformational leadership characteristics such as communicating beliefs and values, stimulating intellectual curiosity, and a deep focus on the values, goals, ethical foundations, cultural identity, and desires of subordinates.[19]

POWER AND INFLUENCE

An effective leader must be able to get followers to follow. In other words, a leader must have the capability to influence others to follow his/her advice, suggestion, or directive in pursuing the common goals of the groups or organizations to which they all belong. Therefore, before we introduce various leadership approaches, we need to briefly discuss the topics of power and influence, which are relevant and important to leadership. **Power** is defined as the capacity to influence others' behavior. When we say Person A has power over Person B, we mean A can get B to do what A wants, rather than what B himself or herself wants. Power is a different concept than authority, which is obtained by a manager when she or he takes a position and has the legitimacy to expect compliance from subordinates. Power refers to A's ability to influence B, not A's right to do so.

Power is no doubt essential to a manager to become a true leader. There are several theories on where power comes from. According to Emerson's **dependency theory**, individual/group A will have power over an individual/group if B is dependent on A.[20] Most of the time, we will find this dependence to be resource-related. A will have power over B if A controls the resources that are desirable to B and B will not be able to gain access to such resources other than through A. The desired resources could be money, materials and space for work, tools and equipment, knowledge and expertise, political networks, etc.

Another theory on the sources of power was developed by psychologists John French and Bertram Raven.[21] According to French and Raven, based on the difference in sources, power can be categorized into the following groups: legitimate power, reward power, coercive power, expert power, and referent power.

Legitimate power is derived from a person's position or job in an organization. Being put in the manager's position, a person is authorized by the organization with the legitimate right to require and demand compliance from his or her subordinates. In today's culture, such compliance by subordinates is well expected. It is understood in today's culture that people have a tendency to comply with the requests and demands of their bosses at work. Traditionally, medical laboratories have functioned under this type of "bossiness." While there is no clear explanation for this, this tendency is believed to have something to do with our life experiences with parents, teachers, and law enforcement officials.

Reward power exists in those who have the capacity to influence others by providing positive rewards. The rewards that are perceived to be valuable may include: raises, promotions, favorable job performance evaluations, assignment of preferred tasks, better working conditions, recognition, and compliments, to name a few. **Coercive power** is the capacity to apply punishments to those who refuse to comply with requests or demands. The punishments in organizations include, but are not limited to, docking pay or other benefits, assignment of unfavorable tasks, blocked promotion, disciplinary actions, criticisms, and being isolated. Both reward and coercive powers are based on the expectation of those supposedly influenced that they may either lose the chance to get desired rewards or simply get punished if they refuse to comply with the demands or requests.

Expert power derives from powerholders' superior knowledge, skills, and abilities. People tend to be influenced by experts who know how to perform and have experience in performing their jobs well. The more crucial and unusual this expertise, the greater the expert power will be. It is not surprising that expert power is especially common in scientific and technical areas such as the medical laboratory. Such power, once obtained, is not easy to lose because of the difficulty in replacing the superior skills, abilities, and knowledge.

Referent power exists when the powerholder is liked, respected, or admired by others. As human beings, we are more likely to be influenced by the people we like and to whom we are attracted. We may easily welcome their opinions, often seek their approval, sometimes even use them as role models, and we tend to ignore their failures. Referent power represents a more profound base of power than those based on incentives or threats. Both referent and expert power are most likely to generate true commitment and enthusiasm on the followers' side with regard to the manager's requests or demands.

In general, the power possessed by a manager is a combination of legitimate power, reward power, coercive power, referent power, and expert power. By taking the manager's position, an individual is given the authority to make demands and requests of the subordinates. Normally with such authority comes the ability in various levels to give rewards or apply punishment to the subordinates. It is also likely that the manager is a true expert in his/her technical area and/or a charismatic person who is greatly admired by his/her colleagues. Oftentimes, this is the major reason for a person being promoted. Therefore, managers can use a variety of strategies to build and accumulate power.

First, newly promoted managers should be willing and feel comfortable to give orders or make demands; realizing that the general tendency of employees is to comply with such orders and demands. By confidently and appropriately exercising the authority to give orders, managers can enhance their legitimate power. Most successful managers should strive to achieve competencies in the domains of self-awareness, self-management, social awareness, and relationship management.[18, 22]

Secondly, managers should constantly absorb new knowledge and develop their skills in the technical areas related to their work. This is particularly important in the medical laboratory setting. If they are already technical experts, managers should be willing to demonstrate their expertise by helping employees to solve technical problems. If they are not yet technical experts themselves, they should be able to delegate a technical specialist, and be ready to listen to and learn from that individual. Repetitive mistakes in making technical decisions will greatly harm a managers' reputation, and ultimately discount the effectiveness of their leadership. Laboratory managers must take swift corrective action to avoid repetitive mistakes, although technical instrument failures, laboratory personnel errors, and erroneous test results may be unavoidable in a medical laboratory arena. Quick corrective action allows a manager to safeguard their patients, clients, and overall reputation of the laboratory. However, development of new knowledge and skills should not be limited solely to technical knowledge, but should also incorporate the study of leadership. Wood, Coppola, and Satterwhite describe the study of leadership as important due to potential stakeholder consequences, which must be considered for a leader to be successful and prosper.[19]

Thirdly, managers should consciously cultivate friendly interpersonal relations with subordinates, peers, bosses, and outsiders to gain the referent power within organizations. Although it is often difficult and sometimes impossible to

be liked by everybody at work, managers should try their best to win as much respect as possible from their colleagues. In contrast, many of the traits that make a
person likable may not be learnable. However, many behaviors that make a person
respectable are indeed learnable; like being loyal and committed to others, treating everyone fairly, being righteous and responsible, and self-sacrificing when
needed. In addition, the self- and social-emotional intelligence competencies that
have been identified as key components of leadership, can be developed through
self-assessment, self-reflection, and self-directed learning, which drive the emotional environment.[22, 23] If you as a manager have these behaviors, you are well
on your way to win the respect of your colleagues.

Finally, managers should use every opportunity on the job to gain control of
resources that are desirable to their employees. In addition to financial resources,
desirable tools and equipment, preferred workspace, and chances for promotion
and career advancement, there are also political connections and professional networks. With more resources under direct control, managers increase their ability
to reward employees. On the other hand, managers should also negotiate wisely
both before and after taking their positions, so that their own employees will not
be prevented from obtaining rewards, and will not be subject to reprisals or sanctions. Although good managers may not necessarily resort to coercive mechanism
to increase their ability to influence employees, it is nice to have such mechanism
available if it is ever needed.

APPROACHES TO LEADERSHIP

During the 20th Century, there has been a significant transformation in the approach to leadership. In the first half of the century, the **trait approach** to leadership
produced varying lists of personal traits that purportedly guaranteed successful
leadership to persons who possessed varying outstanding characteristics such as
height, charisma, intelligence, and the like. The trait approach focused on addressing the question "what a leader is" or "who become leaders." The major problem
of this approach is its assumption that there was a definite set of characteristics
that made a leader and that leadership cannot be learned.

In the 1950s and 1960s, trait theories were disputed by writers such as Ralph
Stogdill, a distinguished leadership researcher, who were more interested in the
behavioral approach to leadership and focused attention on what a leader "does,"
rather than what a leader "is." The behavioral approach took the position that
leadership can be learned through education, training, life, and work experience.
Within this approach, different patterns of leaders' behavior were grouped together and labeled as leadership styles. However, the behavioral approach did not
address the issue of how a manager should select the most effective leadership
style in a specific situation.

Since the 1960s, **situational contingency approach** has emerged, focusing
on the importance of the context of the situation in explaining leader effectiveness.
The central point of the contingency approach is that the leadership style needed

would change with the situation. Various models of the contingency approach have been proposed to help choose the appropriate leadership style for a particular circumstance.[24, 25]

The trait, behavioral, and contingency approaches have traditionally been the foundation of most of leadership theories. This chapter is also firmly based on these approaches in introducing various leadership concepts and principles. However, it is noteworthy that there are other approaches to leadership. From the mid 1920s to the late 1970s, advocates of the influence approach asserted that leadership was an influence, or social exchange process, followed by the present day **reciprocal approach** that leadership is a relational and shared process that includes a strong emphasis on followership. In the book *Exploring Leadership*, Komives and colleagues summarized the chronology, assumptions, criticisms, and theories associated with each of the aforementioned approaches.[2] Other perspectives of leadership have emerged, including those on transformational leadership, transactional leadership, and charismatic leadership.[9, 26, 27, 28]

FULL-RANGE LEADERSHIP THEORY

Leadership is described as the ability to turn vision into reality.[29] Various approaches in applied leadership are combined in full-range leadership theory (FRLT) proposed by Avolio and Bass.[30] FRLT includes three typologies of leadership behavior: transformational, transactional, and non-transactional laissez-faire leadership, represented by nine distinct single-order factors. Transactional leadership focuses on follower goal and role clarification and how leaders reward followers, which Bass suggests only induces basic interactions, and is based on contingent rewards and management-by-exception (active and passive).[31] Laissez-Faire leadership is non-transformational and non-transactional leadership, in which the leaders avoid involvement, and have very limited application. Transformational leadership is described by House et al. as how a vision can be realized through leadership by the ability to influence, motivate, and enable others for the success of the organization.[32] Transformational leadership has five aspects of idealized influence or charismatic leadership (attributed or behavioral), inspirational motivation, intellectual stimulation, and individualized consideration. Therefore, FRLT consists of five transformational leadership factors, three transactional leadership factors, and one non-transactional laissez-faire leadership. The complexity of applied leadership theory is evident.

TRANSFORMATIONAL LEADERSHIP

Wood et al. suggest that transformational leadership is based on the tenets of social exchange theory, in which individuals engage in social interactions with the expectation that they will give and receive a benefit or reward.[19] These benefits or rewards can be intrinsic or extrinsic. In these situations, transformational leadership borrows from previous trait theories as the leader uses motivation techniques, including emphasis on personal charisma, individual attention to the follower, intellectual stimulation of the task, and appeal to strong emotions within the group. In contrast to transactional leadership, transformational leadership uses transactions and interpersonal relations as the means to affect change and not as ends in and unto themselves. Using these principles, change may be catalyzed in an environment in which there exists a crisis or recognized need for change.[33, 34]

Sullivan and Decker suggest that transformational leadership merges the motives, desires, values, and goals of leaders and followers towards a common goal.[35] Therefore, the transformational leader motivates, facilitates, and educates individuals toward a vision. Emotions and feelings, such as admiration and loyalty toward the leader, are mechanisms through which followers strive to exceed expectations, both individually and collectively.[36] Burns identifies this motivation as a basic requirement for leadership; however, Wood et al. emphasize that motivation may differ between individuals and be external or internal in nature.[26, 19]

The effect of transformational leaders on followers is not completely understood. Wood et al. (in press) suggest that a combination of factors must be present, including the possession of various attributes by leaders, receptiveness of followers, and specific environmental conditions that may be necessary or even essential in the development and efficacy of such leadership.[19] In addition, certain personality characteristics are often associated with transformational leaders, such as: intelligence, self-confidence, a positive image, excellent communication skills, and the ability to empathize with followers.[4] These characteristics include a variety of intelligences identified by other authors.[29, 17, 37] Transformational leaders should also possess a highly socialized need for power, strong moral conviction, and high energy levels, which are then used to create and project competence.[19] As a result of these attributes, intelligences, and behaviors, followers have confidence in the leader's direction and develop a strong relationship and emotional bond with the leader and value the leader's vision.[4] The internalization of the leader's values and moral convictions may also be assisted by the perceived need for immediate change as a response to an unacceptable situation.

EMOTIONAL INTELLIGENCE

Goleman, using the qualitative observation of almost 4,000 executives, identified six leadership styles: *coercive, authoritative, affiliative, democratic, pacesetting,* and *coaching*.[37] Goleman concluded that a successful leader has to have several styles to meet the demands of leadership.[38] Goleman et al. also identified the four emotional intelligence (EI) competency domains of a successful leader as: self-awareness, self-management, social awareness, and relationship management, through the analysis of competency models in a study of 188 multinational companies.[18] On analysis of these factors, after data collection, the effects of

EI were found to be twice as important than other skills at all levels of leadership, but became even more important at higher or more senior levels in organizations. Notably, Goleman also reported that emotional intelligence can be learned, thus improving leadership performance.[38]

CULTURAL INTELLIGENCE

Cultural Intelligence (CQ) is a person's ability to function effectively in situations characterized by cultural diversity.[5, 6, 7] Cultural intelligence provides an understanding about individuals' capabilities to be successful within multicultural situations, cross-cultural interactions, and perform in culturally diverse work groups. Ang et al. completed a personality assessment of 338 business undergraduates at two points in time. The assessment used the 20-item, four-factor model for CQ (CQS). After controlling for age, gender, and years of experience, the study demonstrated the relationships between the big five personality factors of openness, conscientiousness, extraversion, agreeableness, and neuroticism, and the four-factor model of CQ, and indicated the ability of the model to deal effectively with cultural diversity.

Lugo explains that CQ also reflects leadership motivation and describes individuals' confidence about their ability and internal satisfaction in cross-cultural interactions.[39] Earley and Ang describe two motivational frames for understanding motivational CQ: self-efficacy and self-consistency.[6] Self-efficacy is based on the ability of an individual to accomplish a certain level of performance, and self-consistency relates to emotional intelligence and the capability to regulate emotional states.

LEADERSHIP AND TEMPERAMENT

As we pointed out previously, the efforts that intended to isolate specific personal traits as determinants of leadership abilities in the early years of leadership research led to the conclusion that no single trait separates leaders from non-leaders. On the contrary, various studies since the 1970s suggested that people of various characters and personalities all have the potential to become effective leaders. Among the studies is the *Keirsey Temperament Theory.*

David Keirsey proposed a modified model of the *Myers-Briggs Type Indicator* questionnaire for identifying actions and *attitudes* associated with 16 personality types.[40] Keirsey's questionnaires, called the Keirsey Temperament Sorter II, are self-scoring questionnaires designed to identify 16 combinations of four temperament types. Following the Myers-Briggs model, Keirsey elected to label each of the temperament types with a combination of letters, seen in parentheses to describe elements of personality traits represented in the four basic types shown in Table 3-2.

TABLE 3-2. Letters and Descriptions of Keirsey's Four Temperament Types[40]

Artisan	(SP)	S stands for Observant and P stands for Probing
Guardian	(SJ)	S stands for Observant and J stands for Scheduling
Idealist	(NF)	N stands for Introspective and F stands for Friendly
Rational	(NT)	N stands for Introspective and T stands for Tough-minded

TABLE 3-3. Keirsey's Sixteen Types of Personality Grouped by Four Temperament Types[40]

A	Artisans	(Promoter, Crafter, Performer, Composer)
G	Guardians	(Supervisor, Inspector, Provider, Protector)
I	Idealists	(Teacher, Counselor, Champion, Healer)
R	Rationals	(Field marshal, Mastermind, Inventor, Architect)

Table 3-3 lists 16 personality types within the four temperament types proposed by Keirsey, who suggests that temperament is an integral part of a person's character and personality that drives one's behavior. Moreover, he provides valuable insight into the self-image, values, interests of, and social roles played by the Artisan (SP), Guardian (SJ), Idealist (NF), and Rational (NT) types.

In his book, *Please Understand Me II,* Keirsey pointed out that, although several great world leaders, including Mohandas Gandhi, Winston Churchill, George Washington, and Abraham Lincoln, are so different from each other in personalities, they are all well recognized for their effective leadership. Keirsey suggested that certain kinds of temperament are needed for certain circumstances to make a leader an effective one.[40] Keirsey and Myers-Briggs questionnaires have served as valuable research tools and sustained public interest over the years, as evidenced by the scores of people who take them each year. The questionnaires and interpretation of the results are both published in Keirsey's book. A modified version of the questionnaire is posted on his website (http://www.keirsey.com). Take the Keirsey Temperament Sorter tests online to ascertain your personality temperament types. Once you complete the questionnaire, you will be provided with an interpretation of the results based on your responses.

ATTRIBUTES FOR EFFECTIVE LEADERSHIP

Whereas we recognize the fact that people of different personalities all have the potential to become effective leaders, we also suggest that there are certain attributes commonly shared by effective leaders. Take a moment to visualize the leaders in your organization who you admire and trust. What are the reasons you would work harder for them rather than someone else? Write down the attributes that you believe they possess. After you are finished, compare and contrast your list with ours. Our list begins with **character**. We may think of character as learning *how to be* rather than *how to act*. It is the essence of being a leader that opens up possibilities. Qualities of character include authenticity, purpose, creating value, trust, congruence, and compassion. Character is the foundation of Win/Win, a philosophy of human interaction and moral strength, on which everything else builds, according to Stephen Covey, an internationally respected leadership authority and teacher.[41] Win/Win is based on the paradigm that there is enough for everyone, that one person's success is not accomplished at the exclusion of the success of others. **Integrity**, the value we place on ourselves and on others, is a key attribute for effective leadership. Integrity, sincerity, and honesty engender trust and respect. In other words, we admire leaders who "talk the talk and walk the walk!" Leaders need to have a **vision**. The leaders need to be visionaries who are able to see the "big picture" and be able to effectively communicate the strategic direction of their vision to the organization. Having self-confidence and a keen understanding of others is essential for being self-empowered and empowering others to be part of a solution or the change process. **Passion** for the job enables great leaders to get through the painstaking tasks of creating change, an inevitable outcome of the leadership process. Passion inspires and creates followership. Effective leaders must be believable. **Credibility** is based on excellent credentials, substantive knowledge, and sound practical experience. Leaders must be willing to assume greater responsibility for changing group outcomes. **Courage** is essential for creating a new vision, taking risks, and challenging the status quo. Personal **insight** and perception into the realities that exist in and outside of the organization are important attributes for effective leadership. **Humility** is a hallmark characteristic of a strong leader, good listener, and a perpetual learner who is willing to admit that others also have good ideas and accept that he/she can be wrong. Next on the list is a **sense of humor**. If you are going to be a leader, a good sense of humor will help you and others. When appropriately used, humor is a valuable tool, especially for ameliorating stress. **Emotional intelligence**, a concept proposed by Daniel Goleman in his book by the same name, consists of basic emotional competencies that describe the abilities needed to manage ourselves and our relationships effectively.[1] These include self-awareness, self-management, social awareness, and relationship management, which underpin six leadership styles, and which may be used according to the situation.[38, 42] Each style has a positive or negative impact on organizational climate. Finally, with a **positive self-esteem**, a leader works selflessly to support people working toward the common good of the organization. A successful leader has positive self-esteem and self-respect, evidenced by the leader's positive behaviors, such as taking risks confidently and communicating with clarity. Rate yourself according to the leadership qualities presented in Table 3-4 and prepare to work on areas in need of improvement. You may wish to use this exercise as an index to monitor your personal growth and professional development as a leader. Leadership development programs are available. Refer to examples of successful programs later in this chapter.

TABLE 3-4.   Key Attributes for Effective Leadership: Self-Assessment

Attribute	I Really Need Help!	I'm Working On It!	I Have It!
1. Character			
2. Integrity			
3. Vision			
4. Passion			
5. Credibility			
6. Empowerment			
7. Courage			
8. Insight			
9. Humility			
10. Sense of Humor			
11. Emotional Intelligence			
12. Positive Self-Esteem			

COMPETENCIES FOR EFFECTIVE LEADERSHIP

Key competencies for effective leadership include: creating and inspiring a shared vision, communicating, diagnosing, problem solving, and adapting, which are consistent with the tenets of transformational and emotionally and socially intelligent leadership.[31, 42] Vision points direction and gives purpose to the organization's work. Effective communication of the vision is an art, and leaders spend more time communicating than performing other activities. The communication process is dependent on varying message forms, including written and spoken words, as well as nonverbal behavior such as facial expressions, body language, and listening. Researchers indicate that people spend approximately 45% of their communication time listening. Nevertheless, the average listener understands and retains only about 50% of what is said immediately after a presentation. This level diminishes to approximately 20% within 48 hours. These data suggest that listening is one of the most crucial skills in the communication process. Other informal survey data suggest that communication is the number 1 problem in the workplace and in interpersonal relationships. The results of a national survey of laboratory directors by the American Society for Clinical Pathology ranked "effective communication skills" on top of the list of preferred skills for potential employees. Being able to understand the situation or a problem you are trying to influence is another important part of the leadership process. The leader must be able to analyze the current situation/problem and develop an effective strategy for intervention. Having the ability to adapt to change is key to successful leadership. The leader must adapt to behaviors and other available resources in such a way as to close the gap between the current situation and what he or she wants to influence.

In applying these competencies in the international or global arena, Matear suggested that cultural intelligence in the forms of metacognition (challenging and revised one's beliefs regarding cultures); cognition (knowledge of different cultures); motivation (willingness and value placed on intercultural relationship success); and behavior (appropriately demonstrating verbal and non-verbal behaviors) were important to the development of global transformational leadership competencies, based on the model in Figure 3-1.[23]

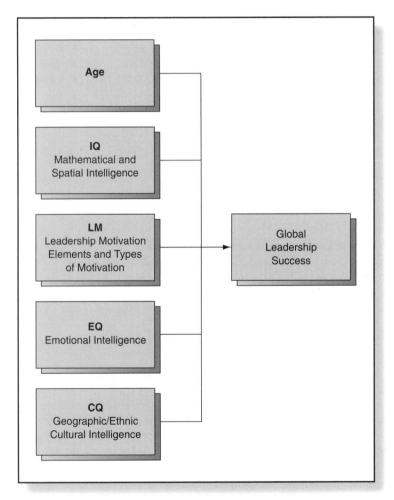

FIGURE 3-1.   **Matear's Conceptual Model of Global Leadership**

Adapted from Matear, DW. "An examination of cognitive, cultural, and emotional intelligences, and motivation in the development of global transformational leadership skills." Ph.D. Diss. Capella University, 2009.[23]

THE LEADERSHIP STYLES

"Becoming a leader is synonymous with becoming yourself. It's precisely that simple, and it's also that difficult."

—Warren Bennis, *On Becoming a Leader*[43]

Although the concept of leadership remains debatable and elusive, there is consensus among researchers that leadership is, and effective leaders are, crucial to the success of an organization. Like parenting, leadership is not an exact science. Leadership must and can be learned. The learning process starts from first understanding various styles of leadership and identifying "what effective leaders do." These styles are different from competencies or responsibilities of leaders. Styles are concerned with the observed manner of the leader's behavior and actions. Until today, much of the research done in the area of leadership styles focused on some combination of high/low production and high/low concern for people.

The Blake-Mouton Model

Robert Blake and Jane Mouton proposed one classic research model on leadership style in 1964 called the managerial grid.[44] They visualized leadership styles in terms of a balance between concerns for getting the job done and the working relationships that must be integrated to achieve effective leadership. In the **Blake-Mouton managerial grid**, five different types of leadership, based on concern for production (task) and concern for people (relationship), are positioned in four quadrants (Figure 3-2). Concern for production is illustrated on the horizontal axis and concern for people on the vertical axis. The strength of a concern is rated on a scale from 1 to 9, with a 9/1 (*Task*) indicating the maximum commitment to working objectives, with little to no concern given to people's feelings. A 1/9 (*Country Club*) suggests a preoccupation with relationships and satisfying the needs of others at the expense of the task that needs to be done. A 1/1 (*Impoverished*) would be characteristic of a low-profile manager, who exerts minimal effort to get the job done and has minimal contact with others. The 5/5 (*Middle Road*) managers tend to maintain a satisfactory balance between the need to get the work done and the morale of the people doing the work. Like McGregor's Y, the belief of the 9/9 manager is that people have an inherent desire to perform well at work provided they are given the opportunity and encouraged to do so. All styles except the 9/9 (Team) suggest an expectation of conflict between keeping people happy and getting the job done.

The Lorenzi-Riley Model

Derived from the task-oriented and people-oriented model developed by Hersey and Blanchard, Nancy Lorenzi and Robert Riley proposed the following styles of

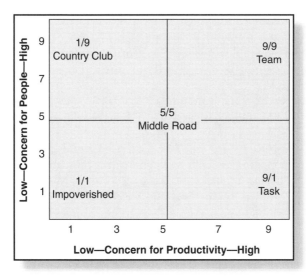

FIGURE 3-2. **Blake-Mouton's Managerial Grid**

Adapted from Hersey P, Blanchard KH, and Johnson DE: *Management of Organizational Behavior: Leading Human Resources.* 9th ed. Upper Saddle River, NJ: Prentice Hall, 2001.[25]

leadership behaviors: the on-the-job retirees, the whip crackers, the schmoozers, and the team builders.[25,45] On-the-job retirees are low on task skills, low on interpersonal relationships, and are usually procrastinators. The whip crackers are usually very task oriented, low on interpersonal skills, and see the task to be done as their primary responsibility, no matter what the cost. The whip crackers motto is "damn the torpedoes, full speed ahead!" Schmoozers, taken from the Yiddish word for, "one who chats and idly gossips," rank low on task and high in interpersonal relationships. They can be enthusiastic about a project, but have a problem getting their group to get the job done. The last category, team builders, rank high in both task and interpersonal skills. They empower their staff and they know what questions to ask and when to offer support.

Theories X, Y, and Z

Another model on leadership styles is the **Theory X-Theory Y** model proposed by Douglas McGregor in 1960. This model is somewhat different and more classic than the two other models introduced previously. McGregor suggests that managers operate from two sets of expectations about employees' attitudes and abilities that ultimately influence their work performance.[46] McGregor's X-philosophy implies that employees are basically lazy, that they detest work, and that they need direction and control to protect them from the anathema of work. The X-oriented manager is likely to have to compensate for the worker's shortcomings. X-oriented managers tend to be dictatorial and autocratic. By contrast,

McGregor's Y-philosophy suggested an optimistic set of expectations that workers view work as natural as play, that they are highly motivated, self-disciplined, and exercise creativity in problem solving. The Y-oriented manager's role then is one of capitalizing on the strengths of the workers. Y-oriented managers have a participative leadership style.

In more recent years, a modified **Theory Z** model has been introduced. Proponents of the Z-model suggest that the self-disciplined and highly motivated characteristic of employees in the Theory-Y model is cultural. This concept evolved from efforts to incorporate some of the Japanese ideas into our American management practices as a possibility for increasing productivity and job satisfaction. The Z-philosophy implies that changing societal goals must be included in the workplace, and that productivity and rewards are not the only objectives of workers, but other issues such as quality of their work lives have a significant impact on their performance. Goldsmith refers to the Japanese Theory Z approach as a "magic potion" that, when applied to ailing U.S. industries and government, can solve problems of turnover, productivity, and alienation.[47] The Japanese magic formula contains elements such as lifetime employment; a company's concern for their employees' total well-being; consensus decision making; and a consistent system of promotions, among other elements. Quality circles and total quality management "TQM" are an outgrowth of the Japanese approach to management taught to them by the American, William Edwards Deming, and others.[48]

Leadership Styles and Situations

Most people have a leadership style that they prefer and feel comfortable with. What you must realize is that different leadership behaviors may be required for different situations in order to get the job done. Leadership is not static, but rather a dynamic, fluidic, complex process involving a combination of three factors: the group, the environment, and the task. The most effective leadership style for a laboratory manager depends on the strength of the leader's abilities, the work environment, the group dynamics and morale, and the motivation of each of the workers. Hence, successful and effective leaders have the ability to adapt their style to fit the requirements of the situation. Table 3-5 lists conventional leadership styles, associated behaviors, and in what situation each style is effective and ineffective.

Goleman, Boyatzis, and McKee describe six leadership styles of commanding/coercive, pacesetting, visionary/authoritative, affiliative, coaching, and democratic.[18] The styles are the tools which leaders can apply according to the situation, in terms of task and maturity of the individual and group involved. Each style is underpinned by emotional intelligence competencies, which may be developed. Each style in the continuum has a positive or negative impact on organizational climate by affecting flexibility, responsibility, standards, rewards, clarity, and commitment. Therefore, a single style is not appropriate for all circumstances and efforts must be made to develop a variety of approaches for effective and successful leadership.

TABLE 3-5. Leadership Style, Behavior, and Situation

Style	Authoritative	Democratic	Laissez-Faire
Behavior	"Telling." Leader identifies a problem, considers solutions, chooses one, and then tells others what they are to do.	"Consulting." Leader gives people a chance to influence a decision from the start; members asked for ideas and leader then selects most promising solution.	"Joining." Leader is "just another member" and agrees in advance to carry out decisions the group makes.
When Style Is Effective	Time is limited; people lack skills; group doesn't know each other.	Time is available; group is motivated; people have some degree of skills.	Group is highly motivated; sense of team exists; routine is familiar to group members.
When Style Is Ineffective	Strong sense of team; people have some degree of skills/ knowledge; group wants spontaneity in work.	Group is unmotivated; people have no skills; high level of conflict present.	Low sense of team; people have low degree of skills; group expects to be told what to do.

LEADERSHIP DEVELOPMENT PROGRAMS

This section consists of just a few examples of successful leadership development programs for those who wish to further explore leadership potential and/or enhance a current leadership role. Further information on each of these development programs may be obtained using the corresponding reference or Internet resources located at the end of this chapter.

Global Transformational Leadership Development

Matear identified the key components of **global transformational leadership** as emotional intelligence and cultural intelligence.[23] As a result, Matear suggested that global transformational leadership can be developed. The basis of the development of global leadership skills are the competencies of these intelligences, which may be achieved through self-reflection, self-assessment, self-directed planning, and mentoring and coaching.

Leadership Learning Laboratory

The University of California, Davis offers a course entitled, "The Leadership Learning Laboratory." This introductory course is designed to explore one's organizational culture and leadership needs, discuss challenges of leading and opportunities for leadership, and identify specific leadership competencies through self-knowledge and awareness.

Leadership Coaching Certificate Program

Georgetown University offers a certificate program for project leaders, mid-level managers, directors, and executives leading organizational changes. The program includes personal assessment of leadership skills, strategies, and tools for implementing change, and development of leadership capabilities.

Chartered Management Institute—Leaders Who Inspire and Motivate

The Chartered Management Institute (CMI) of the United Kingdom offers leadership programs including Creating Inspirational Leaders; three 2-day intensive programs, Strategic Leader, Operational Leader, and Tactical Leader; and a more in-depth 12-month program.

LEADERSHIP STYLES FOR THE FUTURE

"A leader is someone you choose to follow to a place you wouldn't go by yourself."

—Joel A. Barker in *Leadershift*

The challenge for the future is to be able to inspire leadership at all levels and to be comfortable with ambiguity and chaos. As organizations get more complex, structures flatten, and decision making gets closer to the place of the customer interface, leadership characteristics become an expectation throughout. Corporate leaders like Max DuPree of Herman Miller, Inc. and Dee Hock of VISA International see their organizations as communities often exhibiting a high degree of chaos.[49, 50] They create a space for more leaders with inspiring goals and trust that employees guided by vision and goals will do the right thing. Effective leaders use the tools of community building to create an environment in which many leaders can emerge.

Peter Block redefines "leadership" for the future in terms of "stewardship":

> "Stewardship is . . . the choice to preside over the orderly distribution of power. This means giving people at the bottom and the boundaries of the organization choice over how to serve a customer, a citizen, a community. It is the willingness to be accountable for the well-being of the larger organization by operating in service, rather than in control of those around us. Simply stated, it is accountability without control or compliance."[51]

The concept of stewardship fits well with emerging organizational structures, team concepts, and shared accountabilities. It is one thing to describe the concepts and theories; it is another to understand *how leaders shall act* and *how leaders shall be*. Peter Drucker, the acknowledged "father of modern management," has studied leaders and leadership for more than 50 years. In *The Leader of the Future*, he concludes that effective leaders know four simple things:

1. A leader is someone who *has followers*.
2. The effective leader gets followers to do the right things. He/she might not be popular but he/she gets *results*.
3. Leaders are *visible*; they set examples.
4. Leadership is not about rank or title; it is about *responsibility*.[52]

"Get results" is a resounding answer to the question, "What do leaders do?" Using extensive research tools, Daniel Goleman has described six distinct leadership styles that appear to have a direct impact on the performance of an organization.[37] The effectiveness in these styles is not in the exclusive use of any one, but in the mental and emotional agility to choose the right style for the right situation. Table 3-6 delineates the styles and some of their dimensions.

If a leader can use these styles to challenge, support, and inspire members of the organization, they will spark optimum performance and get the desired results. The most effective leaders are those who can be flexible with their style and fluid in action. Mastery of at least four of the six styles—especially visionary/authoritative, affiliative, democratic, and coaching—creates the best organizational climate and best business performance. This can be achieved by developing the underlying relevant emotional intelligence competencies through self-reflection and the five personal stages of discovery, which assess ideal-self against real-self resulting in plans to close the gap using identified practice opportunities and mentoring.

The leaders of the future will need to demonstrate mental and emotional agility, guiding organizations through new and complex situations. It begins with appropriate use of self—self-awareness and self-leadership. Leaders need to take inventory of personal attributes and values and to understand the vision and purpose that motivates them to lead. As organizations move from a mentality of "chain-of-command" management to an attitude of "web-of-influence" leaders, we highlight three fundamental dimensions for leaders:

- *Embrace Vision and Change.* Create an "invisible force" that gives organizational clarity and purpose and future direction. Embrace change and your role as a change agent. Get agreement of goals and values, which will allow people the freedom to develop and make choices for which they will be accountable.
- *Share Information.* We no longer think of Knowledge as Power, but rather applying the knowledge as a means of nourishment for the organization.

TABLE 3-6. Leadership Styles for the Future

Styles:	Coercive	Authoritative	Affiliative	Democratic	Pacesetting	Coaching
The Leader's modus operandi	Demands immediate compliance	Mobilizes people toward a vision	Creates harmony & builds emotional bonds	Forges consensus through participation	Sets high standards for performance	Develops people for the future
What they say	"Do what I tell you"	"Come with me"	"People come first"	"What do you think?"	"Do as I do, now"	"Try this"
Underlying emotional intelligence competencies	Drive to achieve, initiate, self-control	Self-confidence, empathy, change catalyst	Empathy, building relationships, communication	Collaboration, team leadership, communication	Conscientious, drive to achieve, initiative	Developing others, empathy, self-awareness
When to use the style	In a crisis, to kick-start a turnaround	When changes require a new vision, or when a clear direction is needed	To heal rifts in a team or to motivate people during stressful circumstances	To build buy-in or consensus or to get input from valuable individuals	To get quick results from a highly motivated and competent team	To help individuals improve performance or develop long-term strengths
Long-term impact	Negative	Most strongly positive	Positive	Positive	Negative/Positive	Positive

Adapted from Goleman, D. Leadership that gets results. *Harvard Business Review, 78*(2), 82–83, 2000.[37]

- *Develop Collaborative Relationships.* Creating a web of influence through relationship building provides strength and energy to the organization. The quality and diversity of collaborative relationships will help identify resources and foster a learning environment.

Wood et al. recognize that many industries, including the healthcare industry, have adopted a global perspective, which has refocused leadership development towards international applications of leadership.[19] Healthcare executives are expected to lead people and manage resources. However, global leaders must understand and appreciate that the human capital of international organizations is comprised of people with vastly different education, training, and experience. Therefore, it is important for leaders to have cultural awareness, and an ability to analyze and work within the culture of an international organization or system. Cultural awareness allows a global leader to successfully motivate individuals within the organization or system towards goal-directed behavior that supports the leader's vision and organization's mission.

In an examination of global transformational leadership, Matear identified a model in which the key components are defined as emotional intelligence, cultural intelligence, and motivation (Figure 3-1).[23] The development of emotional and cultural intelligence competencies through assessment, evaluation, and personal development planning, will result in the development of transformational leaders with the capacity to lead multicultural groups in international settings.

SUMMARY

In this chapter, we presented definitions, theories, concepts, principles, and styles of leadership in the context of the medical laboratory setting. The themes throughout this chapter support our notion that leadership means change for the common good of the laboratory community. Leadership involves the ability to create and communicate a vision that acts as an invisible guide, to build a rich diversity of relationships that energize teams, and to share information to nurture change. The application of these key leadership skills for effective leadership of multicultural groups and in international settings requires culturally intellectual leaders. We hope that the information and exercises in this chapter will serve as a useful guide while working with others to accomplish change as we face the challenges of living and working in the global workforce of the 21st Century.

SUMMARY CHART:
Important Points to Remember

➤ Management and leadership are not the same and both are necessary for a successful organization.

➤ Managers are primarily administrators who are able to influence decisions and actions; whereas, leaders influence the opinions and attitudes of others to accomplish a mutually agreed-on task, while advancing the group's integrity and moral purpose.

➤ John Kotter, in *Leading Change*, makes the distinction of management versus leadership in the following way. He describes management as a set of processes (such as planning, budgeting, organizing, and problem solving) that can keep a complicated system of people and technology running smoothly.[13]

➤ Leadership creates organizations or adapts them to significant changes in circumstance. Leadership defines the future and establishes direction, aligns the people and processes with a vision, and inspires the organization to make it happen.

➤ Legitimate power is derived from a person's position or job in an organization. Being put in the manager's position, a person is authorized by the organization with the legitimate right to require and demand compliance from his or her subordinates.

➤ Behavioral approach focuses attention on what a leader "does," rather than what a leader "is." The behavioral approach took the position that leadership can be learned through education, training, life, and work experience.

➤ Situational contingency approach has emerged, focusing on the importance of the context of the situation in explaining leader effectiveness. The central point of the contingency approach is that the leadership style needed would change with the situation.

➤ Reciprocal approach—leadership is a relational and shared process that includes a strong emphasis on followership.

➤ Various studies since the 1970s suggested that people of various characters and personalities all have the potential to become effective leaders. Among the studies is the *Keirsey Temperament Theory*.

➤ The Blake-Mouton Model visualized leadership styles in terms of a balance between concerns for getting the job done and the working relationships that must be integrated to achieve effective leadership.

➤ The Lorenzi-Riley Model, derived from the task-oriented and people-oriented model, proposed the following styles of leadership behaviors: the on-the-job retirees, the whip crackers, the schmoozers, and the team builders.[25, 45]

➤ The three conventional leadership styles are Authoritative, Democratic, and Laissez-Faire, as listed in Table 3-5 along with the associated behaviors and in what situation each style is effective and ineffective. Flexibility of leadership styles is important for success.

➤ Behavioral theories such as McGregor's Theory X and Theory Y suggest that managers operate from two sets of expectations about employees' attitudes and abilities that ultimately influence their work performance.[22]

➤ The Japanese Theory Z contains elements such as lifetime employment; a company's concern for their employees' total well-being; consensus decision making; and a consistent system of promotions, among other elements.

➤ Leadership is a collection of qualities that are developed and begin with self-awareness and self-identity.

➤ An effective leader must have the power to influence others to follow his/her advice, suggestion, or directive. In general, the power possessed by a manager is a combination of legitimate power, reward power, coercive power, referent power, and expert power.

SUGGESTED PROBLEM-BASED LEARNING ACTIVITIES

Chapter 3: Principles of Leadership: Past, Present, and Future

Instructions: Use Internet resources, books, articles, colleagues, etc. to present solutions to the problems listed below. There is no correct solution to any problem.

Note to Instructor: Students in class may be divided into groups and given the problem-based learning activity to discuss and solve. Once the group has reached consensus as to a solution, the group may present it to the other students in the class. This activity will provide all students with information regarding solutions to the problem.

Problem #1

Use a personality trait assessment tool (e.g. The Keirsey Four Types Sorter or Myers-Briggs Type Indicator) to type students in your class and stratify them into working groups. Observe the working behaviors of group members during problem-based learning exercises.

Problem #2

Identify a leadership style and use it to explain how it could be used in dealing with a problem employee.

Problem #3

You have implemented a participative management process within your department. When input is requested, you receive minimal if any responses from your supervisors. Discuss what leadership skills may be used to best facilitate and accomplish this process.

Problem #4

You have been assigned to manage a laboratory overseas. Describe the relevant factors of global transformational leadership, identify the key components, and describe your approach to personally develop the relevant competencies.

REFERENCES

1. Goleman D: *Emotional Intelligence: Why It Can Matter More Than IQ.* Bantam Books, New York, NY, 1997.

2. Komives SR, Lucas N, McMahon TR: *Exploring Leadership: For College Students Who Want to Make a Difference,* ed 2, 5. Jossey-Bass, San Francisco, CA, 2007.

3. Thurgood K: *Construct for Developing an Integrated Leadership Model: Linking the Correlates of Effective Leadership, Development and Succession Planning.* Ph.D. Diss. Capella University, 2008.

4. Nahavandi A: *The Art and Science of Leadership,* ed 3. Prentice Hall, Upper Saddle River, NJ, 2003.

5. Ang S, Van Dyne L, Koh C: Personality Correlates of the Four-Factor Model of Cultural Intelligence. *Group and Organization Management* 2006: 31(1); 100-123. doi: 10.1177/1059601105275267

6. Earley PC, Ang S: *Cultural Intelligence: Individual Interactions Across Cultures.* Stanford University Press, Stanford, CA, 2003.

7. Earley PC, Mosakowski E: Cultural Intelligence. *Harvard Business Review* 2004: 82(10); 139-146.

8. Ang S, Van Dyne L: Conceptualization of Cultural Intelligence: Definition, Distinctiveness, and Nomological Network, 3-15. In: Ang S, Van Dyne L, eds. *Handbook of Cultural Intelligence: Theory, Measurement and Applications.* M. E. Sharpe, New York, NY, 2008.

9. Longest BB, Rakich JS, Darr K: *Managing Health Services Organizations and Systems,* 737. Health Professions Press, Baltimore, MD, 2000.

10. Freiberg K, Freiberg J: *NUTS! Southwest Airlines' Crazy Recipe for Business and Personal Success,* 298. Broadway Books, New York, NY, 1997.

11. Snyder JR, Senhauser DA: *Administration and Supervision in Laboratory Medicine,* 93. J.B. Lippincott, Philadelphia, PA, 1989.

12. Maccoby M: Understanding the Difference Between Management and Leadership. *Research Technology Management* 2000: 43(1); 57-59.

13. Kotter J: Leading Change. Harvard Business School Press, Boston, 1996.

14. Zalesnick A: Managers and Leaders: Are They Different? *Harvard Business Review* 1977: 55(3); 67-78.

15. Cashman K: *Leadership from the Inside Out.* Executive Excellence Publishing, Provo, UT, 1998.

16. Gardner L, Stough C: Examining the Relationship Between Leadership and Emotional Intelligence in Senior Level Managers. *Leadership & Organization Development Journal* 2002: 23(2); 68-78.

17. Gill R: Change Management—or Change Leadership? *Journal of Change Management* 2003: 3(4); 307-318.

18. Goleman D, Boyatzis R, McKee A: *Primal Leadership: Realizing the Power of Emotional Intelligence.* Harvard Business School Press, Boston, MA, 2002.

19. Wood S, Coppola MN, Satterwhite R (in press): The Role of Transformational Leadership. In: Harrison JP, ed. *Leadership and Strategic Planning in Healthcare Organizations.* Jones and Bartlett, Boston, MA, in press.

20. Emerson RM: Power-Dependence Relations. *American Sociological Review* 1962: 27; 31-41.

21. French J, Raven B: The Base of Social Power. In: Cartwright D, ed. *Studies in Social Power,* 150-167. University of Michigan Press, Ann Arbor, MI, 1959.

22. Goleman D: *Social Intelligence: The New Science of Human Relationships.* Arrow, London, 2006.

23. Matear DW: "An Examination of Cognitive, Cultural, and Emotional Intelligences, and Motivation in the Development of Global Transformational Leadership Skills." Ph.D. Diss. Capella University, 2009.

24. Fiedler FE: *A Theory of Leadership Effectiveness.* McGraw-Hill, New York, NY, 1967.

25. Hersey P, Blanchard KH, Johnson DE: *Management of Organizational Behavior: Leading Human Resources,* ed 9. Prentice Hall, Upper Saddle River, NJ, 2001.

26. Burns JM: *Leadership.* Harper and Row, New York, NY, 1977.

27. Trishy NM, Devanna, MA: *The Transformational Leader.* John Wiley, New York, NY, 1986.

28. House RJ: A 1976 Theory of Charismatic Leadership. In: Hunt JG, Larson LL, eds. *Leadership: The Cutting Edge*, 1977.

29. Alon I, Higgins JM: Global Leadership Success Through Emotional and Cultural Intelligences. *Business Horizons* 2005: 48; 501-512.

30. Avolio BJ, Bass BM: *The Full Range Leadership Development Programs: Basic and Advanced Manuals*. Bass, Avolio & Associates, Binghamton, NY, 1991.

31. Bass B: *Leadership and Performance Beyond Expectations*. The Free Press, New York, NY, 1985.

32. House RJ, Hanges PJ, Ruiz-Quintanilla SA, Dorfman PW, Javidan M, Dickson M, et al: Cultural Influences on Leadership and Organizations: Project GLOBE. In: Mobley WH, Gessner MJ, Arnold V, eds. *Advances in Global Leadership*, 184. JAI Press, Stamford, CT, 1999.

33. Northouse PG: *Leadership: Theory and Practice*, ed 2. Sage, Thousand Oaks, CA, 2001.

34. Weber M: *The Theory of Social and Economic Organizations* (Parsons T, Trans.). Free Press, New York, NY, 1947.

35. Sullivan EJ, Decker PJ: *Effective Leadership and Management in Nursing*. Prentice Hall, Upper Saddle River, NJ, 2000.

36. Yukl G: *Leadership in Organizations*, ed 5. Prentice Hall, Trenton, NJ, 2002.

37. Goleman D: Leadership That Gets Results. *Harvard Business Review* 2000: 78(2); 78-90.

38. Goleman D: What Makes a Leader? *Harvard Business Review* 1998: 76(6); 93-102.

39. Lugo M: An Examination of Cultural and Emotional Intelligences in the Development of Global Transformational Leadership Skills. *Dissertation Abstracts International, DAI-A* 68(10), 2007 (UMI No. 3283980).

40. Keirsey D: *Please Understand Me II*. Prometheous Nemesis Books, Delmar, CA, 1998.

41. Covey SR: *The 7 Habits of Highly Effective People*. Simon & Schuster, New York, NY, 1990.

42. Goleman D: What Makes a Leader? *Harvard Business Review* 2004: 82(1); 82-90.

43. Bennis WG: *On Becoming a Leader*. Addison-Wesley, Reading, MA, 1989.

44. Blake RR, Mouton JS: *The Versatile Manager: A Grid Profile*. Irwin, Homewood, IL, 1981.

45. Lorenzi NM, Riley RT: *Organizational Aspects of Health Informatics: Managing Technological Change*. Springer-Verlag, New York, NY, 1994.

46. McGregor D: *Leadership and Motivation*. MIT Press, Cambridge, MA, 1966.

47. Goldsmith SB: *Principles of Health Care Management: Compliance, Consumerism, and Accountability in the 21st Century*, 161. Jones and Bartlett Publishers, Boston, MA, 2005.

48. Drucker PP: What We Can Learn from Japanese Management. *Harvard Business Review* 1971: 59(3); 110-122.

49. DuPree M: *Leadership Jazz*. Dell Publishing, New York, NY, 1992.

50. Hock D: *Birth of the Chaordic Age*. Berrett-Koehler, San Francisco, CA, 1999.

51. Block P: *Stewardship*. Berrett-Koehler, San Francisco, CA, 1996.

52. Hesselbein F, Goldsmith M, Beckhard R: *The Leader of the Future*. Jossey-Bass, San Francisco, CA, 1996.

BIBLIOGRAPHY

Bennis WG: *Managing the Dream*. Perseus Publishing, Cambridge, MA, 2000.

Dye CF, Garman AN: *Exceptional Leadership: 16 Critical Competencies for Healthcare Executives*. Health Administration Press, Chicago, IL, 2006.

Hiefetz RA, Linsky M, Grashow A: *The Practice of Adaptive Leadership: Tools and Tactics for Changing Your Organization and the World*. Harvard Business Press, Cambridge, MA, 2009.

Spath P: *Leading Your Healthcare Organization to Excellence: A Guide to Using the Baldrige Criteria*. Health Administration Press, Chicago, IL, 2005.

Wheatley MJ: *Leadership and the New Science*. Barrett-Koehler Publishers, San Francisco, CA, 1999.

INTERNET RESOURCES

Association of Coach Training Organizations (ACTO)
http://www.acto1.com/

The Cultural Intelligence Center (CQC)
http:/www.culturalq.com/about.html

Daniel Goleman's Emotional Intelligence Information
http://www.danielgoleman.info/

Georgetown University's Leadership Coaching Certificate Program, 2009
http://www.acto1.com/Schools/GU.htm

Joel Barker's Leadershift: Five Lessons for Leaders in the 21st Century
http://www.starthrower.com/joel_barker_leadershift.htm

Keirsey Temperament Sorter—Personality Test
http://www.keirsey.com

Southwest Educational Development Laboratory (SEDL)—History of Leadership Research
http://www.sedl.org/change/leadership/history.html

University of California, Davis—Leadership Learning Laboratory
http://www.hr.ucdavis.edu/sdps/catalog/human-resource-management/leadership-learning-laboratory

Management Functions

Christine Pitocco, MS, MT(ASCP)BB
Randall S. Lambrecht, PhD, MT(ASCP), CLS(NCA)
Marie Cato, MBA, MT(ASCP)

CHAPTER OUTLINE

OBJECTIVES

Following successful completion of this chapter, the learner will be able to:

1. Identify the major roles and functions associated with effective laboratory management.
2. Discuss the qualities and style an effective manager should possess.
3. Describe how laboratory management has evolved over the past 20 years.
4. List important basic components of the planning process and be able to explain their role on short-term and long-term goals.
5. Provide a list of steps or functions essential for organizing a plan of implementation.
6. Identify effective means of communication and describe the benefits of taking a collaborative approach to problem solving.

7. Apply key management principles in response to a problem-based case study situation.
8. Outline assessment tools that provide a measurement of successful management and operational performance outcomes.

KEY TERMS

Collaboration
Communication
Controlling
Coordination
Directing
Functions
Goals
Implementing
Management

Mission Statement
Objectives
Organizing
Outcome Assessment
Personnel Development
Planning
Supervisory
Tasks

INTRODUCTION

The effectiveness of any organization is determined by the way work is organized and by the way people work with or against each other. The way in which people cooperate with each other, with management, and with the community, depends on the style of management and the extent of their commitment to their organization. **Management** can be and has been defined in many different ways over the years. The most contemporary rendition of this term in the business world involves the concept of achieving organizational goals in an effective and efficient manner by working with and through people. Management, and in particular healthcare management, has undergone significant changes over the last 10 to 20 years. Historically, laboratory management had a primary function of organizing and directing the staff to ensure the production of quality laboratory results. In today's healthcare environment, the production of quality laboratory results is only one of many expected outcomes that must be achieved for a medical laboratory to attain success. The ability to handle change is one of the most important skills a manager who is a leader can have. As organizations develop, management and leadership traits such as transformational, charismatic, and visionary rise in importance as workforces become more diverse, technology becomes more complex, and competition heightens. Other facets leading to success include marketability, cost management, benchmarking, reengineering, personnel management, **personnel development**, staff empowerment, collaboration, standardization, and providing exceptional service. The competition among healthcare providers today rivals that among the major business corporations.

However difficult the competition becomes, successfully managed organizations invest in their people; and they do so wisely.

The philosophy of management has also undergone a type of metamorphosis and continues to evolve. In the past, management tended to function from a more autocratic and "power of position" focus, often perceived as being controlling, inflexible, and lacking inclusivity. There were, however, important advantages related to this approach, such as firmer and quicker decisions, predictability, and a zone of comfort for the manager. Today's management style has evolved in power derived from leadership, rather than power derived from position. Leadership is a quality that evolves with time and experience, and requires a high degree of confidence in addition to competence. Power from leadership facilitates a more global view and a broad-based approach to issues. Leadership also requires the ability to form and communicate a vision as well as build teams of individuals who work together toward common goals. There is an old axiom that says, "A leader cannot lead if there are no followers." Today's leadership is much more democratic and participatory. It increases the roles of facilitator, coach, and communicator for the manager and has the advantages of greater employee involvement, broader based decisions, and greater creativity. In earlier years, employees were often hesitant to question management authority. In today's environment the employee does not hesitate to ask questions or seek answers. Today's manager must be able to respond to challenges and be prepared to explain decisions, rather than simply being dismissive.

The management of a laboratory is complex and varies depending on its size, geographic location, patient/client population, goals of the institution, and the board that oversees it. Aligning the clinical laboratory's vision, goals, programs, resources, facilities, and expectations with mission, strategic plans, and objectives is critical to its efficiency and performance. Evaluation and assessment should focus on both the planning and achievements that encompass the laboratory's function. Effective management is a process that begins with establishment of goals and ends with assessment of the achievement of those goals. Within this process are functions that enable these goals to be realized. These basic functions include planning, decision-making, and organizing, as well as implementing and controlling (Figure 4-1).

Embedded within each of these functions are more specific and very important responsibilities and activities. The primary task for each of these management functions is listed in Table 4-1. For example, within the management function of organizing are the critical roles of prioritizing and implementing. Similarly, the function labeled implementing contains controlling, monitoring, assessing, and making adjustments when needed. In reality, the boundaries separating each function are somewhat obscure, because there is much overlap and crossover as a result of mutual reliance between functions. Important to the entire process is the recognition that coordination, collaboration, communication, personnel management and development, innovativeness, and vision are critical to the realization of successful outcomes.

As a result of the combination of changes in management style and the tools available to measure success, the functions of today's healthcare manager are much more diverse, complex, and interdependent. It is imperative that a manager is skilled in all of these functions to attain both a job and personal satisfaction.

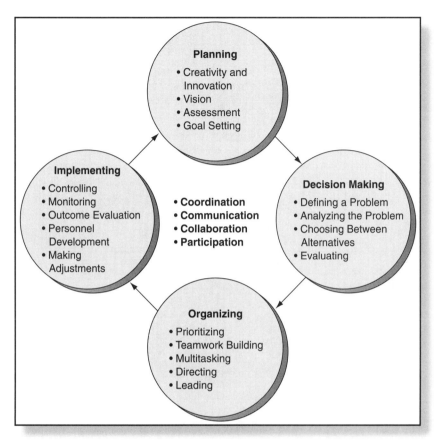

FIGURE 4-1.   The Basic Functions of Management

TABLE 4-1.   Primary Components of the Management Function Process

Planning	Clarifies the process of attaining organizational goals
Decision Making	Decisions are made based on choosing between alternatives
Organizing	Identifies the steps needed to implement a successful plan
Implementing/Controlling	Puts plan into operation and measures implementation and progress

Obtaining management and leadership skills is often a factor of experience. Even though certain individuals may naturally possess some of the building blocks required to manage, expertise and experience must still be developed. A management position requires conceptual (thinking) skills, people skills, and technical skills. As you progress from lower levels of management toward upper levels of management, the mix of these required skills changes. In the lower levels of management (e.g., **supervisory**), the technical skills are more frequently used along with the people skills. In the upper levels of management (e.g., director), conceptual or cognitive skills are more frequently used along with people skills. The increase in conceptual and people skill levels is often a function of experience and not something that can simply be taught. Figure 4-2 shows how time spent on various management functions changes in relation to the management level.

To summarize, the four primary components of the management function process are interdependent and critical to making the laboratory a productive and competitive organization. We have chosen to consider the function of controlling as embedded within implementing because of the high degree of interdependence and because they are often concurrent.

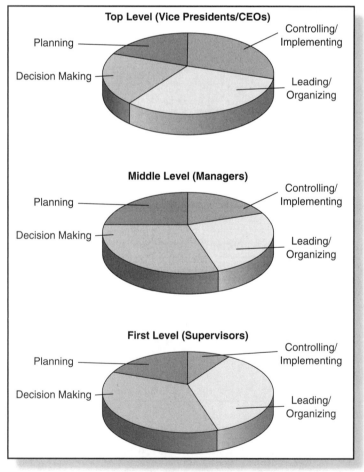

FIGURE 4-2.   Relative Functions within Management Levels

Throughout the management function cycle of planning, organizing, and controlling phases are embedded the 3 Cs (coordination, communication, and collaboration), which invite participation of all stakeholders.

The basic functions of management represent a consistent strategy that can be used when addressing any of the responsibilities that managers face. Management **functions** should not be confused with the **tasks** and responsibilities associated with management duties. The former (functions) describes a process and strategy for dealing with issues of change, whereas the latter (responsibilities) deals with the routine tasks for which laboratory managers are held responsible and accountable. This chapter is designed to introduce the learner to the basic management functions (planning, decision making, organizing, and implementing/controlling) using a case study approach.

Each subsection begins with a case study followed by questions to consider. A discussion of the management function(s) covered provides the learner with background and descriptive information to ponder and use to determine suitable answers to the case questions. It is important to note that more than one answer may be appropriate for a given question. Learners are encouraged to share their thoughts on these cases with their instructors and other students. This approach will allow everyone to consider all of the possible answers.

MANAGEMENT FUNCTIONS

Planning is the management function that clarifies the process of attaining the desired goals of an organization. It includes activities such as data gathering, assessment, calculation of risks, and determination of a strategy. Planning is the most fundamental management function. Planning requires an emphasis on creativity, innovation, vision, and thinking "beyond traditional methods." In other words, a manager should not be constrained by preconceived notions or doing things as they have been done in the past. A simple lesson when trying to effect change is that if you do things the way they have always been done, you will get the same results as in the past. Planning is concerned with the future impact of today's decisions and is the fundamental function of management from which the other functions stem. The need for planning is easy to postpone in the short-run and too often apparent after the fact. The organizing, staffing, leading, and controlling functions stem from the planning function. Planning is a function where goals, vision, core values, and mission are established. The determination of whether or not goals are being accomplished and standards met is based on the planning function. The planning function provides the goals and standards that drive the controlling function.

Planning is important at all levels of management. However, its characteristics vary by level of management. Planning represents the cognitive (thinking) function of management. Management often finds it difficult to allocate sufficient quality time to this phase despite its importance to the entire process. There is a dangerous tendency to immediately jump into action, rather than thinking through the options and impli-

Case Study — Planning

You are the laboratory manager of a medium-sized 120-bed hospital and are called to a hospital leadership meeting by the CEO of the facility. You are told that the hospital is having problems meeting some debt responsibility and there is a possibility that budgetary cutbacks will be needed to alleviate the situation. Each departmental manager is being given one week to plan how to accomplish a cost reduction of 10% within his/her department, should it become necessary. You are also told that this situation is highly confidential because it is not yet known whether the cost reduction will be needed.

Issues and Questions to Consider:

1. *Identify the steps in developing short-term goals to address the potential reduction in resources described above.*
2. *What type of information will you need to gather to assess your current state and develop a plan?*
3. *What criteria will you use to determine the best plan of action?*
4. *What type of long-range planning should be considered?*

cations. Planning requires attention to detail, creativity, globalization, flexibility, logic, predictability, decisive decision-making, and vision, as well as a deep understanding of the organization's purpose. It might be better to refer to strategic planning as *strategic management,* as it is often regarded as the first step in the functional role of management. The major components of the planning function are listed in Table 4-2.

Planning is a process that is essential to:

1. Make advanced rational decisions about the future.
2. Anticipate and react positively to changes.
3. Analyze information and make improvements.
4. Reduce ambiguity and anxiety among staff.
5. Accomplish goals and objectives in a timely and efficient manner.
6. Remain competitive and cost effective.
7. Be proactive rather than reactive.

Planning begins with fully understanding the institution's "purpose for being." Planning has as its components:

Vision: Provides nonspecific, directional, and motivational guidance for the entire organization. Top managers are eager to provide a vision for

TABLE 4-2.　Major Components of the Planning Function

- Mission statements and core principles
- Innovation and vision
- Assessment
- Goal setting
- Tactics

the business. The vision is usually the most emotional of the levels in the hierarchy of purposes.

Mission: An organization's reason for being. It is concerned with the scope of the business and what makes the enterprise distinct from similar operations. Missions reflect the culture and values of the institution or laboratory enterprise.

Objectives: Objectives address key issues within the organizational mission such as market standing, innovation, productivity, physical and financial resources, profitability, management and worker performance and efficiency. They are expected to be general, observable, challenging, and untimed. Objectives are the tangible plans that are usually expressed as results to be achieved. Objectives may be expressed quantitatively or qualitatively.

Goals: Goals are specific statements of anticipated results that further define the organization's objectives. They are expected to be *SMART: Specific, Measurable, Attainable, Realistic, and Timely. They stem from the organizations vision and mission.*

Tactics: Tactics are another level of planning and are the most specific plans that describe how, who, what, when, and where activities will take place to accomplish a goal.

Every healthcare provider and/or medical laboratory service should have a **mission statement** that is clear and consistent. The mission statement articulates the purpose, attitude, and core competencies of the institution in as concise a declaration as possible. The mission statement should highlight what the healthcare organization and the laboratory do best or excel at most. The mission statement should incorporate what the organization is trying to satisfy, who they are trying to satisfy, and how they go about satisfying these needs. Policies, practices, and behaviors should all evolve around the mission statement, and management decisions should be consistent with supporting the mission statement. Although it is common and healthy for changes and adaptations to occur in any organization, the mission statement should remain steadfast because it exemplifies the core principle of why an organization exists, and the assumptions on which the organization was built. The mission statement, together with the assumptions that shape an organization's behavior, should dictate any decisions an organization makes. If an organization has been struggling to survive for a long time, it may need to review its mission statement and assumptions to see if they no longer fit with reality or have become obsolete. For the most part, the mission statement describes the heart of an organization's existence and is therefore nonnegotiable. Peter Drucker, the author of *Managing in a Time of Great Change* coined the phrase, "Theory of the Business" to describe the clear, consistent, and focused assumptions that usually define the principles by which a business or organizational unit operates.[1] The healthcare system in the United States currently exists in a dynamic and rapidly changing environment; thus, healthcare providers who are slow to accept change or are unreceptive to adapting to meet the needs of the future will soon find themselves uncompetitive and struggling to survive. Careful planning and anticipation for the future are essential for an organization to remain in business.

The planning stage should be participatory. This will increase the scope of ideas and will also help with "buy-in" from those who are involved. In addition, it will help identify and dilute any preconceived notions or biases you as an individual may bring to the process. Planning is a critical step of the process and, unfortunately, is often rushed or short-changed. The act of planning will allow you to set a direction. A simple but instructive analogy would be taking a vacation by automobile. You must identify your final destination and then determine a route and direction that will take you there. Planning requires that you have a comprehensive understanding of your starting point. If you misinterpret that point, you may well miss your final destination or target. The plan represents the road map of your automobile vacation.

Planning can take place over different time periods. Short-term goals will usually have fewer benchmarks, but that does not decrease their importance, as you will also have less time for adjustment. The short-term plan often defines less lofty goals, but is much quicker to accomplish than the long-term plan, which is more complex and whose goals are generally more difficult to achieve. Advantages of short-term goals are that they are usually good for morale during the longer planning process, and they provide "quick wins" in terms of witnessing accomplishments in a short period. Irrespective of the period, there are a number of approaches to good effective planning. The first step usually involves an assessment or survey of the organization's strengths, weaknesses, opportunities, and threats. Regardless whether long term or short term, the plan must include goals that are clear and concise, as well as attainable. Plans that are not realistic are nothing more than organized dreams.

A careful study of the assessment survey is necessary to identify areas that need improvement and to help the organization meet its goals, which are usually the endpoint of most management efforts. The assessment tool should look at issues such as: environment, safety, space, equipment and personnel needs, employee morale, productivity output, technology, demographic trends, cost issues and qualitative outcomes, as well as external items such as healthcare trends and government-legal and political climate. The assessment phase should attempt to develop baseline data. For the assessment to be comprehensive and of greatest use, it should involve input from as many groups and individuals as possible, keeping in mind, however, that decision making is both the privilege and the burden of managers.

Establishing **goals** helps the institution define its mission, control its destiny, motivate its employees, and ensure that everyone understands the purpose of the enterprise. Setting goals helps move an institution forward. Goals should be challenging but achievable, visionary but realistic, and supported by available resources with measurable outcomes. A laboratory needs to decide where and what it wants to be in the future. Does it want to have a particular focus or expertise? Can it do all things equally well, or does it have a particular niche whereby it is regarded as an invaluable resource? Long-term goals are broad ambitions that are often met through a series of smaller, more focused **objectives**. Objectives are often developed as directives for accomplishing the established goals.

Planning is the stage in which policies and procedures are put into place. Policies are the guides to action, they spell out the required, prohibited, and the suggested course of action.[2] Procedures may be considered a series of tasks that are placed in chronological order in which the task is performed. Procedures and policies are put in place in order for there to be uniformity of practice and to aid managers in training and performance evaluations.

In addition to identifying opportunities in the planning function, management must identify possible threats, uncertainties, or negative consequences inherent in a plan. These need to be anticipated, as each one can become such an enormous unexpected factor that they may render an institution paralyzed, leaving any future planning futile if not counterproductive. Planning for surprise events involves peering into the future and forecasting potential problems in an attempt to avoid them. Many uncertainties have already occurred and, with experience, can be anticipated and avoided if history is not forgotten. A good plan will also help the manager and staff sharpen their focus, thereby accomplishing goals more quickly and efficiently. Another benefit of planning that should not be underestimated is the value of discussion and preparing those involved for change. Change itself is often less dramatic or stressful than the unknown, and individuals are less resistant to change if the process is clearly outlined. Planning will reduce that fear of the unknown. If open discussions cannot be held in the planning stage, it should be incorporated as soon as possible, and your plan should allow for refinement or revision based on acquired input.

Decision making is the management function in which decisions are made based on choosing between alternatives. When a decision is needed, there must be a choice between at least two alternatives. This function is most closely related to the planning function. In healthcare, the decision-making process has an additional component in that the medical staff may participate in making some of the more major or medically-related decisions.

Case Study

Decision Making

You are the manager of the chemistry department in a large tertiary care hospital. One of your senior technologists, Tina, has had an increase in her lateness and absenteeism. When she is at work, she has a negative work attitude and it seems to be causing problems with her fellow employees. She has not been completing the tasks assigned to her with little regard for patient care. Tina has always been a reliable, conscientious and capable employee in the past. You feel Tina's overall work effectiveness and reliability has been declining. You have spoken to Tina about her performance but her behavior has not changed. Two employees that work with Tina have complained about Tina's work performance and have told you in confidence that they have believe alcohol may be the cause of her change in performance.

Issues and Questions to Consider:

1. *You as the manager must decide how to handle this situation. Define the problem.*
2. *Develop some choices of possible solutions to not only aid in the efficiency of your department but also help your employee, Tina.*
3. *Choose the best choice among those solutions developed.*
4. *Select an alternative solution and explain your decisions.*

Some decisions may need to be made by top level managers while others may not. Top level managers may make decisions that align with the organizational goals, vision, and mission. Top level managers in healthcare may defer their decision making to individual department heads or those with technical competence within their area of expertise.[2]

There are steps in the decision making process which are best carried out in sequence. These steps include: defining the problem, analyzing the problem, developing alternative solutions, evaluating the alternatives and making a decision between the alternatives and follow up after the decision has been implemented. Choosing between alternatives may be influenced by a manager's past experience. Past experience should be viewed with the future in mind.[3] There are quantitative tools available to managers that aid in the decision making process, including linear programming, modeling, probability and simulation. In healthcare these tools aid in problems involving schedules, inventory, and staffing of the various shifts.[3]

It is best to keep in mind when making any decision who and what will be effected by the decision. In healthcare, all departments, employees, and patients should be considered before the decision is made. Decisions that are a major gain for one area or person but are a major loss for another should be avoided.[3]

Some decisions may be made due to factors such as economic conditions, political conditions, or regulatory restrictions. Objective decision making utilizes facts, analyzes alternatives, and rationalizes using all tools available. Taking into consideration the desired consequences as well as the possible ramifications makes the best decision making process.

Decision making is also influenced by the expertise and experience of the person or persons making the decision. Resources and time constraints may factor into the decision making process. The degree of risk and uncertainty must be weighed in the decision-making process.[2]

Organizing is the process of determining the steps needed to implement a successful plan. It includes identifying the various steps that need to take place in addition to determining the appropriate personnel for accomplishing those steps. This step also includes allocating or reallocating resources including equipment, funds, and/or staffing. Staffing is one of the most important managerial activities that ensure qualified people for all positions in the laboratory. Recruiting, hiring, training, evaluating, and compensating are the specific activities included in the function. Directing is another organizing activity that influences people's

Case Study — Organizing

After you have presented your proposal to hospital administration and it has been accepted, you are informed that the impending cost reductions will need to be implemented. You are told to meet with your supervisory staff to organize the implementation of your plan. The CEO will be holding hospital employee briefings beginning the next afternoon to provide the employees with an overview of the situation confronting the hospital. Over the next two to three days you will be meeting with your supervisory staff and then with the laboratory employees to provide additional detail specifically as it pertains to the laboratory and its staff. Your goals are to have your employees fully understand the situation and its implications, allow them to communicate their thoughts and concerns, and to finally accomplish buy-in from the staff regarding the proposal you must implement.

Issues and Questions to Consider:

1. *What steps or functions are key to organizing the plan for implementation?*
2. *Who needs to be included in this process and why?*
3. *What are the various means of communication that could be used in this situation? Which one(s) is chosen and why?*
4. *What areas of collaboration or coordination, if any, will be needed with the supervisory staff, pathology staff, bench staff, medical staff, other hospital staff?*
5. *What situations could require mentoring and/or motivating of staff?*

behavior through motivation, communication, group dynamics, leadership, and discipline. The purpose of directing is to channel the behavior of all personnel to accomplish the organization's mission and objectives while simultaneously helping them accomplish their own career objectives. There are at least four key elements of laboratory organization that include: the assays and tasks to be performed, the individual task performers, teams of laboratory personnel working together, and the physical environment of the workplace. Organization plays an important role in determining the effectiveness of the clinical laboratory by defining the relationship among those key elements. Organizing brings structure to your plan by detailing what has to be done, who has to do it, and how it is going to be done.

Organizing for a specific activity usually entails being cognizant of the organizational structure with which the laboratory operates. There are a number of organizational charts and modeled hierarchal structures that describe many types of organizational management systems in healthcare. These include multilevel pyramids (Figure 4-3) or vertical charts with clear delineation about who's on top and who's not. They profile the lines of authority and communication, as well as illustrate patterns of coordination. Conflict in an organization is inevitable, but may be reduced through clarity of organizational relationships. Although organizational diagrams can sometimes help depict how different units or disciplines relate to each other and to administration, it may be difficult to glean activities between units that are integrated and interdisciplinary. Few areas of a laboratory are independent with the exception of highly specialized laboratories that require

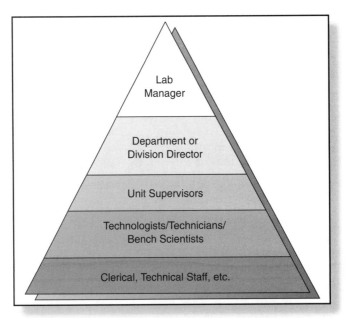

FIGURE 4-3.   Typical Laboratory Pyramidal Hierarchy

segregation and separate treatment for security, safety, or other purposes (drug testing laboratory for example).

A dual form of organization as a result of the traditional dichotomous relationship between medical staff and administrators often characterizes healthcare institutions. The ultimate authority and responsibility for the management of the overall institution rest with its governing board. Because of licensure, medical governance boards, and accreditation policies, there are usually two lines of authority, each with their own hierarchical structure, whereby the board appoints a chief executive officer and a chief of the medical staff. In an attempt to consolidate authority, some institutions will designate a high-level administrative position to whom both the CEO and Chief of the Medical Staff report. The same dual reporting structure (administrative and medical) may hold true within the medical laboratory depending on its size.

Organizational structures have become more flexible recently as institutions and managers have recognized the need to effect change and have witnessed the benefits in having a flexible structure that can respond more readily to external and internal pressures and changing environments. Several successful strategies include forming interdisciplinary task forces, establishing temporary cross-disciplinary teams, encouraging cross-training and multitasking, and using a matrix organization approach. Matrix organizational design involves creating a flexible and adaptable organizational structure by combining workers from several different functional units to form a collaborative group to work on a specific project. The structure is thought of in terms of a lattice or grid because it combines the talents and expertise of individuals across disciplines and improves the communication and understanding among different units.

As a management function, organizing is a skill that contains a number of activities and responsibilities. Effectively organizing and leading a workforce requires prioritizing, coordinating, communicating, collaborating, team building, and directing. The primary tasks for the organizing function are listed in Table 4-3.

When organizing for a specific task at the workplace, there are some underlying premises:

1. Everyone is working toward a common goal.
2. The goal has been articulated in detailed plans in terms of scope and priorities.
3. Responsibilities are clearly outlined and delegated.
4. There is a command structure and an understanding of authority.

Inherent in the organizing function is the prioritizing function. Prioritizing involves ordering the functions or tasks to be accomplished. Priority may be established based on urgency, availability of resources, or foundation (i.e., step a must precede step b). Prioritizing will allow you to more appropriately allocate the resources identified earlier in the organizing function. Clearly, setting priorities for the laboratory is a primary responsibility of the laboratory manager.

TABLE 4-3.   Major Components of the Organizing Function

- Prioritizing
- Coordination
- Communication
- Collaboration
- Team building
- Staffing & Directing

The Importance of the 3 Cs

It is perhaps the organizing function for which the 3 Cs—coordination, collaboration, and communication—are most important. All three are dependent on participation and have profound influence on the "people side" of the equation.

Coordination is the blending of functions so that they are intertwined and build on each other. Coordination ensures that you are minimizing the risks of duplication or redundancy. It will also minimize the risk of allowing something to be overlooked or "falling through the cracks." Coordination requires that various portions of the plan move at specified speeds so they remain synchronized. Coordination requires significant attention to detail and continual monitoring to allow for any needed adjustments.

The second C, **collaboration**, is the act of working together to achieve a common end. Collaboration may be required both internal and external to the department. Collaboration is difficult to attain without cooperation. Collaboration requires definite managerial expertise regarding people skills. Although collaboration is designed to align people, if not carefully planned and implemented, it actually may have the opposite effect.

The third C, **communication**, may well be the most critical element to the success of a manager. Studies have shown that information needs to be communicated a minimum of seven times to ensure that people have actually heard the correct message. There is a saying within management that you can never communicate too much. When appropriate and timely communication is not present, the rumor mill or grapevine will fill the gap. In some ways the grapevine is one of the most effective ways of communication in that it is faster than formal communication and often is clear, accurate, and factual; however, it can be damaging if it is not factual. Experienced managers will find ways to use the grapevine to their advantage. Today's computer technology is, to some extent, making the grapevine obsolete. With electronic mail (e-mail) availability, the manager is able to disseminate accurate information to all personnel in a timely manner. As with any written communication, however, there should be a mechanism for employees to ask for and receive clarification. This type of communication does not eliminate the need for face-to-face discussion; however, it should serve as a foundation for such discussion. Another form of communication that is available to the manager is called the chance encounter. Chance encounters are those times when a manager is walking through the workplace and is approached spontaneously regarding an issue or question. Chance encounters are informal and may involve only a single employee but still provide an additional opportunity for communication. Most employees see chance encounters as positive because they are less formal, tend to be one-on-one with management, are spontaneous, and indicate that the manager is willing to take the time to listen to the employee's concerns.

Organizing is often accomplished through work teams that are brought together based on common responsibility, needed skills, expertise, or some combination of these qualities. It is critical for the manager to solicit involvement from employees at this point if it could not be accomplished previously. The staff and supervisory level know and understand the details of the workplace more thoroughly than upper level management. In addition, the plan and its implementation will in all likelihood affect the staff more directly than management. Inclusion of staff in this function will result in a better-defined organizational plan in addition to increasing the "buy-in" of employees. Good communication among all employees and the sense of belonging and involvement will lead to positive morale, which in turn will result in greater productivity.

Directing, or *leading*, as it is often called, accounts for a large percentage of the organizing function. Depending on the level of management, directing makes up 40% to 50% of a manager's efforts. Directing is vital to organizing and implementing a plan. Managers who are good at directing are capable of matching organizational goals to the abilities and interests of their employees and work groups. A leader can make things happen through inspiring goal-directed behavior and by his/her directing, which is leadership put into action. Directing can reward, punish, strengthen, motivate, and influence individuals, all in support of the task at hand. There are many different types of management/leadership styles, from autocratic to participative, from bureaucratic to laissez-faire. The type of style has a tremendous impact on the amount of effort employees exert toward the organizing process. When working with professionals, a participative leadership style is usually effective at inspiring organization effort. The manager consults with employees concerning goals, work assignments, and directives during the decision-making process. This approach is an attempt to capitalize on the talents and contributions that others have to offer, and it is difficult for participants not to accept the final outcome when they've been a part of it. A leadership style in which the manager is viewed as a facilitator is usually effective when building participation and consensus. Nonetheless the manager is still responsible for giving directives to accomplish the task. This is a major responsibility of the manager and is instrumental to moving the organizing function forward. Issuing directives involves attentions to timing, language, and precision so as to avoid misunderstanding. Directing does not stop with the organization function, but rather is carried through the implementation phase where it becomes part of the controlling function. It should be emphasized that the three primary management functions overlap and their boundaries are not distinct.

It is unlikely that conflict and disagreement can be totally avoided, but if the planning and organizing of a project have been effectively managed, negative and unpleasant events can be reduced.

Every organization should have an organizational structure. By action and/ or inaction, managers provide structure to the organization. Ideally, in developing an organizational structure and distributing authority, managers' decisions reflect the mission, objectives, goals, and tactics that grew out of the planning function. Specifically, they have responsibility for making decisions concerning hiring, division of labor, delegation of authority, departmentalization, scope of responsibility, and coordination.

Organizing depends on good planning, devoted employees, and competent leadership. Staff development and mentorship are qualities that can nurture good employees and make them invaluable to the organization. A manager who is a leader will recognize leadership qualities or other special talents in others and will encourage that individual to take advantage of those skills. Likewise, encouraging a network of individuals who have something in common and are willing

Case Study   Implementing and Controlling

You and your team are ready to begin implementation of your cost reduction plan (see case study in the organizing section for details). The plan will be implemented in phases because of its complexity and the required time lines for some of the ideas.

Issues and Questions to Consider:

1. *Define the managing role in the actual implementation.*
2. *What types of challenges could you encounter during implementation, and how would you address them?*

Your plan has been underway for two weeks. You have been asked by hospital administration to attend a leadership meeting and report on the status of your cost reduction plan.

Issues and Questions to Consider:

1. *What type of monitors would be helpful to ensure that the implementation is progressing according to plan?*
2. *What methodologies or processes might you use to accomplish any adjustments to the implementation?*
3. *What do you consider to be the key factors indicating your plan's degree of success?*

TABLE 4-4. **Major Components of the Implementing and Controlling Functions**

- Monitoring
- Outcomes evaluation
- Personnel management and staff development
- Making adjustments

to promote each other and the organization in a mutually beneficial manner is a win-win situation for everyone. Through a network, recommendations and ideas may be shared, which will benefit the process.

Allowing the staff to seek development and networking opportunities is an investment in their professional growth, enabling them to make contributions to the organization. Investments in staff development will positively influence morale, stimulate enthusiasm, and avoid job stagnation and staff turnover, thereby providing for the retention of good employees and decreasing the need for employee recruitment.

Implementing and **controlling** could be separate management functions but are discussed together under one function because in practicality they should occur simultaneously. The major core components of the implementing and controlling functions are listed in Table 4-4.

Weaved throughout effective control systems are also the following characteristics: control at all levels, acceptability to those responsible for assurance, flexibility, accuracy, timeliness, cost-effectiveness, balance between objectivity and subjectivity. Implementing is the action that starts to put the plan into operation. As implementation takes place, monitoring must be in place to observe plan's performance; otherwise no conclusion will be able to be drawn regarding achieving the desired outcome and goal. Controlling is actually an extension of the directing activity that occurred during the organizing phase, but with the manager playing a much greater role during implementation, as decision making must be swift and deliberate. The control function completes the management function cycle through its outcomes and assessments.

The word *controlling* is often seen as negative, especially in today's work environment. In this context, it is not meant to refer to an exclusive dictatorial or autocratic management, but rather to indicate the process of measuring implementation progress, with the control resting with the manager. Controlling is a performance measurement of implementation whereby adjustments and corrective actions can be made to ensure that organizational goals are achieved. Controlling can take the form of a feed forward (checking ahead of action) to anticipate deviation in implementation and outcomes and prevent it. It can also take the form of concurrent or feedback mechanisms whereby deviations are addressed as they happen or after they occur. The manager is in control of the operation and closely supervises its performance.

The control process should be designed during the organizing to allow for adequate measurement and assessment. It should be done simultaneously with all other management functions. It should have as one phase a set of acceptable standards, a second phase of measurement performance, and a third phase for correcting problems or making adjustments. Standards may be quantitative or qualitative and are actually the outcomes that are to be measured. Examples of standards might be related to speed of performance, economics and cost, greater productivity, higher quality, or enhanced reporting. Standards may include benchmarking of an organization's activities to that of another organization, or it may compare output and productivity to some other respectable target. There are standards that are intangible (not measurable) but provide valuable information. Intangible standards include such things as job satisfaction and employee engagement. A well-organized plan should solicit feedback on all aspects of implementation. Listening to feedback and being open to making adjustments are essential to successful implementation. A common critical mistake is to be so locked into the plan that you jeopardize its entire success because you don't make minor adjustments. Needed adjustments and/or the assessment of outcomes will likely reinitiate the planning function and refuel the continuous management process.

Many organizations have incorporated Six Sigma and Lean manufacturing techniques into their business. Six Sigma, is based on continuous quality performance improvement using statistical analysis. The Greek symbol, Sigma is used in statistics to measure variation. Six Sigma is designed to minimize variation, minimize errors, and increase customer satisfaction. The target for Six Sigma is 99.999% or less variation from the desired level of performance. Lean manufacturing based on the Toyota Production System (TPS) is another method many organizations have implemented to reduce waste. The aim is to reduce defects and to improve quality.

In summary, controlling should be both anticipatory and retrospective. The process anticipates problems and takes preventive action. With corrective action, the process also follows up on problems whereby each person in the business views control as his or her responsibility. Controlling is related to each of the other functions of management and builds on planning, organizing, and leading. Our final **outcome assessment** will be reaching our objectives, and qualitatively (i.e. purposefully and enjoyably) and quantitatively (i.e. costly and timely) evaluating the experience of having attained our goals.

SUMMARY

Although the functions of a healthcare manager can be grouped into four primary categories—planning, decision making, organizing, and implementing/controlling—they do not exist separately but rather are interconnected in a type of concentric circle. If one of the functions is weak or nonexistent, the success of the project may be compromised. Without continuity, the manager may be seen as weak and ineffective and may not be considered a leader by staff, peers, or executive leadership.

One of the most critical attributes of a successful manager is the ability to balance multiple responsibilities. In the most basic interpretation, this refers to the ability to multi-task, prioritize, organize, and keep agendas moving forward. This balancing act becomes more complicated when there are two or more sides to an issue that require the manager to weigh and consider all potential outcomes (Table 4-5).

This can be a delicate balancing act with the manager as the fulcrum straddling the center. Although it would be ideal to keep everything evenly balanced, this goal is not realistic. If the manager is to be successful and keep advancing the agendas of his/her department, she/he will need to maintain flexibility as urgent situations and priorities warrant. Over the longer term however, balance in the organization must be reestablished and in a reasonable time frame.

In addition to the ongoing struggle to maintain a balance of functionality, a myriad of external pressures are also brought to bear on laboratory management. In this example, external refers to those issues not directly related to testing or producing the product. These issues will pull or stretch the manager in one direction or another at various times. The following diagram illustrates some of these "gravitational external forces" (Figure 4-4).

Healthcare management functionality is complex and diverse. It requires formal learned skills, experiential skills, and a high level of dedication and commitment; it presents those involved with significant challenges on a daily basis. In return, however, the successful manager will experience a significant degree of achievement and satisfaction.

TABLE 4-5. Management Balancing Act

People centered	versus	Task centered
Personnel resources	versus	Capital resources
Laboratory issues	versus	Hospital or corporate issues
Financial goals	versus	Service goals
Opportunities	versus	Threats
Speed	versus	Detailed process
Perceptions	versus	Facts

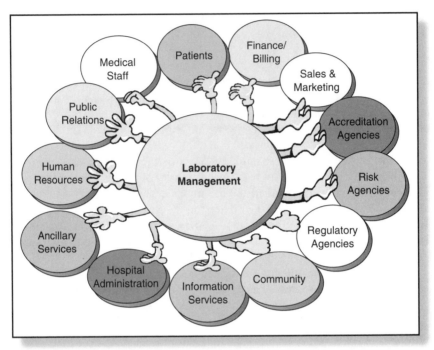

FIGURE 4-4. **Laboratory External Forces**

SUMMARY CHART:
Important Points to Remember

➤ The four basic management functions are: planning, decision-making, organizing, and implementing/controlling.

➤ One of the most critical attributes of a successful manager is, being able to balance multiple responsibilities.

➤ Planning is the most fundamental management function.

➤ In the process of decision making, there must be a choice between at least two alternatives.

➤ The control process should be done simultaneously with all other management functions.

➤ Organizing may best be accomplished through work teams.

➤ A manager must have ability to multi-task, prioritize, organize, and keep agendas moving forward.

➤ A manager must be dedicated, flexible, and positive.

SUGGESTED PROBLEM-BASED LEARNING ACTIVITIES

Chapter 4: Management Functions

Instructions: Use Internet resources, books, articles, colleagues, etc., to present solutions to the problems listed below. There is no one correct solution to any problem.

Note to Instructor: Students in class may be divided into groups and given the problem-based learning activity to discuss and solve. Once the group has reached consensus as to a solution, the group may present it to the other students in the class. This activity will provide all students with information regarding solutions to the problem.

Problem #1

You have just been hired as the manager of a laboratory. How do you introduce yourself? What is your initial plan of action for being in charge? What are the first steps you intend to take in the running of your laboratory?

Problem #2

Suppose you terminated an employee who has now filed a discrimination complaint. How do you handle this situation?

Problem #3

You are requested to set up an offsite laboratory at a community outreach facility. How would you proceed in the implementation of such a laboratory?

REFERENCES

1. Drucker PF: The Theory of the Business. In: *Managing in a Time of Great Change.* Truman Talley Books/Plume, Penguin Putnam, New York, NY, 1998, pp. 21–38.

2. Liebler JG: *Management Principles for Health Professionals,* ed 5. Jones and Bartlett Publishers, Sudbury, MA, 2008.

3. Dunn R: *Haimann's Healthcare Management,* ed 7. Health Administration Press, Chicago, IL, 2002.

BIBLIOGRAPHY

Allen RW: A Behavior Known as Performance. The Dreyden Press, Orlando, FL, 2000.

Bishop JW, Scott KD, Burroughs SM: Support Commitment, and Employee Outcomes in a Team Environment. *Journal of Management* 2000: 26; 1113–1132.

Daft RL: Management, ed 5. The Dryden Press, Orlando, FL, 2000.

DuBrin AJ: *Essentials of Management,* ed 3. College Division South-Western Publishing, Cincinnati, OH, 1994.

Garcia LS, Balselki BS, Burke MD, Schwab DL, eds.: *Clinical Laboratory mManagement.* ASM, 2004.

Hudson J: *Principles of Clinical Laboratory Management: A Study Guide and Workbook.* Prentice Hall, 2003.

Jones GR, Gerorge JM, Hill CW: *Contemporary Management,* ed 2. Irwin McGraw-Hill, Boston, MA, 1998.

Liebler JG, McConnell CR: Part II. The Management Functions: From Theory to Application. In: *Management Principles for Health Professionals.* Aspen Publications, Gaithersburg, MD, 1999: 85-278.

Robbins SP: *Organizational Behavior,* ed 9. Prentice Hall, Upper Saddle River, NJ, 2000.

Snyder JR, Wilkinson DS: Management Functions in the Clinical Laboratory. In: Snyder JR, Wilkinson DS, eds.: *Management in Laboratory Medicine,* ed 3. Lippincott-Raven Publishers, New York, NY, 1998.

Turnbull DC: Communicating Successfully in the Workplace. *Lab Med* 2005: 36(4); 205-208.

Workman RD, Lewis MJ, Hill BT: Enhancing the Financial Performance of a Health System Laboratory Network Using an Information System. *Am J ClinPathol* 2000: 114(1); 9-15.

INTERNET RESOURCES

Barnett T: Management Functions. Reference for Business—Encyclopedia of Business, 2nd ed. http://www.referenceforbusiness.com/management/Log-Mar/Management-Functions.html

CliffsNotes.com, *Functions of Managers.* Wiley Publishing, 2011. http://www.cliffsnotes.com/study_guide/topicArticleId-8944,articleId-8848.html

McNamara C: Free Basic Guide to Leadership and Supervision. Adapted from the Field Guide to Leadership and Supervision. Free Management Library, Authenticity Consulting, LLC. http://www.managementhelp.org/mgmnt/prsnlmnt.htm

"Principles of Management" Management Study Guide http://managementstudyguide.com/management_principles.htm

Managerial Decision Making and Process Improvement

Vicki S. Freeman, PhD, MLS^{CM}(ASCP)SC

CHAPTER OUTLINE

OBJECTIVES

Following successful completion of this chapter, the learner will be able to:

1. Define problem solving and decision making.
2. Differentiate decision making from problem solving.
3. Describe the five steps that managers should take to make the best decisions.
4. Explain the eight traps that affect decision making and lead managers to make poor decisions.
5. Describe the PDCA (plan, do, check, act) cycle of process improvement.
6. Contrast PDCA cycle to LEAN and Six Sigma Methodology for process improvement.

7. Define tools that are used in the decision-making process.
8. Apply the problem-solving process to a laboratory management issue.

KEY TERMS

Benchmarking
Brainstorming
Cost/Benefit Analysis
Decision Making
Decision Tree
Fishbone Diagram

Pareto Chart
PMI (Plus/Minus/Interesting)
Problem Solving
Scatter Diagram
Shewhart Cycle
Spaghetti Diagram

Case Study   Decision Making and Process Improvement

You are the manager of a clinical laboratory at a mid-size (200-bed) community hospital. Physicians and nurses are concerned about the turnaround time for laboratory tests ordered on early morning rounds. It appears that the samples are collected by the phlebotomy team on the 6:00 A.M. rounds. Physicians begin their patient rounds at 7:30 A.M. The physicians prefer to review the results of the laboratory tests ordered at the time they see the patient. They explain to you that they cannot make decisions with regards to further patient treatment or discharge without these results. Time is of the essence, as the hospital is cutting the budget, and it is important to decrease the patient length of stay. You are expected to look into this matter and make recommendations regarding the most efficient and effective way to address this problem.

Issues and Questions to Consider:
1. *What is the best method of addressing this problem?*
2. *What management techniques/styles might be used?*
3. *Who should be included in a team assigned to address this issue?*
4. *What decision traps might be encountered and how can they be avoided?*
5. *What decision-making tools would facilitate the analysis of the problem?*

INTRODUCTION

The day-to-day operation of the laboratory requires strong leadership and management. The laboratory manager must serve as an advocate for the laboratory, providing quality patient care while ensuring an effective and efficient customer-centered operation. As physicians, nurses, and other allied health professionals have come to rely on the laboratory to provide them with timely, accurate information to diagnosis and treat the patient, it is important that the laboratory be responsive to any problems that arise and impede the flow of test results. The laboratory manager must intervene and find ways to solve the problem by researching the problem, identifying the causes, and solving it by making a decision from a cadre of alternatives. A proactive manager will welcome this opportunity as a chance to improve the laboratory process and service rather than viewing it as an intrusion.

Problem solving and decision making are interrelated. **Problem solving** is the process of identifying and defining the problem; determining what happened to cause it, and what steps or possible solutions will be necessary to solve it. Problem solving focuses on solving an immediate tangible problem. It consists of multiple steps, which includes the decision-making process. **Decision making**, on the other hand, is the process of choosing among several alternatives. It may or may not be the result of an immediate problem, but is usually very goal directed. An effective manager uses a systematic process in decision making to choose among the various options using clearly defined criteria. In decision making, the end-result is first defined and then the means to achieve that result are identified.

This chapter is designed to introduce the learner to the problem-solving process. A discussion of the five associated steps is followed by a detailed description of the problem-solving component known as decision making. Two specific methodologies, LEAN and Six Sigma, and their tools are discussed that can be used for process improvement. Traps associated with decision making, tips for using these components in groups, and strategies and tools used in the decision-making process are also discussed.

STEPS IN THE PROBLEM-SOLVING PROCESS

Problems can be structured or unstructured. Structured problems tend to be routine, recurring, and involve an almost automatic process. They have a high degree of certainty with regard to outcome. With structured problems, managers have established rules or guidelines to follow because they have made decisions about the same type of problem many times. Quite often, preplanned actions have been developed to apply to the situation when it arises. An example of a routine problem is the reordering of laboratory supplies on a regular basis or the scheduling of personnel. In contrast, unstructured problems are non-routine, nonrecurring, have an uncertain outcome, and require new and often unique solutions. These are unusual situations that have not been addressed very often. There are no rules to follow as the decision is new. These decisions are made based on information gathered and a manager's intuition and judgment. Examples of unusual problems include the decision to investigate a new technology or instrumentation for the laboratory or the reorganization of a laboratory section.

There are five steps in the problem-solving process: 1) problem identification, 2) problem analysis, 3) criteria establishment, 4) alternative development and decision making, and 5) problem solution feedback.

Problem Identification

Once the manager has identified whether the problem is routine or unique, the problem must be defined. One approach to problem solving is grounded in John Dewey's analysis of the steps of the reflective-thinking process.[1] This process emphasizes the detailed analysis of the problem before a discussion of solutions and then a systematic evaluation of alternatives. In this model, problem solving consists of five steps. The first step is identifying and defining the problem. According to Hersey and Blanchard, a problem exists when there is a discrepancy between what one would like to happen and what is actually happening.[2] This discrepancy may be in the eyes of the manager, a subordinate, or a customer. In the laboratory setting, a common complaint heard from individuals outside of the laboratory is the time it takes for a laboratory result to be generated and returned to the patient's chart (called turnaround time). In the laboratory, technologists may believe that they are completing the laboratory tests in record time, but from a nurse's or physician's standpoint, when patient care is the primary concern, the time may seem much too long. The manager must define what ideally should be happening (How long should it take to get a test result back?) and where the discrepancy lies (Is it really taking too long? Is the problem pre, post, or during the analytical phase?). At this point, symptoms and evidence that a problem exists are looked at, but not the causes or why a problem exists. In addition, information about the problem is collected, potential resources for data collection identified, and unfamiliar terms and concepts defined. It is important that the problem be clarified from the information received before proceeding to the next step.

Problem Analysis

The second step in the problem-solving process is the analysis of the problem. After evidence has been collected, the problem identified and defined, the manager's attention turns to analyzing the evidence more thoroughly, and looking for relevant data that may explain why the problem exists. This step in the procedure is a matter of evaluating the data that has been collected in step one, and the sources from which that data comes. In the turnaround time example, the manager will collect the following data: 1) the time of the request for the test,

2) the time the specimen is obtained and received in the laboratory, 3) how the specimen is processed, 4) when the test is performed, and 5) when the result is reported back to the patient's chart. Managers must determine the actual problem and avoid looking only at symptoms. By using actual data, as well as individuals' perceptions, the manager will get a clearer picture of the real problem. Managers often leave out this step and jump to conclusions without understanding the root problem. They react on and solve the problem based on those visible symptoms, not the actual root causes of the problem. In other cases, managers are distracted by another problem identified in the data gathering process and solve it instead of the original problem. Failure to accurately identify the root cause is one of the major reasons why a solution that is tried is unsuccessful. It is often advantageous to invite individuals from outside the laboratory situation to discuss the issues in order to give an outside perspective and insight into the problem.

Criteria Establishment

Step three in the problem-solving process involves establishing criteria on which potential solutions will be evaluated. Clear specifications of 1) what the decision has to accomplish (this is the most difficult step), 2) what minimum goals must be attained, 3) what objectives the decision has to reach, and 4) what conditions it has to satisfy (boundary conditions) must be determined. Ideally, based on the definition of the problem and analysis of its cause(s), only one objective should be set that any acceptable solution could attain.

In the case of a turnaround time (TAT), considerations may include the following:

1. What criteria are necessary for quality patient care in the turnaround time of a laboratory test? Is 60 minutes soon enough?
2. Does this test result need to be available for physician review in 30 minutes?
3. What data supports this need?

By using this information, the laboratory can set a standard turnaround time against which future turnaround times can be measured for evaluation purposes. The standard may need to be varied based on the type of laboratory test being performed or the situation of the patient. If the problem is too complex to set only one objective to meet the goal(s) (the desired outcomes), another means for establishing criteria to evaluate proposed solutions is to make a list of "must's" and "want's." "Must's" are those basic requirements without which the solution would be unacceptable. "Want's" are those qualities that are desirable in any solution and should be assessed according to their priority. This type of checklist may help to maximize the effectiveness of any solution without omitting any essential requirements. Constraints or unchangeable factors must also be identified, as these will limit the options. By identifying them early, the manager can avoid solutions that waste time and money.

Alternative Development and Decision Making

Next, the manager must develop appropriate solutions to really solve the problem; this is where managerial decision making takes place. The classical model of decision making assumes managers have access to all the information required to reach a decision and that they can make the optimum decision by easily ranking their own preferences among alternatives. However, according to James March at Stanford University, managers do not consider all the alternatives or consequences and do not evoke all preferences at the same time.[3] Instead of considering all the alternatives simultaneously, decision makers consider only a few and look at them sequentially. If good alternatives are missed, the resulting decision is poor. It is hard to develop creative alternatives, so managers are encouraged to look for ways to obtain new ideas. Brainstorming is an excellent method to develop a list of potential solutions. From the list of options that emerge, a realistic range of solutions can be developed. The one that best fits the needs of the laboratory is selected according to the evaluation criteria set in step three. Each alternative can be ranked based on its advantages and disadvantages, weaknesses and strengths, and how well it meets the objective. How each alternative satisfies the must and want requirements from step three should also be analyzed. According to Stephen Covey, a win-win solution, wherein both parties feel good and feel committed to the decision and action plan, is what should be strived for in this situation.[4] To achieve this takes more than time; it takes patience, self-control, and courage balanced with consideration.

Problem Solution and Feedback

The final step in the problem-solving process is to put the solution into place. Converting the decision into action is the most time-consuming step. First, an action plan must be written that details the steps that need to be taken to implement the solution and the resources required to do it. It should be noted that often a decision is made and not implemented; however, utilizing an action plan will ensure that the decision is implemented.

Issues and Questions to Consider:

1. *Who has to know of this decision?*
2. *What action must be taken?*
3. *Who is to take the action?*
4. *How will it be implemented?*

Criteria to measure, observe, or discern progress toward the objectives and goals—that is, the ultimate desired outcomes—must be set to evaluate the effectiveness of the solution. Feedback must be built into the decision to provide a continuous testing against the actual experience and the expectations that underlie the decision. This "feedback" must test the validity and effectiveness of the decision against the actual course of events. Managers must consider what went right and wrong with the decision and learn for the future. Without feedback, managers never learn from experience and make the same mistake again.

DECISION-MAKING PROCESS

Decision making is the process by which managers respond to opportunities and threats by analyzing options, and making decisions about goals and courses of action. This process occurs in step four of the problem-solving process. It is the most important management skill that an individual who aspires to become a leader can acquire. The speed in which a decision must be made will vary based on the problem to be solved. Effective managers must make both quick as well as complicated decisions by drawing on their own experiences, reliable sources of information, good "sounding boards," and a fairly clear sense of purpose. They must also be willing to act and accept necessary risks when making the decision. At times, a manager must make a quick decision such as in the case of a "life and death" or critical situation. The worst-case scenario in these cases may be that not making a decision is worse than making a poor decision. These quick decisions are often made on the run, with limited time, limited information, and limited participation of others. At other times, the decision requires more information to be gathered, more input from others, and lots of alternatives generated and evaluated. These complicated decisions come together in bits and pieces over an extended period of months or even years. Usually, many people are involved. The group decision-making process is discussed later in this chapter.

Decision-Making Traps

Even though making decisions are the most important activities that managers engage in, individuals are generally amateurs when it comes to making the right decision. Because of the numerous internal and external influences that exert pressure on an individual, many hidden traps can be found in decision making.[1] A manager should become aware of these perceptual and behavioral decision traps in decision-making situations to actively avoid them. Eight traps are briefly discussed next.

The first trap, the *anchoring trap*, is an approach that many negotiators use to influence an individual's perception by giving information up-front that later impacts the decision that is made. "When considering a decision, the mind gives disproportionate weight to the first information it receives. Initial impressions, estimates, or other data anchor subsequent thoughts and judgments."[1] An example of this trap is a sales representative giving a price for a product or new instrument and what the contract for that commodity would be. The manager then comes back with a counter offer, which is usually somewhat lower than the price originally offered by the company. However, the company, upfront, has established the negotiation table. A manager should be wary of anchors in negotiations.

Individuals instinctively stay with what seems familiar. Thus, they look for decisions that involve the least change. This is called the *status-quo trap*. To protect their egos from damage, individuals avoid changing the status quo, even in the face of early predictions that change will be safer. They look for reasons to do nothing. Quite often, in business, making an incorrect change (doing something) tends to be punished much more severely than doing nothing. In all parts of life, people want to avoid rocking the boat. Managers can avoid this trap by first thinking about their objectives and goals when preparing to make a decision. They should review how these objectives and goals are served by the status quo, rather than a change and look at each possible change, one at a time. This will prevent them from being overwhelmed, and also prevent them from instinctively wanting to stay "safe" and unchanged.

The *sunk-cost trap* (or the justify-past-actions trap) is the escalation of commitment where an individual, because of past decisions, believes that he/she must continue in that direction, although the reason is no longer valid. The more actions that a manager has already taken on behalf of a choice or direction, the more difficult the manager finds it to change direction or make a different choice. Whenever an individual has invested time, money, or other resources in a decision, or whenever his/her personal reputation is at stake, he/she finds it much more difficult to change his/her decision or course of action. How can a manager avoid this trap? As Warren Buffet, a successful business investor, once said, "When you find yourself in a hole, the best thing you can do is stop digging." A manager can help him/herself and his/her subordinates to make better decisions by setting an example of admitting mistakes when it happens, and then changing course. They will then believe they can do likewise without penalties.

People have a tendency to subconsciously decide what they want to do before they figure out why they want to do it. The *confirming-evidence trap* is a mental bias that leads managers to seek out information to support their existing point of view while avoiding information that contradicts it. This bias affects where they go to collect data to reinforce a current stance or perspective and how they interpret the facts received. It then leads them to give too much weight to supporting information and opinions and too little to those that are conflicting. To avoid this trap, managers should have someone play devil's advocate, or build counterarguments themselves. They should not accept evidence confirming their viewpoint without questioning it, and should make sure that the people from whom they are gaining a perspective can offer independent information and opinions.

The next mental trap, the *framing trap*, deals with how you view your choices or how you frame the questions around the problem. Since the first step in the problem-solving process is identifying and defining the problem, this trap can be especially dangerous. This trap is also perilous, as it can lead to managers bringing other traps into the process. A frame can establish the status quo, introduce an anchor, lead a manager to justify past actions, or highlight confirming evidence. To avoid this trap, a manager should find ways to restate the problem or situation presented to them in their own way, and take the opportunity to see it from different sides in order to envision various outcomes.

The following three traps are based on the ability of a manager to estimate and forecast uncertain events. Managers make decisions under three conditions: 1) certainty—they know the outcome (this never really occurs); 2) uncertainty—they have absolutely no idea what will happen; or 3) risk—they have some degree of understanding in regards to the possible outcomes (most common). By forecasting what might happen, a manager will then have a better chance of making a successful decision.

In the **overconfidence trap**, the manager believes that he/she is better at making forecasts or estimates than he/she actually is. Overly confident about their ability to predict, most managers set too narrow a range of possibilities. Ironically, research has found a positive relationship between overconfidence and task difficulty. In other words, the harder the task, the more people are apt to make decisions with confidence, almost as a self-justification.

Managers can also be overly cautious or prudent in forecasting; this is called the **prudence trap**. When faced with high-stakes decisions, they tend to adjust their estimates or forecasts "just to be on the safe side." A manager will look for the worst-case scenario and make decisions based on this analysis, which can be just as damaging as being overconfident.

The last trap, the **recallability trap**, is an association bias in terms of "it worked before." In this trap, managers get caught using past experiences to forecast the future and become overly influenced by events that left a strong impression on them.

By being aware that these traps can distort their thinking, involving others in the decision-making process, gathering appropriate data, and building checks and balances into their decision-making process, managers can avoid these traps as they make their decisions.

Group Decision-Making Process

"Enlightened leaders and business managers . . . know that when people are meaningfully involved, they willingly commit the best that is in them. Moreover, when people identify their personal goals with the goals of an organization, they release an enormous amount of energy, creativity, and loyalty."[6]

Although managers find that it is often easier to make decisions alone, they also find that decisions made by oneself are often not the best decisions. Therefore, involving other individuals and groups in the decision-making process is best. However, the type of group involvement should be determined by the quality of the decision needed, the amount of information available, and the degree of group acceptance needed for success. The amount of subordinate/group involvement in the decision-making process is referred to as *decision participation*. The leader may follow one of four decision-making styles when involving the group in the decision.[2]

In the **autocratic style**, the leader makes the decision without consulting with others. The leader may use only the information available at the time or may obtain more information from group members. The role played by team members in making the decision is one of providing the necessary information to the leader, rather than generating or evaluating alternative solutions. In the *consultative style*, the leader obtains suggestions and ideas from the team members, but then makes the decision, which may or may not reflect the team members' influence. The third participative style, *joint decision*, is also sometimes called the democratic style. The leader shares the problem with the relevant team members as a group. Together they generate and evaluate alternatives, and attempt to reach an agreement (consensus) on a solution. The leader's role is much like that of a chairperson. The leader does not try to influence the group to adopt a solution and is willing to accept and implement any solution that has the support of the entire group. In the last style, *delegation*, the leader turns the problem over to the group, and lets them generate and evaluate alternatives, in an attempt to reach an agreement on a solution without any leader involvement. When they reach an agreement, they tell the leader what their solution is and then together begin the process of implementation.

PROCESS IMPROVEMENT

Approaches to problem solving and process improvement, such as the Shewhart Cycle of Management, LEAN, and Six Sigma, have common roots and overlapping principles. The roots of process improvement can be traced back to Walter Shewhart, who developed the concept of Statistical Process Control to aid a manager in making scientific, efficient, and economical decisions. He based this process control on Carl Frederick Gauss' work, which occurred during the 19th Century. Gauss introduced the concept of the normal curve (i.e. the Gaussian curve). In the 1920s, Shewhart showed that three sigma from the mean is the point where a process requires correction. Six Sigma as a measurement standard can be traced back to this work. Additionally, Shewhart conceived the Shewhart Cycle of Management Process, based on the traditional scientific method to examine processes and remove undesirable causes and their effects. This Cycle of Management Process, also called the Plan-Do-Check (or Study)-Act Cycle (PDCA), was later modified and applied by Deming.[3]

Many measurement standards (Cpk, Zero Defects, etc.) later came on the scene, but credit for coining the term "Six Sigma" goes to a Motorola engineer named Bill Smith. "Six Sigma" is a federally registered trademark of Motorola. The tools of Six Sigma are most often applied within a simple performance improvement model known as Define-Measure-Analyze-Improve-Control, or DMAIC. The term "LEAN" was first coined by John Krafcik, but is based on principles that were developed by the Japanese manufacturing industry.[9] It is a more generic process management philosophy derived mostly from the Toyota Production System.[1] Both the LEAN and the Six Sigma methodologies have shown that dramatic improvements in cost, quality, and time can be obtained by focusing on process improvement. Whereas Six Sigma is focused on reducing variation and improving process capability by following a problem-solving approach using statistical tools, LEAN is primarily concerned with eliminating waste and improving flow by following the LEAN principles of Value, The Value Stream, Flow, Pull and Perfection, through a defined approach in the implementation of these principles.[4]

Interestingly, Edward Deming applied the problem-solving approach to work processes and team decision making for Japanese companies.[12] He envisioned it as a circular system in which the work and processes are thought of as a continuous cycle, not a linear path with a beginning, middle, and end. There are many overlaps to these models and John Dewey's reflective thinking process. However, the use of problem-solving tools to help group members make decisions is a key part of the Deming group problem-solving approach.

A centerpiece of Deming's vision of an effective team is the use of the consensus method for making key decisions. A consensus requires unity but not unanimity; concurrence but not consistency. A consensus is reached when all members can say they either agree with the decision or have had their "day in court" and were unable to convince the others of their viewpoint. In the final analysis, everyone agrees to support the outcome. The Consensus approach is appropriate when: 1) there is no clear answer, 2) there is no single expert in the group, 3) a commitment to the decision is essential, and 4) sufficient time is available to allow everyone to have input.

The following section will discuss the Shewhart Cycle as a group decision-making model and contrast this cycle with the LEAN and Six Sigma methodologies.

The Shewhart Cycle

As common causes of problems are inherent in every process and are not attributable to the worker, only a data-driven, scientific approach that involves participants in the process can identify and eliminate these causes. The **Shewhart Cycle** (Figure 5-1) is a continuous, circular process which includes the four steps: Plan, Do, Check, Act. The next section will describe the components of each step.

Step 1 – Plan
The team identifies the real problem and spends time defining and analyzing the nature of the problem. They must spend sufficient effort to understand the steps in the process and the causes of the problem. How the problem is defined affects the kinds of solutions that are seen. By describing the process, reviewing available data, and identifying the customers, the team begins to understand the process to be studied. Rather than relying on hunches or historical data, the team develops skills in data collection and analysis to illuminate the root causes of problems and to identify solutions that are meaningful to the customer.

Describe the process. The process to be studied must be described in a step-wise manner, so that each individual contribution is understood and the resources used are identified.

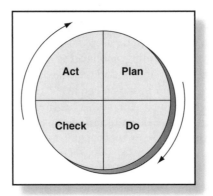

FIGURE 5-1.   The Shewhart Cycle

Example: Laboratory Turnaround Time—Request receipt

1. *Request received from the hospital floor via: telephone call, written communication, computer.*
2. *If the request is from the computer system, it can be directly processed.*
3. *If the request is via telephone or written communication, it must be entered into the computer system before it can be processed by the phlebotomist.*
4. *Request sent to phlebotomist to draw.*

Review existing information. The team must identify potential sources of existing data or information to determine the gaps that need to be filled.

Example: Laboratory Turnaround Time

Information can be gathered from hospital floor, patient charts, LIS, HIS, laboratory work logs. Information available might include: Number of requests received by laboratory, time of requests sent, method of request transmission, time results returned to patient chart, time of call from the hospital floor.

Potential Gaps include:

1. *Personnel time to answer phone calls and send out information.*
2. *How does the laboratory handle requests which are received?*
3. *What is the time frame of the responses (turnaround time)?*

Identify customer. Define all of the internal and external customers for a given process—quality should be defined by the needs of the customer.

Example: Laboratory Turnaround Time

Internal customers: phlebotomists, receptionists, technicians, technologists
External customers: nursing staff, medical staff, patients

Select appropriate strategies to gather meaningful data. The team must begin to identify approaches that will allow them to collect data about the outcomes of the current process, the experiences their customers have with the process, and where the problems in that process may exist. Developing surveys of external and internal customers, collecting information from databases, and developing new databases for collection of information are all methods to gather data. What methods are used will vary with the process being studied.

Interview customers. The teams survey the customer and ask the customer to identify their quality requirements and preferences. This allows the organization to anticipate rather than react to customer needs. Team begins by interviewing their customers, focusing on root causes and barriers to improvement, and base their decisions and actions on real data. The team members survey customers to provide input to process, to define quality, and to identify concerns about the process.

Example: Laboratory Turnaround Time

Interview individual nursing and medical staff about their experiences.
Interview laboratory phlebotomists, technicians, and technologists about their experiences.

Plot the process out on a process flow diagram. The process is then tracked on a flow chart. A flow chart will help to determine the appropriate sequence and to determine what training and resources are needed and which people need to be involved (Figure 5-2).

Brainstorm problem and produce a fishbone diagram. Once the process is mapped out, the cause of the problem is then explored through brainstorming and a tool called a fishbone diagram (Figure 5-3). This allows the team to see all of the factors that might affect the process. The **fishbone diagram** (discussed in detail later in this chapter) is an effective method for studying the process and for planning. It is a pictorial list of the factors with branches representing the main categories of potential causes of problems. Typical categories include: people, methods, equipment and materials, and environment.

Collect data on the process. The team members gather facts by reviewing existing literature, talking with the customers, and collecting data on the process. Data that is gathered is used as a guide to improvement and diagnosis of the problem, not

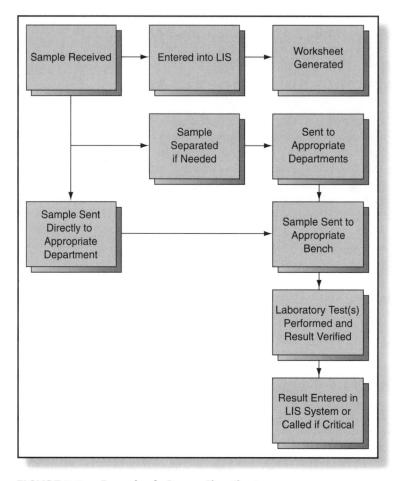

FIGURE 5-2.   Example of a Process Flow Chart

as an accountability device. The team uses the data to define the problem and understand its root causes. They seek to understand the process and how decisions about potential solutions might affect the process.

The team cannot improve a process without data. Data are often numerical, but they might also include characterizations of how a process really works or other kinds of facts. In virtually every process to improve quality, participants learn by using the PDCA cycle that their initial judgments about the nature of the problem and its root causes are, at best, partially supported by the data. Often the data yield surprises.

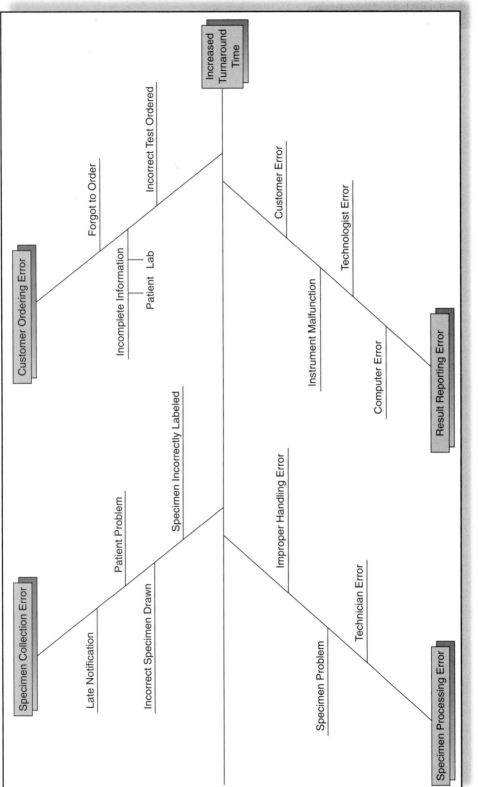

FIGURE 5-3. Laboratory Example of a Fishbone Diagram

127

Data on the nature and magnitude of the problem is collected. Then more data is collected to ensure that the cause or causes are the actual root of the problem.

Example: Laboratory Turnaround Time

Data which might be collected includes:
- *number of requests received by laboratory*
- *time the requests are sent*
- *method of request transmission*
- *time results returned to patient chart*
- *time of call from floor requesting results*

Analyze the data. Data collected may be tallied and analyzed using a chart as shown here. Other tools are also used to diagram the data (e.g., histograms, Pareto charts, scatter diagrams, run charts, statistical process control charts). Scatter diagrams are covered in more detail in the *Decision-Making Strategies and Tools* section later in this chapter.

Example: Laboratory Turnaround Time

Reasons for Delays	Average Time of Delays	Average Number of Delays	Total
A number of requests received by laboratory			
B time the requests are sent			
C method of request transmission			
D time results returned to patient's chart			
E time of call from floor requesting results			

Develop a theory or hypothesis. Team members use the data collected and analyzed to develop a theory or hypothesis about the causes of the problem for process improvement. (If we do such and such, the process will improve in these ways, for these reasons.)

Remember, the plan is to fix the process, not the outcomes. A team must be careful about adding steps to a process, as this adds opportunities for new problems. Teams must make each process as simple as possible to improve quality.

Example: Laboratory Turnaround Time

Patient care is being compromised because essential information that should be received by the laboratory is missing. A training session for physicians and nurses should be arranged.

Step 2 – Do

In this step, the team implements the improvement effort they planned using a small-scale test. The individuals responsible for implementation need to know what the goal of this change is, how they impact the implementation process, and receive training in the process.

Test the hypothesis. In the *Do* step, the hypothesis that was developed is tried out. A solution is determined and implemented. The team tries out the solution in a limited way to be sure that it works. The question to be asked is: Did the solution work as intended, or does it need revision?

Example: Laboratory Turnaround Time

- *Develop and implement a training program for physicians and nurses.*
- *Track laboratory requests through the process, from ordering to the reporting out of test results.*
- *Gather data on turnaround times.*
- *Send out a follow-up survey to customers.*

Step 3 – Check

The results of the improvement effort are measured in this step. The data collected is analyzed and the results studied to see if the process was improved. This gives the team a chance to see if the correct components of the process were measured. It allows team members the opportunity to examine and evaluate any variables that may be present in the process.

Check by collecting data. The team tests the hypothesis by collecting data as they did earlier in the processes. The results are monitored against the original data to ascertain if the desired outcome is achieved. Data are collected at this stage to be sure that the new process is better than the old one.

Step 4 – Act

If the results showed the expected improvement, the team should standardize and document all actions with the intention of making the changes permanent. Otherwise, the team's next step would be to reevaluate by returning to the "plan" step and starting the cycle over with the newly acquired knowledge.

Implement. When the team is satisfied with the results, the solution is implemented permanently in all areas where it is relevant.

Monitor. Periodically, the process is monitored to ensure that the root cause does not reoccur and to examine other opportunities for improvement. It is important that the team returns to the customers and obtain continuous feedback on the process and how the change is working.

The PDCA cycle enables team members of work groups to identify customer expectations, determine the standards and measurements which will be used to meet these expectations, and continuously evaluate and improve the quality of the work they perform. As issues or problems arise in the application of the process, the systematic problem-solving process ensures the thorough analysis of the problem, the determination of the true cause, and the careful planning and implementation of the optimum solution.

LEAN Methodology: Cut waste, make work easier, and simplify systems[9]

The purpose of LEAN is to standardize the way that a group works and to eliminate waste, i.e. "non-value-added" steps in the laboratory's processes to improve efficiencies. By doing this, it uses less of everything, by focusing on the elimination of wasted motion, space, and supplies, as well as reducing errors and improving safety. LEAN is not an acronym. According to the Mayo Clinic's Medical Laboratories white paper, "Innovations in the Clinical Laboratory," LEAN is a continual process of improvement that when applied to the laboratory has as its main objective, "to deliver quality patient laboratory results, at the lowest cost, within the shortest time frame while maintaining client satisfaction."[13] "LEAN is basically a set of techniques used to manage a work environment by eliminating waste, organizing the workplace, streamlining procedures and establishing clear, visual standards."[5] LEAN is a descriptive process that uses less of everything—space, time, investment in equipment, inventory, and staffing resources. LEAN's five principles (Figure 5-4) which guide the implementation of lean techniques include:[11]

1. *Identify Value*—specify what creates value from the customer's perspective.
2. *Map the Value Stream*—identify all the steps along the process chain, eliminating, whenever possible, those steps that do not create value.
3. *Create Flow*—make the process flow so the product or service will flow smoothly toward the customer.
4. *Establish Pull*—introduce a continuous flow of events between all steps of the process where possible. In a well-defined pull system, the process lets you know by inherent triggers when something needs to be done and the process manages itself.

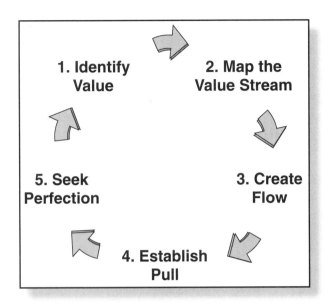

1. Identify Value

2. Map the Value Stream

5. Seek Perfection

3. Create Flow

4. Establish Pull

FIGURE 5-4.   LEAN Principles

5. *Seek Perfection or Continuous Improvement*—begin the process again and continue it until a state of perfection is reached in which perfect value is created with no waste.

According to Nelson, there are four tactics that are essential to removing the waste and establishing a LEAN laboratory: value stream mapping, 5S workplace organization, visual workplace, and work cell specimen processing.[12] *Value stream mapping* is an early step that provides an overall assessment of the process. The mapping should be carried out as a unified team, which will increase the buy-in for the improved process. To carry out the mapping process, three steps are undertaken. First, there is direct observation of the laboratory process and identification of where waste is found in the process. From this observation, the current process is examined and documented from start to finish. Finally, future-state maps are developed to show how the operation would look, if staff did only that which was necessary to complete the work based on high-quality standards. To carry out this step, it is important that the necessary stakeholders for each process are involved—those who work throughout the process, as well as those involved with its input and output.

5S workplace organization tactic emphasizes the maintenance of an orderly workplace.[15] The five workplace practices used in this organization originate from Japanese words. The practices (in English and Japanese) include:

Seiri – Sort: sorting, i.e., proper arrangement of all items, storage, equipment, tools, inventory, and traffic.

Seiton – Set (or Simplify): orderliness, i.e., determine the best place to keep the items that are used regularly.

Seiso – Shine: cleanliness, i.e., keep the work area clean, return items that were used during the day to their proper location.

Seiketsu – Standardize: i.e., make things common and consistent where possible.

Shitsuke – Sustain (or Self-Discipline): i.e., make a habit of maintaining this system.

Visual workplace is the concept of creating a workplace that is entirely visually instructive.

Visual cues—such as labels, signs, or colors—are used to reduce the amount of wasted time that is spent searching, looking, and waiting. These cues are vital to sustaining the LEAN practices. They ensure that the improvements are clearly visible, easily understood, and adhered to by all employees.

Work cell specimen processing is the physical or logical layout of all testing and processing equipment, technicians, machines, and materials through which a specimen flows. Work cells minimize movement, reduce batch sizes, decrease set-up time for testing, improve lab safety, and standardize work processes with visual cues.

Six Sigma DMAIC Methodology[6]

The Six Sigma DMAIC methodology can also be thought of as a roadmap for problem solving and product/process improvement. DMAIC, as does the PDCA cycle, refers to a data-driven quality strategy for improving processes, and is an integral part of the Six Sigma Quality Initiative. DMAIC is an acronym for five interconnected phases: Define, Measure, Analyze, Improve, and Control. Each step in the cyclical DMAIC process is required to ensure the best possible results. The first three steps of the DMAIC process are encompassed in the planning step of the PDCA cycle. These process steps include: 1) defining the project goals/ customer, 2) measuring the current process performance, and 3) determining the root causes of the problem. Each step is detailed next:

In *Step 1,* define the project goals and customer (internal and external) deliverables, it is important to first define who the customers are, what their requirements are for products and services, and what their expectations are. Then the project boundaries, the stop and start of the process must be defined. Finally, the process to be improved must be determined by mapping the process flow.

Step 2 measure the process to determine current performance. In step 2, the method to measure the core business process involved is developed. This includes developing a data collection plan for the process, collecting data from many sources to determine types of defects and metrics, and comparing to customer survey results to determine shortfall.

Step 3 analyze and determine the root cause(s) of the defects. This step includes: analyzing the data collected, determining the root causes of defects and opportunities for improvement, identifying gaps between current performance and goal performance, prioritizing opportunities to improve, and identifying sources of variation.

Step 4 in the Six Sigma methodology is similar to the "Do" and "Check" steps in the Shewhart cycle. In step 4, the process is improved by eliminating defects. Creative solutions are used to fix and prevent problems, creating innovative solutions using technology and discipline, and developing and deploying an implementation plan to the targeted process.

Finally, *Step 5,* control future process performance, is the "Act" step of the Shewhart cycle. In step 5, the improvements are controlled to keep the process on the new course and to prevent reverting back to the "old way." This step involves the development, documentation, and implementation of an ongoing monitoring plan. The improvements are institutionalized through the modification of systems and structures (staffing, training, incentives) in this final step.

Six Sigma uses many of the same tools as the Shewhart Cycle discussed previously, but its focus is a more structured application of tools and techniques and tends to be on the financial aspect of the business and the dollars saved through its process improvement. This methodology, when applied on a company-wide scale, becomes part of the culture of the organization.

Using LEAN and Sigma Six together can have added value. Each alone has limitations. Six Sigma eliminates defects but does not address the question of how to optimize process flow. The LEAN principles create a flow to decrease waste, but exclude the advanced statistical tools often required to achieve the process capabilities needed to be truly 'lean'. Therefore, most practitioners consider these two methods as complementing each other.

DECISION-MAKING STRATEGIES AND TOOLS

Data analysis is an essential part of any problem-solving team. Problem areas are identified and useful solutions are determined based upon data collected and analyzed. The process can be simplified with the use of several helpful tools. Through use of such tools, team members can work with their customers through situations or problems that arise. By the team focusing on the processes used in a laboratory environment, a system to address a situation or problem can be created that allows everyone involved to feel like they have some control. Further, individuals involved in the process will feel a responsibility for the success of the laboratory, as well as for their own role in the process. Eight analytical tools are described below: 1) benchmarking, 2) brainstorming, 3) scatter diagrams, 4) Pareto charts, 5) PMI-plus/minus/interesting, 6) decision tree, 7) fishbone diagram/honeycomb cause and effect, and 8) cost/benefit analysis.

Benchmarking

An organization can determine a measure of its processes against those of recognized leaders in the field and how it measures up to the standard set by those leaders. This provides an opportunity to identify where improvement will be most beneficial and is called **benchmarking**. Both quantitative and qualitative performance measures can be used to benchmark an organization. Organizations usually establish performance indicators in four categories: 1) cost effectiveness, 2) staff productivity, 3) process efficiency, and 4) cycle time. Some examples of performance indicators that benchmarking practitioners can use, depending on the needs of their specific benchmarking task, are listed in Table 5-1.

Brainstorming

Brainstorming is a method for developing creative solutions to problems. It works by focusing on a problem, coming up with many unbounded solutions, and then pushing the ideas as far as possible. The idea of brainstorming is to generate, clarify, and evaluate a sizable list of ideas, problems, or issues. Brainstorming is a popular technique for enlisting the creative thinking of an individual to meet the purpose of the team. During the brainstorming session there is no criticism of ideas: the idea is to open up as many possibilities as possible, and break down preconceptions about the limits of the problem. Once this has been done, results of the brainstorming session can be analyzed, and the best solutions can be explored, either through further brainstorming or through solutions that are more conventional.

In the generation phase, the team leader reviews the rules for brainstorming and the team members generate a list of items. The objective is quantity, not quality of ideas. In the clarification phase, the team reviews the list to be sure everyone understands each item. Discussion is scheduled for a later time. In the evaluation phase, the team examines the list to remove duplicative, non-relevant, or forbidden (on basis of agreed upon ground rules) items.

TABLE 5-1.   Performance Indicators

Performance Indicator	Data to Gather and Analyze
Usage and Usefulness	Does a given activity add value?
Productivity, Responsiveness	Are calls returned within the same business day?
Working Environment	How does the work environment differ from your operation?
Accessibility	How accessible is the operation to its clients?
Quality	How many errors are made? What is the customer satisfaction rating?
Coverage	This pertains to the comprehensiveness of service provided.
Timeliness	Were specified timelines and commitments met?
Cost	What are comparative costs? Are they within the budget allotted?
Monitoring and Reporting	How often and specific are reporting procedures?

Adapted from the *American Productivity & Quality Center*, http://www.apqc.org.[18]

Scatter Diagrams

A **scatter diagram** is a plot of one variable versus another to see if there is any relationship between the two (e.g. customer turnaround time and time of day). Variable A is plotted on one axis and Variable B is plotted on the other axis. Different factors can affect the process and the people doing the work. The combination of two factors can have a positive or negative effect on the process. When there is no correlation, no apparent relationship between the two variables is found. If positive correlation is found, there is a defined, predictable relationship between the two variables. An increase in one variable is accompanied by a predictable increase in the other variable. On the other hand, although there is a defined, predictable relationship between the two variables, in a negative correlation each increase in one variable is accompanied by a predictable decrease in the other variable. See Figure 5-5.

Pareto Charts

Pareto Charts help to identify major factors and distinguish between the "vital few" causes and the potentially less significant ones. They are used to rank order causes from most to least significant. Such a graphical technique is based on the Pareto Principle, which states that just a few of the causes often account for most of the effect. It is often referred to as the 80-20 Rule. (80% of the problems can be attributed to 20% of the causes.) The Pareto Chart displays, in decreasing order, the relative contribution of each cause to the total problem. Relative contribution may be based on the number of occurrences, the cost associated with each cause, or another measure of impact on the problem. See Figure 5-6.

PMI—Plus/Minus/Interesting

PMI stands for **plus/minus/interesting**. It is a valuable development (by Edward de Bono) of the *pro's* and *con's* technique which has been used for centuries. PMI is a basic decision-making tool. When you are facing a difficult decision, simply create a table with the categories *Plus*, *Minus*, and *Interesting*. In the column

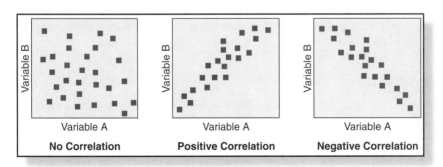

FIGURE 5-5. **Example of Scatter Diagrams**

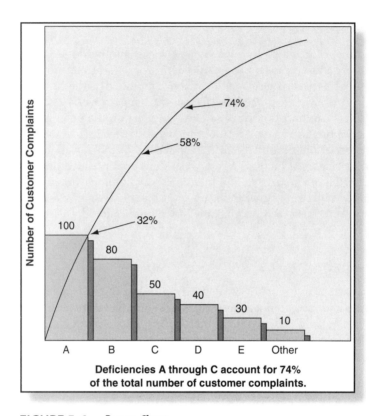

FIGURE 5-6.   Pareto Chart

underneath the *Plus* heading, write down all the positive points of taking the action. Underneath the *Minus* heading, write down all the negative effects. In the *Interesting* column, write down the extended implications of taking the action, whether positive or negative. Scoring your PMI table. You may be able to make a decision from the table alone. Alternatively, consider each of the points you have written down and assign a positive or negative score to each appropriately. The scores you assign can be entirely subjective. Once you have done this, add up the score. A strongly positive score indicates that an action should be taken; a strongly negative score indicates that it should be avoided. See Table 5-2.

Decision Trees

Management invariably encounters situations in which uncomfortable decisions must be made. In some cases, the difficulty may be that, although certain alternative choices are clear, the consequences of these choices are not readily apparent. One possible tool for a manager in such a situation is decision tree analysis. A **decision tree** is a graphical diagram consisting of nodes and branches. The nodes are of two types. The first is a rectangle that represents the decision to be made.

The branches emanating from decision nodes are the alternative choices with which the manager is faced. Only one alternative can be implemented. The second type of node is a circle. Circles represent chance nodes. That is, the alternatives emanating from chance nodes have some element of uncertainty as to whether or not they will occur. The primary benefit of a decision tree is that it provides a visual representation of the choices facing the manager. See Figure 5-7.

Fishbone/Honeycomb Cause and Effect

A Fishbone diagram (Figure 5-8) systematically analyzes cause and effect relationships and identifies potential root causes of a problem. Cause-and-effect or fishbone diagrams are used to display the relationships between a given effect and its potential causes. Such a graphical technique is used to sort out and relate the interactions among the factors affecting a process. A well-detailed cause-and-effect diagram is shaped like a fishbone.

Cost/Benefit Analysis

Cost/Benefit Analysis refers to the several approaches for determining and comparing the forward looking, incremental costs, benefits, and values of solution alternatives. It determines whether the results of a particular course of action are of sufficient benefit to justify the cost of taking the action. Ideally, precise, in-depth economic analyses should be performed by examining the cash flow impact of each alternative, taking into account the time value of money. However, less rigorous evaluations may be appropriate if there are no significant amounts of up-front investment and/or ongoing cash outflows involved.

TABLE 5-2.   Example of a Plus/Minus/Interesting Table Used in Decision Making

Should the laboratory send a test out to be performed at another laboratory?			
Plus	**Minus**	**Interesting**	**Total**
Less expensive (+5)	High turnaround time (−6)	Newer technology? (+1)	
High volume (+3)	Less exposure for MT students (−3)	Learn more about new technology in-house? (+2)	
Chance of sample misplacement greater (+5)	Less technologists needed (−3)	More difficult to get sample to laboratory? (−4)	
	Loss of technologist's expertise (−3)		
Totals +13	−15	−1	*−3

* Added Total = (−3)—It would be best to keep the test in-house.

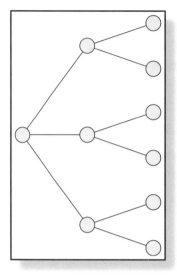

FIGURE 5-7.   Decision Tree

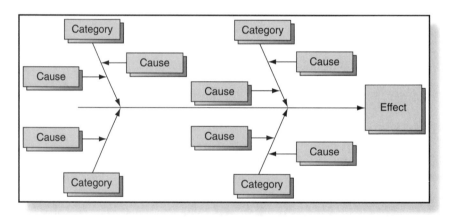

FIGURE 5-8.   Fishbone/Honeycomb Cause and Effect

Standard Work Chart (or Spaghetti Diagram)

A Standard Work Chart (or Spaghetti Diagram) (Figure 5-9) is tracking, on paper, the path of the person or persons performing the process tasks. Called a **Spaghetti Diagram** because of the lines drawn to trace the operation sequence, this step-by-step documentation is a visual creation of the flow and describes the actual activities, distance from the last step, estimated task time, observations, and return rate.

These are just a few of the many analytical tools available to teams and managers to detail out processes to make an informed decision. The value of the tools lies in the ability of the team to look at various pieces of data in different

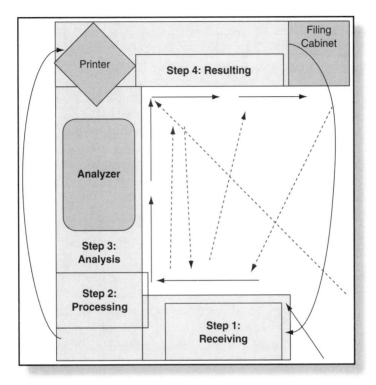

FIGURE 5-9. Spaghetti Diagram[17]

perspectives and frames of reference. It helps the team members to move from their departmental biases to a more neutral point of view; however, it is also important for the team to not focus so much on the use of these tools that it delays their decision making.

SUMMARY

Problem solving and decision making are important functions of a laboratory manager to ensure the smooth operation of the laboratory and to ensure quality patient care. By using John Dewey's reflective thinking process, managers should identify the problem, analyze it using data gathered, establish criteria for making a decision and develop alternatives, and finally, implement the solution. By following this process, they can avoid the many traps, both internal and external, that exist in the decision-making step of the problem-solving process. Involving individuals in the problem-solving process can be important to the buy-in of the final decision. Using a systematic problem-solving process, such as the PDCA, and analysis tools, such as scatter diagrams and Pareto charts on the data gathered, ensures the thorough analysis of customer expectations and concerns with a detailed view of the entire problem.

SUMMARY CHART:
Important Points to Remember

➤ The five steps in the problem-solving process: 1) problem identification, 2) problem analysis, 3) criteria establishment, 4) alternative development and decision making, 5) problem solution feedback.

➤ The Consensus approach is appropriate when 1) there is no clear answer, 2) there is no single expert in the group, 3) a commitment to the decision is essential, and 4) sufficient time is available to allow everyone to have input.

➤ Data analysis is an essential part of any problem-solving team.

➤ The Shewhart Cycle is a continuous, circular process, which includes four steps: Plan, Do, Check, Act.

➤ The LEAN methodology includes the five principles: Value, Value Stream, Flow, Pull, and Perfection.

➤ The Six Sigma DMAIC methodology includes five interconnected phases: Define, Measure, Analyze, Improve, and Control.

➤ Using a systematic problem-solving process, such as the PDCA; mapping tools such as spaghetti diagrams; and analysis tools, such as scatter diagrams and Pareto charts on the data gathered, ensures the thorough analysis of customer expectations and concerns with a detailed view of the entire problem.

SUGGESTED PROBLEM-BASED LEARNING ACTIVITIES

Chapter 5: Managerial Decision Making and Process Improvement

Instructions: Use Internet Resources, books, articles, colleagues, etc. to present solutions to the problems listed below. There is no correct solution to any problem.

Note to Instructor: Students in class may be divided into groups and given the problem-based learning activity to discuss and solve. Once the group has reached consensus as to a solution, the group may present it to the other students in the class. This activity will provide all students with information regarding solutions to the problem.

Problem #1

Suppose you are a laboratory director and one of your supervisors resigns. Create a work group to share supervisory responsibilities over that laboratory section until a new individual can be hired and trained.

Problem #2

You are the manager of a clinical laboratory at a mid-size (200-bed) community hospital. Physicians and nurses are concerned about the turnaround time for laboratory tests ordered on early morning rounds. To determine where there might be "waste" in the laboratory process, which is causing increased turnaround time, create a Spaghetti diagram of the process from the time that a test is ordered to the time that the test result is reported out.

Problem #3

Imagine yourself as a laboratory supervisor or manager. How would you delegate authority? How would you organize this process?

REFERENCES

1. Dewey J: *Problem Solving Tasks (Reflective Problem-Solving) How We Think.* D.C. Heath and Company, Boston, MA, 1933.

2. Hersey P, Blanchard K: *Management of Organizational Behavior,* ed 8. Prentice Hall, Englewood Cliffs, NJ, 2000.

3. March JG: A Pioneering and Respected Expert on Decision Making at Stanford University, Jack Steele Parker, Professor of International Management, Emeritus.

4. Covey SR: *Principle-Centered Leadership.* Simon & Schuster, New York, NY, 1991.

5. Hammond JS, Keeney RL, Raiffa H: The Hidden Traps in Decision Making. *Harvard Business Review* 1998: Sept/Oct.

6. Covey SR: *Principle-Centered Leadership.* Simon & Schuster, New York, NY, 1991.

7. Yukl GA: *Leadership in Organizations.* Prentice Hall, Englewood Cliffs, NJ, 2009.

8. The History of Six Sigma, iSixSigma, 2010. Accessed from: http://www.isix sigma.com/library/content/c020815a.asp

9. Womack JP, Jones DT, Roos D: *The Machine That Changed the World: The Story of Lean Production.* Rawson Associates, NY, 1990.

10. Holweg M: The Genealogy of Lean Production. *Journal of Operations Management* 2007: 25(2); 420-437.

11. Womack JP, Jones DT: *Lean Thinking: Banish Waste and Create Wealth in Your Corporation.* Simon & Schuster, New York, NY, 1996.

12. Deming WE: *Out of the Crisis,* ed. 1. The MIT Press, 2000.

13. Innovations in the Clinical Laboratory: An Overview of Lean Principles in the Laboratory. Aug 2007. http://www.mayomedi-callaboratories.com/mediax/outreach/resources/whitepapers/overview-of-lean-principles.pdf

14. Nelson N: Easy Lean Lab Exercises. Laboratory Daily News. Laboratory Equipment. http://www.laboratoryequipment.com/article-safety-Easy-Lean-Lab-Exercises-1209.aspx

15. Hirano H: *5 Pillars of the Visual Workplace.* Productivity Press, 1995.

16. Brue G: *Six Sigma for Managers.* McGraw-Hill, NJ, 2005.

17. Salazar J, Piazza MD: *Spaghetti Diagram.* University of Texas Medical Branch, Galveston, TX, 2009.

18. Higgins L, Hack B: *Measurement in the 21st Century.* American Productivity & Quality Center, 2004. http://www.apqc.org

BIBLIOGRAPHY

Birnbaum R, Deshotels J: Has the Academy Adopted TQM? *Planning for Higher Education* 1999: 28; 29–37.

Brue G: *Six Sigma for Managers.* McGraw-Hill, New York, NY, 2005.

Chaffee EE, Sherr LA: *Quality: Transforming Postsecondary Education.* Washington DC, George Washington University, 1992.

Chaffee EE: Assessing Impact: Evidence and Action. Presentations from the AAHE Conference on Assessment & Quality, Miami Beach, FL: 11-15 June 1997.

Covey SR: *Principle-Centered Leadership.* Simon & Schuster, New York, NY, 1992.

Covey SR: *The 8th Habit: From Effectiveness to Greatness.* Simon & Schuster, New York, NY, 2004.

Dewey J: *Problem Solving Tasks (Reflective Problem-Solving) How We Think.* D.C. Heath and Company, Boston, 1933.

Going Lean in Health Care. IHI Innovation Series white paper. Institute for Healthcare Improvement, Cambridge, MA, 2005. www.IHI.org

Grant LF, Kelley JH, Northington L, Barlow D: Using TQM/CQI Processes to Guide Development of Independent and Collaborative Learning in Two Levels of Baccalaureate Nursing Students. *Journal of Nursing Education* 2002: 41; 537–540.

Hammond JS, Keeney RL, Raiffa H: The Hidden Traps in Decision Making. *Clinical Laboratory Management Review* 1999: Jan/Feb; 40.

Helms MM, Williams AB, Nixon JC: TQM Principles and Their Relevance to Higher Education: The Question of Tenure and Post-Tenure Review. *International Journal of Educational Management* 2001: 15; 322-331.

Hersey P, Blanchard K, Johnson D: *Management of Organizational Behavior*, ed 8. Prentice Hall, Englewood Cliffs, NJ, 2000.

Masters RJ, Leiker L: Total Quality Management in Higher Education: Applying Deming's Fourteen Points. *CUPA Journal* 1992: Summer; 27–31.

Munoz MA: Total Quality Management and the Higher Education Environment: Impact on Educational Leadership Theory and Practice. 1999: Eric Document ED462880.

Patterson M, Baker D, Gable C, et al: Faculty Research Productivity in Allied Health

Settings: A TQM Approach. *J Allied Health* 1993: Summer; 249–261.

Reagan LA, Kiemele MJ: *Design for Six Sigma—The Tool Guide for Practitioners*. Air Academy Press, 2008.

Richardson WC: Introduction to the Final Draft Report of the Advisory Panel for Allied Health. *J Allied Health* 1992: Fall; 25–28.

Seymour D, Chaffee EE: TQM for Student Outcomes Assessment. *AGB Reports* 1992: Jan/Feb; 26–30.

Soetaert E: Quality in the Classroom: Classroom Assessment Techniques as TQM. *New Directions for Teaching and Learning* 1998: 75; 47–55.

Streibel BJ, Joiner BL, Scholtes PR: *The Team Handbook*. Joiner/Oriel, Inc., Madison, WI, 2003.

Vazzana G, Elfrink J, Bachmann DP: A Longitudinal Study of Total Quality Management Processes in Business Colleges. *Journal of Education for Business* 2000: 76; 69–74.

Yukl GA: *Leadership in Organizations*. Prentice Hall, Englewood Cliffs, NJ, 2005.

INTERNET RESOURCES

American Productivity & Quality Center
http://www.apqc.org/

Decision Tree
http://www.eskimo.com/~mighetto/lstree.htm

iSix Sigma
http://www.isixsigma.com/

Problem Solving. Free Management Library, Authenticity Consulting, LLC.
http://managementhelp.org/prsn_prd/prob_slv.htm

Problem Solving Techniques, Mind Tools LTD.
http://www.mindtools.com/pages/main/newMN_TMC.htm

Human Resource Management

Managing people is one of the key responsibilities of laboratory managers. The ability to understand and follow human resource guidelines and regulations, as well as to perform job analyses, write job descriptions, and manage work groups, is critical to success. Laboratory managers must also participate in performance evaluation and development issues with their employees. An introduction to the basic aspects of education and training also assists laboratory managers to achieve good human resource skills.

Section II consists of four chapters based on human resource issues. Because of the overlap of select terms and concepts in each of the topics covered, discussions of them occur in multiple chapters, where appropriate.

Section II Contents:

Human Resource Guidelines and Regulations

Christine V. Walters, MAS, JD, SPHR
George M. Chuzi, ESQ

CHAPTER OUTLINE

OBJECTIVES

Following successful completion of this chapter, the learner will be able to:

1. List and define at least two key legal issues and at least one proactive measure an employer may take in the area of recruitment.
2. List and define at least two key legal issues and at least one proactive measure an employer may take in the area of compensation.
3. List and define at least two key legal issues and at least one proactive measure an employer may take in the area of leave benefits.
4. List and define at least two key legal issues and at least one proactive measure an employer may take in the area of employee/labor relations.
5. List and define at least two key legal issues and at least one proactive measure an employer may take in the area of termination.

6. Accurately describe the minimum legal duty imposed on an employer for each of these areas.
7. Compare and contrast various approaches to managing conflicts in each of the areas covered in this chapter.

KEY TERMS

Affirmative Action
Age Discrimination in
  Employment Act of 1967 (ADEA)
Americans with Disabilities Act (ADA)
Bona Fide Occupational
  Qualifications (BFOQ)
Equal Employment Opportunity
  Commission (EEOC)
Equal Pay Act (EPA)

Fair Labor Standards Act of 1938
  (FLSA)
Family and Medical Leave Act of 1993
  (FMLA)
Human Resource Management
  (HRM)
Title VII of the Civil Rights Act of 1964
Unlawful Harassment

INTRODUCTION

Human resource management (HRM) is an element critical to the successful operation of any department in any industry. Managers, directors, and supervisors who are not familiar with the basic elements of HRM, serve as a potential liability for their own organization, rather than an asset, and are likely to find themselves embroiled in costly litigation. This chapter is intended to provide an overview of the fundamental concepts of HRM in five basic areas: recruitment, compensation, leave benefits, employee relations, and termination. Case studies and subsequent discussions are incorporated into this chapter as appropriate to illustrate key points. It is not intended to serve as nor constitute legal advice. Managers should always contact their human resources practitioner, or legal counsel, before making any decision that may adversely affect any employment relationship. Other chapters in Section II of this text will provide readers with more detailed information about these and other areas involved in HRM. This chapter is intended to familiarize those responsible for the supervisory duties within a department or laboratory with the issues that are most frequently problematic to employers.

RECRUITMENT

Success in any business requires success in competition. Thus, every company within various industries strives to recruit and retain the most highly qualified personnel. Companies are constantly challenged to create new and better services, programs, and benefits with which to entice the most qualified candidates to work for their organization. In the excitement of that competitive spirit, however, many managers have not been provided the opportunity to learn the basics of the recruitment process. What questions may properly be asked in an employment interview? What information should be divulged when answering a call for an employment reference? If a candidate for employment discloses the existence of a disability or need for a religious accommodation, how should you respond? Understanding the basic requirements of the recruitment process is key to creating a high quality, stable workforce.

Table 6-1 lists federal laws that most frequently affect the employment relationship, the number of employees an organization must employ before each law is applicable, and some websites of the federal agencies that regulate the particular statute.

Affirmative Action

Executive Order 11246 (Order), entitled "Equal Employment Opportunity," was issued by President Lyndon Johnson on September 24, 1965. This order, generally known as **Affirmative Action**, prohibits federal contractors, subcontractors, and federally assisted construction contractors and subcontractors (contractors), who conduct more than $10,000 in government business in a year, from discriminating in employment decisions on the basis of race, color, religion, sex, or national origin. Certain government contractors or first-tier subcontractors with 50 or more employees and $50,000 or more in government contracts are required to develop and maintain a written affirmative action plan. In November 2000, the Office of Federal Contract Compliance Program, of the Department of Labor, published a rule that clarified that, except in limited circumstances, the contractor must maintain a separate plan for each of its establishments. Contrary to popular belief, affirmative action is not a quota system or a system that gives preference to certain candidates. Affirmative action does require an employer to measure and assess three areas that may be envisioned as concentric circles (Figure 6-1).

For example, an employer is not required to hire a member of a minority group or a female when a more qualified candidate is available. Affirmative action is a commitment by the employer to proactively reach out into various employment pools and continue to seek the most qualified candidate. However, the employer reaches out to a variety of sources, rather than from the same sources they have always used, such as ads in local newspapers, community publications, or recruitment from colleges and universities.

The outermost circle represents the applicant pool, that is, the pool of all qualified candidates in the employer's geographic labor market. This information is available through federal, state, and local departments of labor. The second circle represents the pool of candidates who actually apply for employment with any particular company. Employers obligated to maintain an affirmative action plan must track all applications received, including the race and gender of applicants and the position(s) for which they have applied. Currently

TABLE 6-1. Federal Laws That Most Frequently Affect the Employment Relationship

Federal Law	Covered Employers	Website
Americans with Disabilities Act (ADA), 1990	Employers with 25 or more employees	http://www.eeoc.gov/laws/statutes/ada.cfm
Age Discrimination in Employment Act (ADEA), 1967	Employers with 20 or more employees	http://www.eeoc.gov/laws/statutes/adea.cfm
Civil Rights Act of 1991	Employers with 15 or more employees	http://www.eeoc.gov/laws/statutes/cra-1991.cfm
Drug Free Workplace Act, 1988	Organizations with federal contracts of $100,000 or more and all individual, federal contractors, and grantees	http://www.dol.gov/elaws/drugfree.htm
Equal Pay Act (EPA), 1963	Same as FLSA	http://www.access.gpo.gov/nara/cfr/waisidx_10/29cfr1620_10.html
Executive Order 11246	Certain federal contractors and subcontractors	http://www.dol.gov/ofccp/regs/compliance/ca_11246.htm
Fair Credit Reporting Act	All	http://www.ftc.gov/os/statutes/fcrajump.shtm
Fair Labor Standards Act (FLSA)	Almost all	http://www.dol.gov/whd/flsa/index.htm
Family and Medical Leave Act of 1993 (FMLA)	Employers with 50 or more employees	http://www.dol.gov/whd/fmla/index.htm http://www.dol.gov/whd/fmla/
Revised Final Regulations under the Family and Medical Leave Act		http://www.dol.gov/whd/regs/statutes/fmla.htm http://www.dol.gov/whd/fmla/finalrule.htm
Immigration Reform and Control Act of 1986 (IRCA)	All	http://www.justice.gov/crt/osc/pdf/oscupdate_nov_06.pdf
Occupational Safety and Health Act (OSHA)	Employers with 2 or more employees (exclusive of self-employed)	http://www.osha.gov/
Title VII, Civil Rights Act of 1964	Employers with 15 or more employees	http://www.eeoc.gov/laws/statutes/titlevii.cfm
Uniformed Services Employment and Re-employment Rights Act (USERRA), 1994	All	http://www.dol.gov/compliance/laws/comp-userra.htm

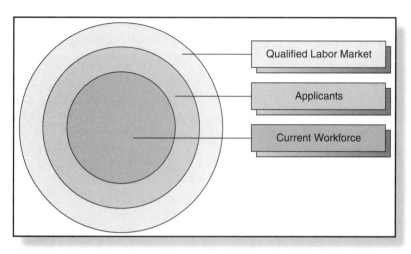

FIGURE 6-1.   Three Areas of Assessment Required by Affirmative Action

this information must be tracked for all applicants, as the employer defines an applicant. In March 2004, a number of federal agencies published proposed regulations that would limit or clarify the definition of an E-applicant, which is one who applies for employment through electronic means such as the internet. The third circle represents the employees who are employed by the company. This data should be tracked through an internal human resources information system (HRIS). If any of the numbers in these three groups are statistically disparate from the general labor market, the employer should audit the company's outreach, recruitment, and hiring practices to ensure those practices are not having an adverse impact on women, minorities, persons with disabilities, or protected veterans.

Many employers maintain voluntary affirmative action plans or programs, even though they are not required to do so under the Order. Affirmative action programs have faced many legal challenges in the last decade. It is currently recommended that voluntary affirmative action programs or plans be implemented only to remedy a history of past discrimination. Programs or plans used as a proactive measure to enhance diversity within an organization have come under legal scrutiny in the last several years.

Position Descriptions

The recruitment process should begin with the writing of the job description. The best job description lists the *essential functions* of the job, defined as those that are most important and/or performed with the greatest frequency of all required tasks within a job. The job description should also include a listing of the requirements with regard to education and experience. Although an employer may want or prefer candidates with a college degree for a particular position, it is important to list only those factors that are **bona fide occupational qualifications (BFOQ)**. Ordinarily, an employer may not limit employment in a particular job to persons of a particular sex, religion, or national origin unless the employer can show that sex, religion, or national origin is an actual qualification for performing the job. This principle will result in scrutiny if a particular qualification is not necessary for a position, but screens from consideration a large number of applicants from an under-represented group. For example, although a clinical laboratory scientist may need a specialized degree or training to conduct certain laboratory tests, it is likely that comparable education (although helpful) is *not* required for a person to successfully perform the duties of a laboratory assistant. However, the use of this criterion may eliminate members of a protected class from consideration. A sample job description is provided in Table 6-2.

After the job description is completed, the employer will need to attach an appropriate pay or salary range to that job. It is generally the duty of the human resources department to conduct market surveys and ensure their compensation structure is both internally equitable as well as market competitive. Maintaining internal equity requires comparing the current wages paid to each person currently employed within a particular job classification with regard to a number of factors such as each incumbent's level of education, years of experience in the field, and years of experience in the job with that employer. Hiring a new candidate at a rate of pay higher than current incumbents with comparable education and experience in the field, may require an upward wage adjustment for every other worker in that job classification. If these wage adjustments are given, it can be very costly to the employer, and must be weighed against the return on the investment of bringing in the new candidate. If the candidate is hired at the higher rate, and no adjustment is made, the likely result is not just a reduction in employee morale and resentment toward the new worker, but also potential claims of wage discrimination. Additional information on and samples of job/position descriptions are located in Chapter 7.

Equal Pay Act (EPA)

The **Equal Pay Act (EPA)**, which is part of the Fair Labor Standards Act of 1938 and is administered and enforced by the EEOC, prohibits wage discrimination between men and women in the same establishment who are performing similar work under similar working conditions. For example, imagine that a healthcare clinic has just opened a new cancer research center. The market is competitive in this area, and the clinic finds that it cannot hire a highly qualified clinical laboratory scientist for less than $25.00 per hour. Several candidates apply and a male is selected and paid the appropriate rate. In the Department of Histology, however, a female scientist is paid only $20.00 an hour. The work the two scientists perform is similar as are their working conditions. In this case, while there is clearly a difference between the wage being paid to the male and female scientists, it most likely would not be a violation of the EPA, as the higher rate is (1) driven by the market demand based on

TABLE 6-2.   Sample Job Description

Position Title: Laboratory Technician

Job Group: Laboratory-Technical   Pay Grade: _____ Position Number: _____

Summary of Duties

Following routine protocols under the close supervision of a faculty investigator or a senior technician, performs laboratory tests utilizing requisite laboratory equipment and instruments, making minor adjustments as required. Typically works with biohazardous and/or radioactive materials. Responsible for laboratory maintenance, preparing solutions and media, and ordering supplies. May be responsible for care of laboratory animals.

Essential Job Functions

- Performs laboratory tests and/or experiments that may include various assays and specialized techniques, following established procedures or protocols.
- Operates required laboratory equipment and instruments, records data, performs quality control and equipment maintenance.
- Uses universal safety precautions to protect self and co-workers from biohazardous materials, including blood-borne pathogens.
- Complies with biohazard/radiation safety standards through the proper handling of potentially hazardous chemical and biological agents, and/or radiation sources in the workplace.
- Completes annual university biohazard/universal precaution/radiation safety training, as appropriate.
- Prepares sterile media such as agar in plates, jars, or test tubes for use in growing bacterial cultures.
- Prepares solutions, reagents, and stains following standard laboratory formulas and procedures.
- Uses sterile techniques to avoid contaminating laboratory experiments.
- Prepares, cleans, sterilizes, and maintains laboratory equipment, glassware, and instruments used in research experiments.
- Monitors inventory levels, orders materials and supplies in accordance with established policies and procedures, counts orders on receipt.

Scope of Responsibility

Knows the informal policies, procedures, and practices necessary to conduct the normal function of a specific section, unit, or work area. Is aware of the role of the position and its potential impact on the working unit.

Decision Making

Carries out duties and responsibilities with limited supervision. Makes decisions and establishes work priorities on essentially procedure-oriented operations.

Authority

Does not direct the activities of staff or a function.

Communication

Exchanges routine information in an appropriate manner requiring good oral and written communication skills.

(Continued)

TABLE 6-2.   Sample Job Description (*Continued*)

Education

Associate degree in medical laboratory science or a laboratory science from an accredited institution.

Experience

Gained through college level classwork in the sciences or summer employment. Biological science coursework or experience in a biological laboratory is preferred.

Certification

MLT(ASCP) or equivalent.

Physical Requirements

- Work produced is subject to precise measures of quantity and quality
- Work environment may include areas of unpleasant extremes of cold or heat
- Biohazardous conditions such as the risk of radiation exposure, fumes or airborne particles, and/or toxic or caustic chemicals may be present in this work environment, which mandates attention to safety considerations
- Near vision to see objects clearly within 20 inches
- Sharp focus to adjust vision when doing close work that changes in distance from eyes
- Full spectrum vision to identify and distinguish color
- Finger dexterity required to manipulate objects with fingers rather than with whole hand(s) or arm(s), for example, using a keyboard
- Handling by seizing, holding, grasping, turning or otherwise working with the hand or hands, but without finger dexterity
- Sitting in a normal seated position for extended periods
- Occasionally lifting, carrying objects weighing 10 lb or less
- Occasionally pushing, pulling objects weighing 30 lb or less
- Ability to move about

the area of research and (2) would be paid to any incumbent in the cancer research laboratory, male or female. If, however, market data did not support that the higher rate was required or competitive in the area of cancer research, or if it was discovered that female scientists in the new cancer research center were paid less than $25.00 per hour, the employer may be found guilty of wage discrimination and violation of the EPA. It is also important to remember that wage discrimination is blind to gender. A male employee may bring charges of wage discrimination just as well as a female. A male scientist working in a predominantly female work environment, should not receive a lower wage than his female counterparts, just because he is more easily recruited. This description is a general statement of required major duties and responsibilities performed on a regular and continuous basis. It does not exclude other duties as assigned.

Interviewing

One of the greatest pitfalls in recruitment is interviewing. Human resource professionals are usually trained in current employment practices, such as

TABLE 6-3.   Questions to Avoid During the Interview Process

What is your date of birth?
When did you graduate from high school?
Are you married?
How many days did you miss from work last year?
Are you currently taking any prescription medication?
Do you currently have, or do you have any history of a disability?
What is your country of national origin?
Are you a U.S. citizen?
Have you ever been arrested?
Have you ever filed a claim for workers' compensation?

how to develop interviewing questionnaires and templates, and what questions are not appropriate to ask during interviews. Front line supervisors and managers, however, do not receive this training very often. As a result, supervisors and managers unintentionally may ask questions that are at best offensive and at worst unlawful. Table 6-3 lists questions that should be avoided during the interview process and removed from job applications. Keep in mind that many states and local jurisdictions provide legal protections for members of certain classes that go beyond those provided by federal law, such as marital status or sexual orientation.

The Americans with Disabilities Act will be discussed in more detail later; but it is worth noting here that an employer has a duty to provide a reasonable accommodation for a job applicant as well as employees who have a disability. For example, some companies have a rule that all applications for employment are to be completed in the human resources department. An employer may have to grant an exception to that rule as a reasonable accommodation for a candidate with a visual impairment who arrives in the human resource office and asks to take the application home to use a reading device to complete the application. Learners are encouraged to read Chapters 7 and 8 for more information on conducting job analyses and interviews, as well as related issues of evaluating an employee's performance of assigned duties and responsibilities.

COMPENSATION

Fair Labor Standards Act (FLSA)

The **Fair Labor Standards Act of 1938 (FLSA)** is the federal law that defines the minimum wage, overtime, and other requirements related to how certain employees are to be paid. The term *nonexempt* refers to employees who are to be paid for every hour in which the employee performs work for, or is under the control of, the employer. With few exceptions, the FLSA also requires that nonexempt employees receive wages at the rate of 1.5 times the employee's regular rate of pay for any hours worked beyond 40 hours in one work week. Note that there are limited exceptions for companies in some industries, such as health care, that have established an 80-hour work week. These situations should be evaluated on a case-by-case basis as well as in conjunction with state laws that may impose greater requirements. This law can be quite complex and its interpretation convoluted, but if a supervisor follows a few basic rules, complications should be easily avoided.

Some employees are exempt from the provisions of the FLSA and are therefore, considered, "exempt" employees. Generally, these employees are classified as executive, administrative, or professional. A number of parameters must be used in determining whether any particular job should be classified as exempt or nonexempt. Because these exemptions are narrowly defined, employers should carefully check the exact terms and conditions for classification and work in conjunction with the company's human resources department and compensation experts to ensure proper classification.

Improperly classifying a nonexempt employee as exempt, as well as any other violation of the FLSA, can have serious financial consequences as a result of fines or penalties imposed by the Department of Labor. These fines may be imposed against an individual supervisor as well as the company, in amounts up to $10,000, in addition to civil money penalties plus damages for back pay, liquidated damages, and more.

Many companies have rules that overtime must be approved in advance of being worked. What if the employee is very dedicated to the job and chooses to come in early, performs work, and tells the supervisor that the company need not pay the employee for this extra time because the employee understands that permission was not granted in advance? Does the employer have to pay the employee for the extra time worked? What if an employee continues to work through his or her lunch period to catch up on some work? Does the employer have to pay the employee for what would otherwise be an unpaid lunch period? The answer is, "yes," in both cases. Even if the work is performed without the permission or knowledge of the employer, the employee is still due appropriate compensation. The employer may, however, limit the compensation that is due under the FLSA by granting the nonexempt employee some time off later in the same work week to avoid incurring hours worked in excess of 40 in that work week.

Employers may also fail to properly pay nonexempt employees when an employee is on the employer's premises during his or her scheduled shift but not performing work.

The intent of the FLSA, as drafted more than 65 years ago, was to provide compensation for an employee who performs work or remains under the employer's control. Thus, in the first and third scenarios the answer is "No." The employer is obligated to compensate employees only for the time they performed work in the laboratory, not for the time spent eating breakfast or parking the car. Keep an eye out for the common practice of nonexempt employees who eat lunch at their desk while working. If a nonexempt employee is not relieved of his or her duties during a scheduled, unpaid meal period, then the employer owes that employee compensation for the time worked, even if while

> ## Case Study
>
> ## Three Scenarios Involving Compensation
>
> *An employee in Laboratory A is scheduled to work from 8:00 AM to 4:30 PM, with one break for lunch from 12:00 to 1:00 PM. The employee accurately records her arrival at work at 8:00 AM. The employee then walks to the company's cafe, gets breakfast, and returns 15 minutes later and begins working. Is the employer obligated to pay the employee for the period covered from 8:00 AM to 8:15 AM?*
>
> *An employee arrives to work at 8:00 AM and is scheduled to conduct blood specimen testing. The equipment, however, is not working and cannot be repaired until at least 9:30 AM. In the interim, the supervisor instructs the employee to stay in the department until the repair specialist arrives. While waiting, the employee does some studying for a course he is taking at the local community college. Is the employer obligated to pay the employee for the time the employee studies?*
>
> *An employee drives into the employer's parking lot at 7:58 AM. He is scheduled to work from 8:00 AM to 4:30 PM. To avoid recording a late time of arrival for work, the employee parks his car outside the door, walks into his department, and records an 8:00 AM arrival time and then leaves to park his car, returning to the department at 8:10 AM. Is the employer obligated to pay for the period from 8:00 AM to 8:10 AM?*

simultaneously eating lunch. In the second scenario, even though no work was performed, the reason for the work stopping was beyond the employee's control. In addition, he remained under the control of the employer until the equipment was repaired. As a result, the employer may be obligated to pay that employee for that idle time. A proactive manager will find other work an employee may perform during down time.

Another common practice in which many employers engage is the granting of compensatory time off from work for nonexempt employees in lieu of overtime wages. At this time, the FLSA generally prohibits private (nongovernmental) employers from granting nonexempt employees compensatory time off from work. For example, imagine that you have a research grant due this Friday. You need your laboratory assistant to work some overtime to help get some last minute administrative details put together. When you convey this news to the employee, he says that would be fine because he would also like to take off early one day next week to take care of some personal business. If you and the employee both agree to this arrangement, can you grant the employee the compensatory time off from work next week in exchange for the additional hours worked this week? The answer is "No." To do so would be a violation of the FLSA. Note that legislation has been proposed for a number of years to permit this type of voluntary arrangement if the employer and employee both agree. As of this writing, those efforts have been unsuccessful.

Compensatory time off from work is also a strategy that employers use with exempt employees with the intent of enhancing the flexibility of work schedules. The new federal regulations that became effective in August 2004, expressly permit the additional payment so long as the exempt employee is still paid the required minimum salary on a salary basis.

All of your employees are compensated for their services. There are two aspects of compensation with which employers should be concerned: 1) that employees performing substantially similar duties are compensated substantially equally; and 2) that the employer complies with applicable laws regulating minimum wages, overtime, and the like. The Equal Pay Act, which specifically prohibits paying men and women differently for the performance of substantially similar work under similar working conditions, has been previously addressed.

In addition, the other discrimination statutes, including Title VII of the Civil Rights Act; the Americans with Disabilities Act; and the Age Discrimination in Employment Act, also prohibit disparate compensation on the basis of age, disability, gender, etc. Significantly, the Lily Ledbetter Fair Pay Act was signed into law in January 2009. As the result employees complaining of compensation discrimination under Title VII, the ADA, and the ADEA may file a charge with the EEOC counting from the date they received their last discriminatory paycheck. The Act reverses a Supreme Court decision which held the employees had to count from the date they received their first discriminatory paycheck.

LEAVE BENEFITS

While the overall administrative oversight of leave benefits (e.g., sick leave, vacation, personal, military) is generally regulated by the human resources department, problems most frequently arise at the departmental level when a request for some form of leave is initially denied, or misapplied by a manager or supervisor. For the purpose of this discussion, the leave benefits covered are presented under two categories: the Family and Medical Leave Act, and the Military and Other Leave.

Family and Medical Leave Act (FMLA)

The **Family and Medical Leave Act of 1993 (FMLA)** provides eligible employees with up to 12 weeks of leave (paid or unpaid) for the employee's own serious health condition, for the care of an immediate family member who has a serious health condition (spouse, child, parent), and for the care of the employee's child following birth or adoption. The FMLA is applicable to any employer in the private sector who is engaged in commerce or in any industry or activity affecting commerce, and who has 50 or more employees each working day during at least 20 calendar weeks or more in the current or preceding calendar year. In addition, all public agencies (state and local government) and local education agencies (schools) are covered. These employers do not need to meet the 50-employee requirement. The FMLA guarantees the employee the right to return to the same or comparable position he had when the leave commenced, upon his or her return to work. A comparable position is one that provides the employee with the same wages, hours, and conditions of employment as the position originally held.

An eligible employee is one who has worked for the employer for at least 12 months (not necessarily consecutively) and at least 1,250 hours in the last 12 months. The employee must work at a worksite with at least 50 employees employed within 75 miles of that site. Although there is more than one definition of what conditions constitute a serious health condition, and they are quite detailed, the general definitions are those conditions that require inpatient care or continuing treatment by a health care provider. The nuances of administrating leave under the FMLA are very broad and easily warrant a chapter unto themselves. Here, we cover those areas of the FMLA that most often result in misinterpretation or misapplication.

Highly anticipated changes to the FMLA took effect on January 16, 2009. These changes involve, among other rules, a clarification of the definitions of "serious health condition" and an improvement in communications between employees, employers, and health care providers to help the law operate more smoothly. Employers must abide by and post the updated FLMA in order to avoid fines for non-compliance.

The U.S. Department of Labor administers the FMLA and has published interpretive guidelines that require an employer to give an employee notice that an absence is being counted towards FML within at least two business days of learning that the employee may have a qualifying event under the Act. In this case, the employer learned this on the first Tuesday, the employee's second day of absence from work. What happens if the employer knew that the leave may have qualified under FMLA, failed to give the employee proper notice, and the employee has returned to work? The leave may be designated retroactively but some penalty may apply, so held the U.S. Supreme Court in March 2002.

It is also important to note that while the FMLA provides employees the right to unpaid leave, the employer is permitted to run paid leave benefits, such as sick leave, vacation pay, workers' compensation, and other benefits concurrently with FMLA. This is a sound business practice to prevent employees from taking up to 12 weeks of unpaid leave and returning to work with full, paid leave banks.

Military and Other Leave

Employers have certain duties to provide some limited benefits and protections to employees who take time off from work to perform a variety of social obligations, such as those required for military service, including weekend reservists units. Separate federal laws cover nearly all employers, including federal contractors. The law provides employees and candidates with certain rights to be free from discrimination based on their military obligations, including a conditional right

Case Study   Leave Benefits

An employee calls in on Monday and tells you that he will be absent that day. On Tuesday, the employee calls in again and tells you that he is very sick and will be out for at least three more days, if not the entire week. The following Monday, you have not heard back from the employee so you call him at home. He says that he saw a physician on Friday afternoon and has been conditionally diagnosed with pneumonia, is scheduled for diagnostic testing, and will be out, at least until the test results come back at the end of the week. The following Monday, following a two-week absence, the employee returns to work. What should you do? What portion of the absence, if any, may be applied to FMLA?

to return to the same or a comparable position when they return from military service, as granted under the *Uniformed Services Employment and Reemployment Rights Act (USERRA)*.

Employers should also become familiar with the laws in their state and local jurisdictions. Many provide further protections for employees taking leave to vote, respond to a subpoena for jury duty, or to serve as a witness at a trial. For example, Maryland law requires employers to grant employees at least two consecutive hours off from work while the polls are open to vote on Election Day.

The FMLA updates that went into effect on January 16, 2009, implemented statutory amendments that allow eligible employees to take up to 26 weeks of unpaid leave to care for a family member who was wounded while on active duty. Eligible employees are also entitled up to 12 weeks of unpaid leave for "qualifying exigencies," to help manage the affairs of a soldier, of the soldier's family before, during, and after deployment.

EMPLOYEE RELATIONS

The arena of employment legislation and litigation is replete with challenges to employers' practices relating to a myriad of issues under the law. Federal, state, and local administrative agencies such as the **Equal Employment Opportunity Commission (EEOC)** and its counterparts are continually challenged to meet the demands of burgeoning case loads alleging discrimination in employment based on a person's membership in a legally protected class. Although the 1990s brought the enactment of several pieces of federal legislation imposing additional duties on employers, Title VII remains the most commonly cited law under which persons file charges with the EEOC. During fiscal year 2004, Title VII charges accounted for the greatest percentage of charges received by the EEOC, as compared to any other single statute.

Title VII of the Civil Rights Act of 1964

Title VII of the Civil Rights Act of 1964 prohibits discrimination based on race, color, creed, religion, national origin, and sex. Keep in mind that a plaintiff may file a claim of discrimination alleging discrimination under more than one federal statute as well as more than one protected class. The burden of proof in such cases rests first with the person bringing the charge to show that: (1) he belongs to a protected class; (2) he was qualified for a job; (3) though qualified, some adverse employment action was taken against him (fired, not hired, demoted, etc.); and (4) thereafter the employer continued to seek applicants with the plaintiff's qualifications. If the plaintiff is able to establish each of these threshold elements, the burden then shifts to the employer to show a legitimate, nondiscriminatory reason for taking the adverse employment action. If the employer can do so, then the plaintiff is afforded one more opportunity to show that the reason given by the employer is a pretext and not the real reason for the decision. On June 12, 2000, the Supreme Court held that a plaintiff was not required to provide any evidence that the real reason for the adverse action was based on some unlawful, discriminatory intent, but only that the reason given by the employer was not true. The Court held that so long as the plaintiff was able to rebut the reason the employer gave as pretextual, then it may be appropriate for a jury to infer that the employer's motive was unlawful discrimination.

Would the laboratory be able to lawfully advertise for only female applicants for this position to monitor female donors? The answer is "Yes." When the work being performed may be reasonably perceived as private or personal in nature (security guards conducting searches of persons, video monitors in department store dressing rooms), then gender may be considered a BFOQ. It is important to note, however, that the courts have held that race may never be used as a BFOQ.

Unlawful Harassment

No issue under Title VII has received more attention over the last decade than issues related to unlawful harassment. From 1986 to 1993, the Supreme Court heard two landmark cases that laid the foundation for sexual harassment litigation under Title VII. From March 1998 to May 1998, however, the Court heard three cases (plus two under another federal statute) that further refined the definition and liability standards for unlawful harassment. The EEOC then followed suit and published new guidelines in June 1999, stating that **unlawful harassment** includes behaviors "based on race, color, sex (whether or not of a sexual nature), religion, national origin, protected activity, age, or disability. Thus, employers should establish anti-harassment policies and complaint procedures covering *all* forms of unlawful harassment."

Case Study

Employee Relations—Civil Rights

A private laboratory has contracts with several companies to conduct "for cause" testing of employees whom the employer suspects have reported to work under the influence of drugs or alcohol. To ensure the donor does not tamper with the urine sample, employees must be monitored when giving a sample. The laboratory has a technician who currently conducts these tests. They have run into a problem, however, the clinical laboratory technician is male. Although employees sent for testing are permitted to give a urine specimen behind a curtain, many female employees refuse to do so with the male laboratory technician in the room. On these occasions, the laboratory has to call a female laboratory technician from another area to oversee the specimen collection process.

Both the definition and liability standards for employers have changed a great deal. As a result of these decisions, it is important for managers and supervisors to understand the new duties and responsibilities that have been imposed on employers.

The Supreme Court has declared that the distinction between the former classifications of *quid pro quo* sexual harassment and hostile environment claims is of "limited utility." In cases in which an employee alleges a personnel action resulting in some tangible economic harm (e.g., lost job, demotion, reduction of overtime or compensation), the employer may be held liable or strictly liable, meaning the employer will have no opportunity to put forward a defense. Only in the case of an allegation of harassment with no tangible economic harm may the employer be permitted to put forward an affirmative defense. That affirmative defense is basically a three-prong defense that requires the employer to show: (1) that the employer took reasonable care to prevent the harassment from occurring, (2) that the employer took reasonable care to promptly correct the harassment, and (3) the employee unreasonably failed to pursue these preventive or corrective measures or otherwise avoid harm. If the employer can meet all three elements, the company may escape liability for a claim of unlawful harassment. As a result, it is imperative that employers provide and document thorough training for managers and employees on unlawful harassment prevention, multiple resources for reporting complaints, and respond promptly to any questions, concerns, or complaints related to unlawful harassment.

In addition, the demographic landscape of harassment claims has changed quite dramatically after 9/11. In the year following the 9/11 attacks, the percentage increase in the number of claims of religious discrimination and harassment that were filed with the U.S. Equal Employment Opportunity Commission (EEOC) were more than double the preceding year. From 2000 to 2001, claims increased about 9.7%; from 2001–2002 the same claims increased at a rate of nearly 21%. They became so prevalent the EEOC named them "Post-9/11" and/or "Backlash" cases. Thus, employers are wise to follow the EEOC's guidance and develop policies and training programs that prohibit all forms of unlawful harassment, not just sexual.

Age Discrimination in Employment Act (ADEA)

The **Age Discrimination in Employment Act (ADEA)**, passed in 1967, prohibits discrimination against any person 40 years old or older. Clinical laboratory managers and supervisors should also note that courts have held that even if both persons are 40 years old or older (a candidate not hired and the candidate hired, for example) the employer may still be guilty of age discrimination by not hiring the older worker. For example, if there are two applicants for a position, one is 42 years old and the other is 52, the 52-year-old candidate may have a *prima facie* case of age discrimination if she can present some evidence that the employer did not hire her because she was older than the other candidate, even though the other candidate was also over 40 years old.

It is important to check with your human resources department or legal counsel, as many states also have laws that prohibit discrimination against persons of any age, including those less than 40 years old.

Americans with Disabilities Act (ADA)

The **Americans with Disabilities Act (ADA)** was passed in 1990 and prohibits discrimination based on a number of classifications of disabilities: a person who presently has a disability, has a past history of a disability, is perceived to have a disability, or associates with a person who has a disability. The Act defines a disability as any physical or mental impairment that substantially limits a major life activity. Major life activities originally were defined as, among other things, walking, talking, maintaining active employment, and conducting daily hygiene. Effective January 1, 2009, however, Congress amended the definition of "major life activities" and it now includes major bodily functions such as, "functions of the immune system, normal cell growth, digestive, bowel, bladder, neurological, brain, respiratory, circulatory, endocrine, and reproductive functions." The Act requires an employer to provide a qualified candidate or employee with a *reasonable accommodation*. A qualified candidate or employee is one who is qualified to perform the essential functions of the job with or without a reasonable accommodation. The employer does not, however, have to provide the candidate or employee with the best accommodation, or one preferred by the candidate or employee.

Can the supervisor transfer the employee to work in Laboratory B part-time and hire a full-time replacement, at least temporarily? The answer is most likely, "Yes." The scenario actually involves the potential application of two federal laws.

Case Study I — Employee Relations—ADA

A clinical laboratory has a vacancy for a medical transcriptionist. The job requires candidates to be able to type at least 60 words per minute with an error rate of no more than 5%. Candidate A has more than 10 years in medical transcription, types 65 words per minute with a 2% error rate. She also has a very strong work record; however, she has been diagnosed with strong indications of carpel tunnel syndrome in her right wrist. To limit the tingling sensation and pain she occasionally experiences, she wears a wrist brace that extends over the lower portion of her hand on both sides and is visible even when she wears long sleeves. Candidate A applies in person for the job. She completes the application and takes a typing test. Impressed with her application, resume, and score on the typing test, the recruiter offers to immediately interview Candidate A for the position. One week later, Candidate A calls the employer to determine her status for employment. The recruiter tells her that, although she was highly qualified for the position, another candidate, whose qualifications were equally impressive, was selected. Candidate A has now filed a charge of discrimination with the EEOC alleging discrimination based on both perceived and present disability. Assuming Candidate A did have qualifications equal to those of the person hired for the job, did the employer discriminate against Candidate A based on a real or perceived disability?

If the employee is eligible for Family and Medical Leave (FML), that law permits an employer to at least temporarily transfer an employee to another, comparable position, while taking intermittent FML. Under the ADA, the employer would also be providing the employee with a reasonable accommodation, assuming the condition qualifies as a disability under the ADA, although not the accommodation preferred by the employee. Note, however, if the employee requested a transfer to Laboratory B as a reasonable accommodation for a disability, the employer may be required to grant the request, even if a more qualified candidate is available for the job. In addition, keep in mind that if using the remedial device, such as medication, results in some other condition that substantially limit a major life activity, such as an inability to stay awake at work, then the employee may fall back under the purview and protection of the ADA.

Is a person with a disability (high blood pressure or poor eyesight) who is no longer substantially limited in a major life activity when he uses a remedial device (medication or contact lenses), still covered under the ADA? While the Supreme Court earlier held that certain disabilities would not be covered by the ADA if they could be corrected with a remedial device, that is no longer the case. In the 2009 Amendments to the ADA, Congress stated that corrective measures other than

---

Case Study II — Employee Relations—ADA

A laboratory's busiest day is Monday. An employee tells his supervisor that he is currently undergoing medical treatment for a serious health condition. The treatment includes dialysis, which can only be conducted on Mondays, and will require him to be absent from work for the entire day. The employee is asking to have his job reduced to a part-time position, Tuesday through Friday, at least until the treatment is completed. At this time, his doctor projects the treatments will continue for at least 12 weeks. The supervisor knows that he cannot properly run the laboratory with one fewer person every Monday. Laboratory testing and results will be delayed, affecting patient care. The supervisor also knows there is a vacant position in Laboratory B that can accommodate the employee's request. Transferring the employee to Laboratory B would enable the supervisor to hire at least a temporary, full-time replacement.

"ordinary eyeglasses or contact lenses" shall not be considered when determining whether an individual has a disability.

TERMINATION

A common basis of the employment relationships is the **at-will employment doctrine**. This doctrine maintains that the employment relationship is terminable at the will of either party. An employee may leave his or her job, at any time, for any reason. Likewise, an employer may terminate the employment relationship at any time for any reason, including no reason. The limitation is that an employer may not terminate the employment relationship for an unlawful (discriminatory) reason.

Often, however, employers limit this relationship either intentionally through the use of written employment contracts, or unintentionally, through the creation of employment policies, practices, or statements inadvertently made during the interview process; which are later, construed to create an employment contract.

All policies, procedures, and handbooks should be reviewed and approved by your human resources department and general counsel, before being published and distributed to employees or candidates for employment.

When it comes to terminating the employment relationship, a myriad of claims can arise including invasion of privacy, breach of contract, wrongful discharge, and more. Here are five tips to follow. Each tip addresses one of five elements, often referred to as the elements of **just cause**. Although they are not generally required without a collective bargaining (union) agreement or other written contract, they serve as a reasonable foundation by which to assess the thoroughness of your reasons for discharging any employee.

1. Forewarning: Can you show that the employee in question has received some notice, either through instruction, coaching, a policy manual, or training, regarding the standard or expectation that he has failed to meet? Is this an assumption on your part, or do you have documentation to show that the employee received such notice?

2. Proper investigation: Have you spoken to all parties who can reasonably be expected to have knowledge regarding the information that has led to your decision to discharge? Most important, have you spoken to the employee to get his or her side of the story? Even if you believe there is no reasonable explanation the employee could provide, it is still imperative to give the employee that opportunity to present his or her case.

3. Evidence: Can you show that the information on which you are basing your decision to terminate is factual and not just perception or hearsay? Are there records to support your findings? If there are no tangible records, are there witnesses who are willing to give either a verbal or a written statement supporting your decision? Are these witnesses credible?

4. Lack of discrimination: An employer should determine whether any single decision to discharge is consistent with comparable scenarios and past practice. If another employee engaged in the same wrongful conduct in another department and was *not* discharged, the employer should be able to justify why discharge may be appropriate in one department and not another. For example, lateness or absenteeism may be a much more serious offense in a critical care unit, owing to the potential, negative impact to patient care than it would in the office of volunteer services or gift shop.

5. Penalty meets the offense: Better known as "the punishment fits the crime," it is important to assess whether the employee's behavior is salvageable and might be corrected with a lesser penalty. Discharge is often perceived by arbitrators and courts as economic capital punishment and a measure of last resort. If it is reasonable that the employee might modify his or her behavior with a disciplinary suspension, consider that in lieu of discharge. Very serious or repeated infractions, however, deserve concomitant sanctions.

Managers should also become familiar with the basics of labor law and employees' rights under the National Labor Relations Act. One example was recently illustrated by a decision of the National Labor Relations Board in July 2000. This decision held that if a manager or supervisor interviews an employee as part of an investigation that may lead to disciplinary action of the employee being interviewed, and the employee states that he or she does not want to meet with the management without a representative, the manager must grant the employee's request before continuing with the interview.

REPRISAL/RETALIATION

Managers and supervisors must understand that employees have a virtually unfettered right to claim discrimination, and therefore a violation of that right can lead to liability even if the claim has no merit. Specifically, the EEOC has issued guidance instructing employers that they may not fire, demote, harass or engage in any other reprisal against an individual for filing a charge of discrimination, participating in a discrimination proceeding or investigation, or opposing discrimination. This prohibition against reprisal arises under the same laws that prohibit discrimination on any basis, including race, religion, gender, age, and disability.

Particularly under Title VII (race, color, gender, national origin, and religion), there is a broad definition of the kinds of personnel actions which are considered retaliatory. The Supreme Court has recently held that retaliation can take the form not only of suspension, demotion, or termination, but can be any action by the employer that is likely to deter another individual from claiming or participating in a proceeding involving discrimination. Such actions can include less attractive assignments, involuntary shift changes, and similar actions.

Managers or supervisors naturally may be angered and disappointed to learn that he or she has been accused of discrimination. Nevertheless, these officials must be trained to accept such accusations as part of the job and to avoid treating the complaining employees differently because of the charges. At the same time, employees cannot—and cannot expect to—use the prohibition of reprisal as a shield to engage in conduct that is otherwise subject to discipline.

SUMMARY

The employment relationship can be as rewarding as it is fraught with pitfalls for liability. It has been the goal of this chapter to provide clinical laboratory managers and supervisors with some of the basics of the employment relationship. This knowledge will help them proactively identify issues in the workplace that have the potential to disrupt business operations, and begin generating alternatives for avoiding a problem, rather than trying to negotiate the settlement of a problem after it has arisen.

The best manager and administrator need not be an expert in any of these areas but should be familiar with the basic concepts. They are then able to serve as a resource to the organization in seeking more information and asking questions before making any decision that affects any employee in the organization.

SUMMARY CHART:
Important Points to Remember

➤ The Equal Employment Opportunity Law of 1965 prohibits federal contractors from discriminating in employment decisions on the basis of race, color, religions, sex, or national origin.

➤ Affirmative Action is a commitment by the employer to proactively reach out into various employment pools to find the most qualified candidate.

➤ Three Areas of Assessment Required by Affirmative Action:

1. Qualified Labor Market—Applicant pool of all qualified candidates in the employer's geographical area.

2. Applicants—Pool of candidates who actually apply for employment with any particular company.

3. Current Workforce—Employees who are employed by the company.

➤ Employers obligated to maintain an Affirmative Action Plan must track all applications received for race, gender, national origin, and position for which they have applied.

➤ The Fair Labor Standards Act of 1938 (FLSA) is a federal law which defines the minimum wage, overtime, and other requirements related to how certain employees are paid.

➤ Part of the Fair Labor Standards Act of 1938, enforced by the EEOC, prohibits wage discrimination between men and women working in the same establishment who are performing similar work under similar working conditions.

➤ The Family and Medical Leave Act of 1993 (FMLA) provides eligible employees with up to 12 weeks of job-protected leave (paid or unpaid) for the employee's own serious health condition, for the care of an immediate family member's serious health condition (spouse, child, parent), and for the care of a child following birth or adoption.

➤ In the private sector, the FMLA applies to employers engaged in commerce or industry, and fifty or more employees working at least 20 calendar weeks or more in the current or preceding calendar year.

➤ FMLA provides the right to return to the same or comparable position the person would have had, had he/she not taken leave, upon his/her return to work.

➤ FMLA Eligibility—an eligible employee is one who has worked for the employer for at least 12 months (do not have to be consequently), and at least 1250 hours in the last 12 months. The employees must work at the worksite with at least 50 employees employed within 75 miles of that site.

➤ Taking effect January 17, 2009 the FMLA statue entitles eligible employees up to 26 weeks of unpaid leave to care for a family member who was wounded while serving in the military. Eligible employees are entitled to take up to 12 weeks of unpaid leave for "qualifying emergencies" to help manage the affairs of a soldier or the soldier's family before, during and after deployment.

➤ Title VII of the Civil Rights Act of 1964 prohibits discrimination based on race, color, creed, religion, national origin, and sex.

➤ The Age Discrimination in Employment Act (ADEA), passed in 1967, prohibits discrimination against any person 40 years or older.

➤ The Americans with Disabilities Act (ADA), passed in 1990 and applying to businesses with 15 or more employees, prohibits discrimination to qualified individuals based on a number of classifications:

1. A person who presently has a disability,
2. A person with a past history of a disability,
3. A person who is perceived to have a disability,
4. A person who affiliates with a person who has a disability.

SUGGESTED PROBLEM-BASED LEARNING ACTIVITIES

Chapter 6: Human Resource Guidelines and Regulations

Instructions: Use Internet resources, books, articles, colleagues, etc., to present solutions to the problems listed below. There is no one correct solution to any problem.

Note to Instructor: Students in class may be divided into groups and given the problem-based learning activity to discuss and solve. Once the group has reached a consensus as to a solution, the group may present it to the other students in the class. This activity will provide all students with information regarding solutions to the problem.

Problem # I

Suppose your department has shown a 25% turnover rate. As manager, you must develop a plan to encourage employee retention. In your plan, identify factors associated with excessive turnover.

Problem #2

Identify and define motivational techniques used in your institution to foster effective team interaction.

Problem #3

Suppose you are a laboratory manager and have an employee who is habitually late to work. Develop an action plan to remedy this behavior.

BIBLIOGRAPHY

Fisher & Phillips LLP. *Meet the New ADA: Massive Changes Ahead for Nation's Employers.* 18 Sept. 2008. http://www.laborlawyers.com/shownews.aspx?Show=10879&Type=1122

Thompson Hine LLP. *Employment @lert: New FMLA Regulations Require Major Changes to Existing Policies.* 17 Nov. 2008. http://www.thompsonhine.com/publications/publication1605.html

United States Department of Labor: Wage and Hour Division (WHD). *Revised Final Regulations Under the Family and Medical Leave Act (RIN1215-AB35).* http://www.dol.gov/whd/fmla/finalrule.htm

United States Equal Employment Opportunity Commission: *Notice Concerning the Americans With Disabilities Act (ADA) Amendments Act of 2008.* http://www.eeoc.gov/laws/statutes/adaaa_notice.cfm

INTERNET RESOURCES

Department of Labor: OSDBU's Small Business Resource Center. http://www.dol.gov/oasam/programs/osdbu/sbrefa/

elaws: employment laws assistance for workers & small businesses. United States Department of Labor. http://www.dol.gov/elaws/

Equal Employment Opportunity Commission (EEOC): Charge Statistics FY 1997 Through FY 2009. http://www.eeoc.gov/eeoc/statistics/enforcement/charges.cfm

Equal Employment Opportunity Commission: Enforcement Guidance: Vicarious Employer Liability for Unlawful Harassment by Supervisors. http://www.eeoc.gov/policy/docs/harassment.html

Equal Employment Opportunity Commission: Notice Concerning the Lilly Ledbetter Fair Pay Act of 2009. http://www.eeoc.gov/laws/statutes/epa_ledbetter.cfm

Equal Employment Opportunity Commission: Revised Enforcement Guidance: Reasonable Accommodation and Undue Hardship Under the Americans with Disabilities Act, October 2002. http://www.eeoc.gov/policy/docs/accommodation.html

HR Tools. http://www.hrtools.com

National Labor Relations Board, National Labor Relations Act (NLRA). http://www.nlrb.gov/about_us/overview/national_labor_relations_act.aspx

United States Department of Labor: Find It! In DOL. http://www.dol.gov/dol/findit.htm

Workplace Laws Enforced by Other Federal Agencies. U.S. Equal Employment Opportunity Commission. http://www.eeoc.gov/laws/other.cfm#fmla

Job Analysis, Work Descriptions, and Work Groups

Janet Hall, MS, CC(NRCC)
Jill Dennis, MEd, MLS

OBJECTIVES

Following successful completion of this chapter, the learner will be able to:

1. Describe the importance of a clear, detailed job description.
2. Describe how job descriptions are developed.
3. List the components of a job description.
4. Describe the process of worker selection.
5. Describe the key components of evaluating performance.
6. Describe the difference between criteria-based and competency-based performance evaluations.
7. Describe the basic components of a work group.
8. Describe the dynamics of work groups.

KEY TERMS

Competency-Based
  Performance Evaluation
Criteria-Based Performance
  Evaluation

Job Analysis
Job Description
Performance Evaluation
Work Groups

Case Study — Job Analysis, Work Descriptions, and Work Groups

Katie has recently accepted a position as laboratory supervisor at a large suburban hospital. Although she is thrilled with her new position and working environment, Katie's laboratory manager has indicated that there is a major conflict in her laboratory that she needs to resolve as quickly as possible. The employees whom Katie supervises have been working as an efficient team for more than five years. In the past few months, however, turnaround time for laboratory tests has increased and the laboratory has been filled with tension and resentment toward Helen, a medical laboratory scientist, who joined the team approximately six months previously. Helen is an experienced scientist with exceptional knowledge and skills. She is energetic, hardworking and she possesses a positive attitude. Katie and Helen enjoy a good working relationship. Helen's co-workers, however, have complained that Helen tries to "stick her nose into everyone else's job" and that she slows the output of the other staff members with her unwanted involvement.

Issues and Questions to Consider:

1. How can Katie use her knowledge of the development of work groups to analyze the interpersonal dynamics of the work group under her supervision?
2. How can Katie use job analysis and existing job descriptions to improve the productivity of the work group and reduce the tension among its members?
3. In particular, what approach could Katie use to retain Helen's enthusiasm and commitment to the laboratory while curtailing Helen's negative effect on turnaround time for laboratory testing?

INTRODUCTION

Effective management requires the thoughtful analysis and measurement of job tasks and the careful evaluation of how employees perform those tasks to achieve the goals of the organization. To accomplish this, a job analysis should be performed to determine exactly what management expects from the employee. A **job analysis** is an evaluation and documentation of the tasks, conditions, requirements, and authority arrangements of a working situation. A **job/work description** is defined as a written document describing the tasks, expectations, reporting relationships, and other information relative to the employment of an individual. Ideally the job description should be a concise yet comprehensive summary of the findings of the job analysis. Too often, however, because of time constraints or lack of experience, managers write job descriptions based on historical documents or on a quick analysis of the current situation or on a specific person currently in the job to be described.

Managers are often faced with selecting individuals who meet the criteria determined from a job analysis and subsequent job description to fill open positions. A good understanding of the selection process is critical for a manager to successfully fill such job openings. Once an individual is hired, managers continue to monitor the employee through performance evaluations that may be competency or criteria-based. Further, managers may elect to use the assistance of their employees in the formation of work groups to accomplish designated tasks.

This chapter is designed to first introduce the learner to the specifics of conducting a thorough job analysis and creating an appropriate job description. An in-depth discussion of the selection process that includes job application, regulatory and internal criteria (see Chapter 6 for additional regulatory information) and conducting an effective and legal interview are then presented. Then an overview of the performance evaluation aspect of a laboratory manager's job is presented including a discussion of the two types of such evaluations, competency-based and criteria-based (see Chapter 8 for more information on performance evaluation). The final section is an introduction to the principle and uses of work groups.

JOB ANALYSIS

Job analysis may be done either formally or informally. Most often it is done informally, with a very general knowledge of the expectations of the employee and the working relationships of the employee with fellow employees and with management. Although an informal analysis is frequently adequate, it is not the best way to approach the issue. A formal job analysis involves observation and measurement of tasks and relationships with others, and a thorough documentation of the information gathered.

When performing a job analysis, many factors must be considered (Table 7-1).

1. *Working conditions:* should be analyzed. Working conditions include the physical environment in which the employee performs the work (e.g., temperature, lighting, noise level, physical requirements such as whether or not the employee is seated or standing and for what percentage of the time, requirements for lifting, whether or not the employee is working alone or

TABLE 7-1.   Factors Considered in Job Analysis

- Working Conditions
- Task Analysis
- Technology
- Scope of Labor
- Legal Issues
- Interaction with Co-Workers

with other employees). This is important to note because certain working conditions may not be suitable for certain people.

2. *Task analysis:* The actual tasks being performed should be evaluated to determine the amount of time required to perform them and whether there are specific requirements for space, equipment, etc.

3. *Technology:* The instrumentation or other equipment, including computers, used in the performance of the job should be listed along with any special requirements or skills needed to operate them.

4. *Scope of labor:* The knowledge, skills, and abilities (KSAs) required to perform the job should be evaluated. The availability in the marketplace of persons with these specific qualifications should be assessed. It may be necessary to adjust the KSAs to the availability of the required employees.

5. *Legal issues:* The legal requirements for specific licensures or training should be included.

6. *Interaction with co-workers:* The method and extent of the interaction of the employee should be evaluated both in terms of efficiencies and ensuring that the skill mix and communications with co-workers is adequate.

Although the items to be evaluated may be the same, the analysis of every job will be unique, based on its individual characteristics and requirements.

The job analysis can be accomplished by one or multiple individuals and can involve a number of approaches. Most frequently it is performed by the Department of Human Resources of the institution, only because they have the skills, knowledge, and experience of having done it in many settings. The specific criteria used vary widely, but are consistent in content and scope. Occasionally an industrial engineer may be engaged to do the analysis. The focus of the engineer is in ergonomics and motion, and they are most valuable when developing positions in a new environment. Another resource, at least in classifying the job, is the Department of Transportation's coding system. Their system assigns a 9-digit code based on the type of occupation, the functional level of difficulty with respect to data, people and things, and other criteria. Although it is useful academically, it is not particularly useful when the analysis is used to develop a job description. A more recent resource for occupational descriptors and data is the Occupational

Information Network (O*NET) developed under the sponsorship of the U.S. Department of Labor/Employment and Training Administration. It is continually updated and provides a content model that can be used as a framework to identify the most important types of information about occupations and people and integrates them into a theoretically and empirically sound system. More information can be found here: http://www.bls.gov/oco/oco2007.htm.

JOB DESCRIPTION

After performing the job analysis, a job description is developed. The purpose of the job description is twofold. First, it documents the characteristics of the job and the requirements of the candidates. Equally important, it acts as a measure against which employee performance can be assessed.

The job description, also referred to as a work or position description, should be concise yet thorough. One-line job descriptions may be concise but do not clarify or give the confidence to both management and staff that they know what is expected and what will be used to determine whether the employee is meeting job expectations. The description should contain measurable criteria to be used in the performance evaluation. Ideally, the job description document should be the evaluation tool.

The format of the job description varies widely, but in general it should address a number of facts, nine of which are described here (Table 7-2).

1. *Job title and classification:* The specific title of the position should be stated (e.g., Medical Laboratory Scientist II). This title includes the name of the position and the level of the position within that category (II).

2. *Exempt status:* The description should indicate whether the employee is exempt (salaried) or nonexempt (hourly).

3. *Education/experience:* The description should indicate the specific level or range of education required to perform the job. It may be stated in terms of

TABLE 7-2.   Format for a Job Description

- Job Title and Classification
- Exempt Status
- Education/Experience
- Knowledge
- Duties
- Interactions
- Safety
- Reporting Lines
- Approvals

"required" or "preferred" or a combination of the two. The same is true of experience (e.g., a minimum number of years of experience in the same or relation position). Note that the American Society of Clinical Laboratory Science has outlined levels of practice that list specific skills associated with education, relevant experience and certification. This could be used as a guide to describe specific skills needed for the associate degree level versus the bachelors and masters degree level. It is only a guide; each employer would make their own determination as to what skills, education, relevant experience, and certification are needed for the job.

4. *Knowledge:* The description should spell out the specific skills required to perform the job. These skills may be broad (knowledge of medical terminology) or very specific (experience with Analyzer X required). Generally it is better to be less specific, as equipment changes over time while basic skill sets do not. The degree of specificity is determined by a number of factors including the size of the facility and the scope of the job.

5. *Duties:* The description should list specific duties and tasks to be performed. The extent of detail will depend on the complexity of the job and the number of tasks to be performed. This area of the description lends itself to quantification of performance of the specific tasks when doing a performance appraisal.

6. *Interactions:* The description should indicate with whom the employee will have interaction, whether daily or periodic. Examples are nursing, admitting department, and housekeeping.

7. *Safety:* The description should clearly indicate what possible exposures the employee may encounter and classify the employee as a "contact" (likely to come into contact with hazardous materials) or "noncontact."

8. *Reporting Lines:* The description should indicate the line of authority and where the employee falls in that line. The employee may only report upwards (e.g., "reports to the Supervisor of the Chemistry Laboratory") and/or may have other employees as direct reports to them ("oversees technologists and technicians in the Chemistry Laboratory").

9. *Approvals:* The description should be reviewed and have approval signatures of the person who wrote the description, the Laboratory Manager, and the executive to whom the Laboratory Manager reports. It is also helpful to have the Human Resources Department sign to indicate their review and approval of the contents and intent of the description.

Once formulated and approved, the job description should be reviewed periodically (at least annually) to be certain that it continues to reflect the job, as it exists in real time. This is particularly important if it is to be used as an evaluation tool in addition to a simple description. Appendix 7-A contains an example of a job description for a medical laboratory scientist in a community-based hospital.

SELECTION PROCESS

Once the job is analyzed and documented and the description is developed, it is time to hire the best person. With the pool of qualified personnel shrinking rapidly, it becomes even more important to carefully hire and retain people who both "fit" the institution and who can grow and develop to the benefit of both the employee and the institution. Turnover in the healthcare market has always been problematic, as has the perception of limited chance for advancement. These factors make it even more critical to hire with care and make every effort to create job satisfaction so that employees will stay.

The Job Application

Once the job has been "posted," either within the institution or in print or electronic media outside the institution, the first step in the hiring process is the job application. The format of the **job application** is not accidental. A number of regulations require the asking of certain questions, while others forbid the asking of other questions. Appendix 7-B is an example of a typical job application form.

The provisions of Title VII of the Civil Rights Act enacted by Congress in 1964 are the basis of many of the hiring practices used by employers. Title VII forbids employers of more than 15 persons to discriminate against anyone on the basis of race, color, religion, sex, or national origin. The original Title VII law was expanded to include persons with disabilities, Vietnam veterans, and persons between 40 and 70 years old. For these reasons job applications do not request information about these qualities.

Regulatory and Internal Criteria

Once the application is in hand, regulatory and internal criteria must be met.

1. *Regulatory criteria:* As indicated by the job description, the applicant requires a certain level of education or a certification. The Clinical Laboratory Improvement Amendment of 1988 (CLIA'88) cites specific educational and certification requirements for different levels of employees. In addition, there may be local or state requirements that must be met, or the hiring institution may have its own, more stringent criteria based on its individual needs.

2. *Internal criteria:* Without violating the equal rights provisions, the hiring institution may have written or unwritten criteria related to the particular dynamics of a work group or individual characteristics that are deemed necessary to succeed in the position.

The next step in the process is to review applications received and narrow the field to a handful of candidates who appear to be most qualified for the job. This process is sometimes handled by the human resources department, at least for screening purposes. If this is the policy, the appropriate laboratory manager/ supervisor should then review those applications that have survived the initial screening process and schedule interviews with as many candidates as necessary, but preferably not more than five.

Interviewing

A formal or informal interview is the next step. The interviews may be done by a group of persons who will be working closely with the candidate, or by one or more individual interviews. How this is handled may depend on availability of interviewers and/or past history and/or personal preference. Whatever method is chosen, it is important to keep questions asked as consistent as possible to be able to accurately evaluate the candidates in relation to each other. Developing a list of questions that is reviewed by all interviewers and asked of all candidates works well and allows for such consistency. Questions may be specific or part of a behavioral interview during which the candidate is asked more about how they would react in certain situations rather than direct questions about skills. The behavioral assessment is more commonly used for managerial positions than the specific skills questions, which are used for more technical types of positions. Table 7-3 shows examples of questions that may be asked. Table 7-4 outlines questions that *cannot* be asked during an interview.

Finally, there should be some type of objective rating tool indicating specific characteristics/qualifications and a quantifiable rating scheme so that a total number of "points" can be assigned to each candidate. Table 7-5 is an example of such a scale. A combination of a quantifiable rating tool and a more subjective, narrative evaluation may also be used with the understanding that the selection result may not be totally quantifiable. Once the selection is made, the employee is offered a position. If the employee accepts the position, thus completing the hiring/selection process, a start date is determined.

TABLE 7-3.   Commonly Made Inquiries During a Job Interview

1. Tell me about your educational background.
2. What experiences led you to choose your career path?
3. How has your previous work experience prepared you for this job?
4. Tell me about your most significant accomplishments.
5. What type of problems have you solved in accomplishing your work assignments?
6. What has been your current job's biggest challenge?
7. Describe the most common problems you encounter at your (previous/ current) job.
8. What happens when two priorities compete for your time?
9. Describe two things that motivate you at work.
10. How do you determine if you are successful?

TABLE 7-4.   Things That Cannot Be Asked During a Job Interview

Generally any questions designed to elicit information as to race, color, age, sex, religion, handicap, or arrest and court records, unless based on a documented occupational qualification, should not be asked. Inappropriate questions include:

- Questions about the applicant's name that would indicate applicant's lineage, ancestry, national origin, or descent or marital status.
- Questions about whether an applicant is married, single, divorced, or engaged and questions regarding number and age of children, potential children, or child care arrangements.
- Questions regarding age or date of birth. The Age Discrimination in Employment Act of 1967 forbids discrimination against persons between the ages of 40 and 70 years old.
- Questions regarding the nature or severity of any handicap. The Rehabilitation Act of 1973 forbids employers from asking job applicants general questions about whether they are handicapped.
- Questions regarding the applicant's sex, race, birthplace or origin of parents, spouse, or other relatives.
- Questions regarding applicant's religious denomination or affiliation, church, parish, pastor, or religious holidays observed.
- Questions relating to arrests or convictions of applicant.

PERFORMANCE EVALUATION

Evaluation of job performance is a task that few managers relish, but it is extremely important to employees and can be made reasonably painless by following a few simple guidelines. **Performance evaluation** really starts during the orientation period, when a trainer is teaching the new employee the details of the job, and continues to a more formal stage at the end of the probationary period, when a formal performance appraisal is completed and documented. Two types of performance evaluation are defined and discussed in this section: competency-based and criteria-based.

Competency-Based Versus Criteria-Based Evaluations

Competency-based performance evaluations are helpful during the orientation period because they require the new employee to actually perform tasks while being observed so that the trainer knows that he/she is performing them to documented standards. Competency-based performance evaluation is an evaluation based on a limited number of specifically defined tasks that are taught and assessed by direct observation during the orientation period and periodically thereafter. Direct observation can be beneficial in that it provides formative feedback and evaluation rather than a summative evaluation. The number of tasks assessed during orientation is considerably greater than those assessed at an annual performance appraisal. Observing the new employee as he or she is being trained

TABLE 7-5. Sample Interview Rating Scale

INTERVIEW EVALUATION FORM

Candidate Name: _____

Rate the candidate on the criteria below using a scale of 0 to 5, with 0 indicating that the candidate cannot be rated on the specific attribute, 1 indicating the lowest score, and 5 indicating the highest possible.

Evaluative Criteria	Ranking	Comments
Educational Background		
Work Experience		
Research/Professional Activities		
Laboratory Experience		
Communication Skills		
Interpersonal Skills		
Overall Rating		

Comments:

_____

_____

_____

_____

Interviewer Signature   Date

and documenting on an orientation checklist the satisfactory completion of a learned task assures both the trainer and trainee that the task has been completed successfully. The hard copy documentation serves as proof to inspectors that the individual was, indeed, evaluated on specific tasks and that the individual was deemed proficient at those tasks. The orientation checklist should include a list of specific tasks, the date they were certified/completed, and the signature or initials of the person documenting the training. The checklist, once completed, should be kept indefinitely in the employee's personnel file.

A second means of performance appraisal is the **criteria-based performance evaluations.** This method uses an evaluation based on rating the performance of the employee on specifically defined criteria such as knowledge, judgment, attendance, reliability, and interactions with fellow employees. Ideally the checklist of criteria to be considered will be a part of the job description. In addition to the checklist, however, is a series of standards and criteria used to determine the rating given on the evaluation. For example, for rating attendance, the laboratory may use the standards listed in Table 7-6. Criteria-based performance standards permit satisfactory ratings to be developed for entry-level employees as well as for seasoned scientist.

TABLE 7-6.   Rating Standards for Attendance

Exceeds expectations	No unexcused absences. No more than 2 sick frequencies with a total of 3 days used.
Meets expectations	One unexcused absence. No more than 4 sick frequencies with a total of 7 days used.
Does not meet expectations	More than 1 unexcused absence. Greater than 4 sick frequencies with a total of 8 days used.

The standards are objective and measurable and leave no doubt from the records about the performance of the employee. Both the employee and the employer have documented proof of why a particular rating was given.

Many institutions have adopted an evaluation process that is a hybrid of the criteria-based and competency-based methods. Frequently these have measurable standards for each task, one of which is that all competencies were performed at an acceptable level. In addition, there may be a place for narrative comments by the employer and by the employee.

Some institutions have adopted a policy of 360-degree evaluations for managers, where both the person to whom the manager reports and those who report to the manager complete the evaluation form either together or separately. There are pros and cons for the 360-degree evaluation. Sometimes the input from those being managed is more narrative than quantifiable, but the employees feel that they have some input into the evaluation. The most important feature is that input from those who are managed be strictly confidential so that there is no opportunity for biasing the manager's opinions toward the employee.

However they are handled, performance evaluations should not draw any surprises for the employee. Monitoring of performance is an ongoing process, not a once a year event. Communication must be fostered so that both the employee and the manager are aware at all times of the level of performance being achieved. The goal is guarantee that the excellent employee will continue to be productive and the weaker employee knows what needs to be done to improve.

WORK GROUPS

Most laboratories are staffed by employees with diverse skill sets and capabilities. This is true because there are many different types of tasks that make up the operation of a laboratory. In a very small laboratory, a few employees with similar, broad skill sets will operate the laboratory. In most laboratories, however, the work is broken down into tasks that require different levels of skills. For example, phlebotomists collect the specimens and deliver them to the laboratory. They use a different set of skills from the processing people who receive the specimens, log them in, and prepare them for analysis. Another group includes the medical laboratory technicians and scientists who analyze the specimens and report the results. Yet another group may be clerical and handle reporting and results distribution. The smooth operation of the laboratory requires that all of these employees with different skill sets work closely together to accomplish the tasks required to achieve timely and accurate results needed by the patient's caregiver. Work groups provide the opportunity for shared responsibility from all members of the laboratory team resulting in a better understanding and acceptance of final decisions.

Work groups may be formal or informal. Formal work groups are usually assigned to a particular area to perform different pieces of the process. Staffing and scheduling define these work groups. Informal work groups tend to develop within these groups based on the personalities and priorities of the persons in the groups. Certain role expectations are gained in formal groups and are defined by the task sets of the individual members. Other role expectations develop over time in the informal work groups, but are just as important to the way in which the group functions as is the formal definition of the group.

Work groups tend to take on personalities of their own. Some are efficient and operate smoothly; others are disjointed and dysfunctional. Taking the same group of people from one work site to another, even though the surroundings and tasks may be different, does not generally change how well the group works together. There is a certain bonding that occurs among members, and, indeed, the dynamic of the group does tend to change. Groups go through developmental stages (Table 7-7). When a new employee enters the group, the balance achieved in the old group shifts to accommodate the particular skills and personality traits of the new member. The group first goes through a forming stage. It is a tentative time when the members are getting to know one another, the hierarchy of the group may be established, and mutual accommodation of tasks and priorities takes place. The group then enters a storming stage, where any imbalances come to the forefront and must be resolved. Some groups never get beyond the storming stage, and the manager needs to either step in and smooth out the process or rearrange the group by adding or deleting members to strike a balance.

During the third stage, the norming stage, members have come to agreement on how things are done and who does them and a general leveling off occurs. Finally, the group may reach the performing stage, where all members are comfortable with the dynamics and are productive and happy.

Turnover, which is an ongoing problem in healthcare, has a profound effect on the efficient functioning of work groups. Each time a member leaves and is replaced, the group starts over at the forming stage and must progress through the other stages before it again becomes an efficient work organization. The task of the manager is to expedite this process through open communication and fostering of good relationships among employees so that the time required to reach the performing stage is as short as possible.

Changing the structure and tasks of work groups is sometimes a lesson in management by trial and error. Generally the formal groups will remain relatively

TABLE 7-7.   Developmental Stages of Work Groups

- Forming stage
- Storming stage
- Norming stage
- Performing stage

stable unless process problems indicate that the group needs to restructure. It is the influence of the informal groups, however, that usually causes problems that must be addressed by the manager. Two or more individuals, for example, may attempt to undermine the integration of another individual, either openly or covertly.

The most effective way to manage work groups is to have clear guidelines for employees as to what is expected, select employees carefully, have a quantifiable and reasonable evaluation process in place, and communicate openly with employees at all levels.

SUMMARY

Effective management requires the thoughtful analysis and measurement of job tasks and the careful evaluation of how employees perform those tasks to achieve the goals of the organization. Managers should follow the steps outlined in this chapter as a guide to acquiring and maintaining an effective and efficient laboratory team (Figure 7-1). A job analysis is an evaluation and documentation of the tasks, conditions, requirements, and authority arrangements of a working situation. The factors assessed in performing a job analysis include the working conditions, tasks, technology, scope of labor, legal issues, and interactions with co-workers that affect a particular position. After performing the job analysis a job description is developed. The purpose of the job description is twofold. First, it documents the characteristics of the job and the requirements of the candidates. Equally important, it acts as a measure against which employee performance can be assessed. Once formulated and approved, the job description should be reviewed periodically (at least annually) to be certain that it continues to reflect the job, as it exists in real time. A number of regulations, established by the provisions of Title VII of the Civil Rights Act, govern the interview and selection process. In addition, the hiring institution will develop internal criteria, in accordance with equal rights provisions, to guide the selection and hiring processes. Developing a list of questions before the interview to be asked of all candidates and reviewed by all interviewers works well and allows for such consistency. There should be some type of objective rating tool indicating specific characteristics/qualifications and a quantifiable rating scheme so that a total number of "points" can be assigned to each candidate. Performance evaluation really starts during the orientation period, when a trainer is teaching the new

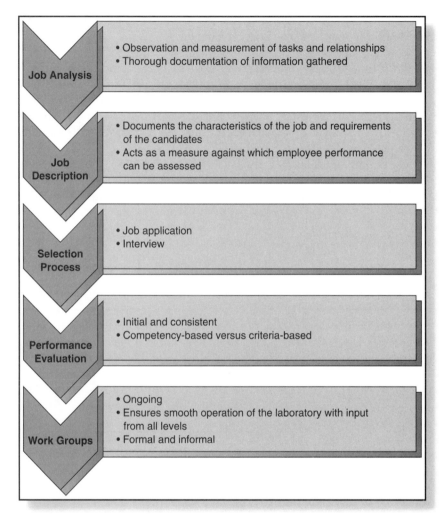

FIGURE 7-1.   Steps to Effective Management of the Laboratory Team

employee the details of the job and continues to a more formal stage at the end of the probationary period when a formal performance appraisal is done and documented.

Competency-based performance evaluations are helpful during the orientation period because they require the new employee to actually perform tasks while being observed so that the trainer knows that they are performing them to documented standards. A second means of performance appraisal is the criteria-based performance appraisal. This method uses an evaluation based on rating the performance of the employee on specifically defined criteria such as knowledge, judgment, attendance, reliability, and interactions with fellow employees.

Ideally the checklist of criteria to be considered will be a part of the job description. Monitoring performance is an ongoing process, not a once a year event.

Work groups may be formal or informal. Certain role expectations are gained in formal groups and are defined by the task sets of individual members. Other role expectations develop over time in the informal work groups, but are just as important to the way in which the group functions as is the formal definition of the group. The most effective way to manage work groups is to have clear guidelines for employees as to what is expected, select employees carefully, have a quantifiable and reasonable evaluation process in place, and communicate openly with employees at all levels. The job analysis and description process is critical to the accurate evaluation of employees. The entire process enhances productivity of the laboratory reaping benefits for the entire healthcare team.

SUMMARY CHART:
Important Points to Remember

➤ The purpose of a job analysis is to establish and document the job relatedness of employment procedures such as training, selection, compensation, and performance appraisal.

➤ The purpose of a job description is to document the characteristics of the job and the requirements of the candidates. Job descriptions also act as a measurement of which employee performance can be assessed.

➤ It is important that job descriptions are written based on the job, not a current situation or specific person currently in the job.

➤ The selection process involves creating an appropriate job application that follows nondiscriminatory regulations. Interviews should be as consistent as possible for all interviewees to enable accurate evaluation of the candidates in relation to each other.

➤ Consistent performance evaluations are necessary to keep the lab operating efficiently.

➤ Competency-based performance evaluations are based on defined tasks that are taught and assessed by direct observation, during the orientation and periodically thereafter.

➤ Criteria-based performance evaluations may also be used. This method uses an evaluation based on rating the performance of the employee on specifically defined criteria such as knowledge, judgment, attendance, reliability, and interactions with fellow employees.

➤ Work groups may be formed to provide the opportunity for shared responsibility from all members of the laboratory team resulting in a better understanding of final decisions.

➤ Work groups may be formal or informal, but should be carefully constructed by the lab manager, so that the right people are in the right groups and there are clear guidelines as to what is expected, with accountability measures in place.

SUGGESTED PROBLEM-BASED LEARNING ACTIVITIES

Chapter 7: Job Analysis, Work Descriptions, and Work Groups

Instructions: Use Internet resources, books, articles, colleagues, etc., to present solutions to the problems listed below. There is no one correct solution to any problem.

Note to Instructor: Students in class may be divided into groups and given the problem-based learning activity to discuss and solve. Once the group has reached consensus as to a solution, the group may present it to the other students in the class. This activity will provide all students with information regarding solutions to the problem.

Problem #1

Suppose the medical director of your institution has requested a STAT laboratory to be placed in the emergency department. You have been charged with researching and reporting on your recommended plan of actions to make this request a reality. Include the aspects of job analysis, work descriptions, and work groups into your plan.

Problem #2

Select a position in the laboratory and write an appropriate job description and corresponding work description for this position.

Problem #3

Suppose the night shift personnel have quit and as laboratory manager, you must devise a plan of action to provide coverage of this shift until a replacement has been hired and trained. (Learners are encouraged to review Chapter 16 of this text for additional information helpful in devising your plan.) Indicate provisions in your plan for incorporating work groups, a thorough shift job analysis, and revised work descriptions for the open night shift positions.

BIBLIOGRAPHY

Bacal R: *Manager's Guide to Performance Reviews.* McGraw-Hill, New York, NY, 2004.

Belker LB, Topchik GS: *The First-Time Manager.* AMACOM, New York, NY, 2005.

Bozzo P: *Cost Effective Laboratory Management.* Lippincott Williams and Wilkins, Philadelphia, PA, 1998.

Brannick MT, Levine EL: *Job Analysis: Methods, Research, and Applications for Human Resources Management in the New Millennium.* Sage Publications, Thousand Oaks, CA, 2002.

Cohen EG: *Designing Groupwork.* Teachers College Press Columbia, New York, NY, 1994.

DeMarco T, Lister T: *Peopleware: Productive Projects and Teams,* 2nd ed. Dorset House, New York, NY, 2000.

Grote, D: *The Performance Appraisal Question and Answer Book: A Survival Guide for Managers.* AMACOM, 2002.

Mathis RL, Jackson JH: *Human Resource Management.* South-Western Publishing Company, Cincinnati, OH, 2008.

Nigon DL: *Clinical Laboratory Management, Leadership Principles for the 21st Century.* McGraw-Hill Health Professions Division, New York, NY, 2000.

Rees F: *How to Lead Work Teams: Facilitation Skills,* 2nd ed. Jossey-Bass Inc, New York, NY, 2001.

Travers EM: *Clinical Laboratory Management.* Lippincott Williams and Wilkins, Philadelphia, PA, 1996.

Turner M: *Groups at Work: Theory and Research* (The Applied Social Research Series). Lawrence Erlbaum Associates, Inc., Mahwah, NJ, 2001.

Varnadoe LA: *Medical Laboratory Management and Supervision.* F.A. Davis Company, Philadelphia, PA, 1996.

Veruki P: *The 250 Job Interview Questions: You'll Most Likely Be Asked . . . and the Answers That Will Get You Hired!* Adams Media Corporation, Avon, 1999.

INTERNET RESOURCES

American Society for Clinical Laboratory Science (ASCLS), Practice Levels and Educational Needs for Clinical Laboratory Personnel. 25 July 2009. http://www.ascls.org/position/Levelsof Practice.asp

BLS – Business & Legal Resources. *Human Resources Management Website.* Business & Legal Reports, 2011. http://hr.blr.com

HR Guide to the Internet: *Job Analysis:* Overview. http://www.hr-guide.com

HR Systems Group. Performance Evaluation Information. HRSG, 2010. http://hrsg.ca

International Federation of Biomedical Laboratory Science. http://www.ifbls.org/

Occupational Information Network (O*NET) http://online.onetcenter.org

Occupational Outlook Handbook, 2010–11. Occupational Information Network (O*NET) Coverage. United States Department of Labor, Last modified 17 May 2010. http://www.bls.gov/oco/oco2007.htm

APPENDIX 7-A: SAMPLE JOB DESCRIPTION

STATE CLASSIFICATION JOB DESCRIPTION

Salary Group B3   Class No. 4400

MEDICAL LABORATORY SCIENTIST I

GENERAL DESCRIPTION

Performs entry-level clinical laboratory work. Work involves performing medical testing procedures and reporting the results to the appropriate medical authority for evaluation, diagnosis, or treatment. Works under close supervision with minimal latitude for the use of initiative and independent judgment.

EXAMPLES OF WORK PERFORMED

Performs newborn screening procedures such as neonatal T4, TSH, and similar tests.

Performs serological tests for medical screening such as RPR, rubella, and similar tests.

Performs erythrocyte protoporphyrin screening assay.

Performs diagnostic procedures in urinalysis and in hematology.

Performs identification procedures on samples submitted for parasite, fungal, and mycobacterial studies.

Reads bacterial bioassay inhibition test plates.

May conduct bronchospirometric studies to determine lung function.

May analyze blood and gas samples; evaluates and reports findings.

May plan, arrange, and assist with cardiac catheterizations.

Performs related work as assigned.

GENERAL QUALIFICATION GUIDELINES

Experience and Education

Experience in clinical laboratory work. Graduation from an accredited four-year college or university with major course work in the natural sciences or a related field is generally preferred. Experience and education may be substituted for one another.

Knowledge, Skills, and Abilities

Knowledge of medical technology concepts and practices, clinical laboratory methods and procedures, and quality assurance methodologies.

Skill in the use of laboratory equipment.

Ability to conduct clinical laboratory tests to determine deterioration or change in reagents or equipment which might influence test results; and to keep abreast of new testing techniques and procedures.

Registration, Certification, or Licensure

Must be registered as a Medical Laboratory Scientist

APPENDIX 7-B

PLEASE TYPE OR PRINT

Administrative Services

INDICATE POSITION(S) AND POSITION NUMBER(S) APPLIED FOR:

_____

_____

OFFICE OF HUMAN SERVICES
737 WEST LOMBARD STREET
BALTIMORE, MARYLAND 21201
AN EQUAL OPPORTUNITY / AFFIRMATIVE ACTION / ADA EMPLOYER
JOBLINE (410) 706-5JOB

_____

_____

APPLICATION FOR EMPLOYMENT

LAST NAME	FIRST	MIDDLE

FOR OFFICE OF HUMAN RESOURCES MANAGEMENT USE ONLY

STREET ADDRESS

POSITIONS QUALIFIED FOR:

CITY	STATE	ZIP CODE

1. _____

2. _____

SOCIAL SECURITY NO.

PHONE NUMBERS

HOME: ( )

3. _____

ARE YOU CURRENTLY AUTHORIZED TO WORK FOR ALL EMPLOYERS IN THE UNITED STATES ON A FULL TIME BASIS?
☐ YES ☐ NO
OR ONLY FOR YOUR CURRENT EMPLOYER?
☐ YES ☐ NO

BUSINESS: ( )

OTHER: ( )

4. _____

5. _____

☐ INTERNAL
☐ EXTERNAL

EMPLOYMENT RECORD   BEGIN WITH YOUR CURRENT OR MOST RECENT POSITION AND WORK BACKWARD. INCLUDE ALL PERTINENT MILITARY AND VOLUNTEER WORK WHICH WILL BE CREDITED AS PAID EXPERIENCE. INCOMPLETE APPLICATIONS MAY NOT BE ACCEPTED. ANY OTHER SURNAME DIFFERENT FROM ABOVE SHOULD BE INDICATED NEXT TO THE APPROPRIATE EMPLOYER.

Employer				DATES EMPLOYED		Your Duties and Responsibilities:
Street Address	City	State	Zip Code	FROM	TO	

Telephone ( )

	MO	YR	MO	YR

Last Position Held

First Position Held

Name and Title of Supervisor   BASE SALARY

Reason for Leaving   Explain

Did You Work Full-Time? ☐ Yes ☐ No

☐ Resignation
☐ Layoff
☐ Termination
☐ If Still Employed, Why Leaving?

FIRST	LAST

If "No," Percent of Time Worked: _____ %

Number of Employees Supervised: _____

$ $

Employer				DATES EMPLOYED		Your Duties and Responsibilities:
Street Address	City	State	Zip Code	FROM	TO	

Telephone ( )

	MO	YR	MO	YR

Last Position Held

First Position Held

Name and Title of Supervisor   BASE SALARY

Reason for Leaving   Explain

Did You Work Full-Time? ☐ Yes ☐ No

☐ Resignation
☐ Layoff
☐ Termination
☐ If Still Employed, Why Leaving?

FIRST	LAST

If "No," Percent of Time Worked: _____ %

Number of Employees Supervised: _____

$ $

Employer				DATES EMPLOYED		Your Duties and Responsibilities:
Street Address	City	State	Zip Code	FROM	TO	

Telephone ( )

	MO	YR	MO	YR

Last Position Held

First Position Held

Name and Title of Supervisor   BASE SALARY

Reason for Leaving   Explain

Did You Work Full-Time? ☐ Yes ☐ No

☐ Resignation
☐ Layoff
☐ Termination
☐ If Still Employed, Why Leaving?

FIRST	LAST

If "No," Percent of Time Worked: _____ %

Number of Employees Supervised: _____

$ $

11.00041 (Rev. 5/95)
CONTINUATION SHEETS AVAILABLE
UMAB IS A DRUG FREE, NON-SMOKING ENVIRONMENT

(Courtesy of University of Maryland.)

(Continued)

APPENDIX 7-B *(Continued)*

Schools	Name and Address of School	Dates From / To	Number of Years and Credit Hours Completed	Major or Type of Program	Type of Degree or Certification and Date Received
High School or Grade School					
College					
Graduate School					
Vocational / Business School					

DO YOU POSSESS ANY OF THE FOLLOWING SKILLS? CHECK "YES" OR "NO."

Data Entry	☐ Yes ☐ No	Legal Terminology	☐ Yes ☐ No	Shorthand	☐ Yes ☐ No
Word Processing	☐ Yes ☐ No	Medical Terminology	☐ Yes ☐ No	Typing	☐ Yes ☐ No
Machine Transcription	☐ Yes ☐ No	Scientific Terminology	☐ Yes ☐ No	Approximate Typing Speed _____	

LIST ADDITIONAL SPECIAL QUALIFICATIONS AND SKILLS (E.G. OFFICE MACHINES / COMPUTER EQUIPMENT OPERATED, SOFTWARE PACKAGES USED, FOREIGN LANGUAGES SPOKEN, LABORATORY EQUIPMENT USED, ETC.)

IF THE POSITION(S) YOU ARE APPLYING FOR REQUIRES A LICENSE (INCLUDING DRIVER'S LICENSE), CERTIFICATION OR OTHER AUTHORIZATION TO PRACTICE A TRADE OR PROFESSION, COMPLETE THIS SECTION.

Type / Class	License Number	Expiration Date	Granted By (Board or Commission)	State

U.S. Military Service	Date of Entrance	Date of Discharge

IF YOUR ANSWER IS "YES" TO ANY OF THE FOLLOWING QUESTIONS, EXPLAIN IN BOX TO RIGHT. PLEASE NOTE THAT "YES" ANSWERS TO ANY OF THESE QUESTIONS DO NOT AUTOMATICALLY DISQUALIFY YOU FROM EMPLOYMENT.

a. Have you ever worked for the State of Maryland or the University of Maryland? ☐ Yes ☐ No

b. Have you been interviewed for a position with the University of Maryland at Baltimore within the last twelve months? ☐ Yes ☐ No

c. Have you ever been convicted in court for anything other than a minor traffic violation? (Please be advised that we may check records through the Criminal Justice Information System Central Repository). ☐ Yes ☐ No

d. Are you under 18 years of age? ☐ Yes ☐ No

e. Have you been discharged from military service within the past 90 days? ☐ Yes ☐ No

MAY WE CONTACT YOUR PRESENT EMPLOYER? IF "NO" PLEASE EXPLAIN. ☐ Yes ☐ No
YOUR FORMER EMPLOYERS / SCHOOLS WILL BE CONTACTED FOR REFERENCES.

PLEASE INDICATE AVAILABILITY BY CHECKING ONE OR MORE OF THE FOLLOWING,
☐ Full-Time ☐ Day Hours Only
☐ Part-Time ☐ Any Hours Considered

APPLICANTS WITH DISABILITIES REQUIRING ACCOMMODATIONS SHOULD CONTACT THE EMPLOYMENT DIVISION AT (410) 706-7171 OR MD RELAY SERVICE 1-800-735-2258.

"UNDER MARYLAND LAW AN EMPLOYER MAY NOT REQUIRE OR DEMAND ANY APPLICANT FOR EMPLOYMENT OR PROSPECTIVE EMPLOYMENT OR ANY EMPLOYEE TO SUBMIT TO OR TAKE A POLYGRAPH, LIE DETECTOR OR SIMILAR TEST OR EXAMINATION AS A CONDITION OF EMPLOYMENT OR CONTINUED EMPLOYMENT. ANY EMPLOYER WHO VIOLATES THIS PROVISION IS GUILTY OF A MISDEMEANOR AND SUBJECT TO A FINE NOT TO EXCEED $100."
This provision does not apply to applicants for law enforcement positions pursuant to Labor and Employment Article, Section 3-702 (b) (Annotated Code of Maryland).

I certify that all information on this application is accurate and complete and recognize that it is subject to verification. I also understand that any offers of employment and / or continuance thereof may be contingent upon its accuracy and completeness. I understand that I may be required to pass a physical examination upon an offer of employment.

Signature of Applicant	Date

THE UNIVERSITY OF MARYLAND AT BALTIMORE IS AN EQUAL OPPORTUNITY/AFFIRMATIVE ACTION EMPLOYER

Performance Evaluation and Development

Paul Labbe, NMT, MCLT
Lani Barovick, MS
Denise M. Harmening, PhD, MT(ASCP), CLS(NCA)

CHAPTER OUTLINE

OBJECTIVES

Following successful completion of this chapter, the learner will be able to:

1. Promote two-way communications between the supervisor and employee regarding employee's job performance.
2. Provide an opportunity for increased job effectiveness and development.
3. Demonstrate an understanding for promoting a win-win relationship with the employee.
4. Apply skills in:
   - Communications
   - Feedback
   - Guidance
   - Evaluation
   - Development planning
5. Develop a performance development evaluation approach using basic principles of professional development.
6. Describe and demonstrate the importance of learning, independent thinking, and sharing expertise for individual pride in performance and development.
7. Describe the use of the evaluation model developed to support the basic principles of professional development and evaluation.

KEY TERMS

Collaborative Management
Competency Modeling
Feedback Skills

Performance Development
Performance Objectives
Task/Production Management

Case Study

Performance Evaluation and Development

Thomas Hancock has been the administrator of the clinical laboratories of a large urban hospital for many years. He excels at fiscal management and he has been successful in acquiring a state-of-the-art laboratory information system to increase efficiency in the laboratories. However, he is reluctant to hold department meetings or provide feedback to staff. Staff evaluations are seldom completed and his department team is unmotivated.

Mr. Hancock primarily communicates to his staff through memos. All processes must be handled according to his rules and he is unwilling to accept input from others. No one is allowed to make decisions on their own (no matter how small). When a staff member does something Mr. Hancock does not like he sends a memo to everyone pointing out the problem and how it should have been handled. The result is that everyone thinks he/she made the mistake and yet they are not sure what is wrong.

Staff members are given job/position descriptions when they are hired, but they have not been reviewed or updated in several years. Therefore, they do not clearly define the core responsibilities, making individuals feel frustrated because many of their accomplishments are not recognized or rewarded. Each year, cost of living allowances (COLAs) and a merit pool increase ranging from 2–5% are provided. Mr. Hancock gives everyone the same rating and the same increase because he prefers not to differentiate between his outstanding and average performers. The individuals needing improvement in their performance usually end up in the employee relations department with a grievance that is resolved on the side of the employee because there is no record of disciplinary action taken by Mr. Hancock.

Mr. Hancock's turnover in the laboratories is high. Staffing analysis shows that the top performers leave at a consistent rate while average performers stay longer. Staff stated that they felt unappreciated as well as distrustful of their supervisor and others in the department. The hospital's top management is concerned about the turnover and the high costs associated with recruiting qualified clinical laboratory professionals.

Issues and Questions to Consider:

1. *Is Mr. Hancock using management by task/production or collaboration? Describe examples of his management characteristics.*
2. *Describe how Mr. Hancock could create an atmosphere of growth and learning and decrease turnover of his top performers.*
3. *How can Mr. Hancock improve department communications and trust?*
4. *What first step is necessary for effective performance evaluation? Why?*
5. *How can Mr. Hancock effectively reward his top performers and improve performance for those whose work is below standards?*

INTRODUCTION

Most managers shrink from their most important task—managing the performance of others. Opposition to performance evaluation is not new. Seventeen hundred years ago, the following observation was recorded about a man appointed to evaluate the performance of the imperial family in China's Wei dynasty: "The Imperial Rater seldom rates men according to their merits, but always according to his likes and dislikes."

Performance evaluation is an important aspect of laboratory management, but most employees and managers often dread it. Creating and establishing a fair, just, and equitable evaluation process, as a positive experience for both the employee and the supervisor, is a challenging task. By establishing a performance development program, the evaluation process can be turned into a "win-win" situation for both the employees and the managers by becoming a tool for professional development. A clear understanding of performance development, including its benefits and how it works, is essential for both employees and supervisors. The employee in consultation with his or her supervisor should establish performance expectations and measurements at the beginning of the process. The supervisor should guide employees in recognizing and developing the competencies required to meet the organizational or laboratory's objectives. A successful performance development program and subsequent evaluation must be a collaborative effort with the employee.

In this chapter on performance evaluation and professional development, we hope to provide a proactive approach to the process. We begin with building relationships and mastering feedback skills. Our focus is on self-evaluation and development with management feedback. This approach provides for collaboration and partnership in the performance evaluation process for professional development and a win-win relationship.

MANAGEMENT TOOLS FOR PAINLESS PERFORMANCE EVALUATIONS AND PERFORMANCE DEVELOPMENT

Performance development is an ongoing two-way process for communicating about the employee's job performance and helping them achieve excellence in their position and job satisfaction. It involves many processes: goal setting, feedback, guidance, motivation, evaluation, and development planning. It is an ongoing process that both supervisors and employees actively use throughout the year.

"Though no one can go back and make a brand new start, anyone can start from now and make a brand new ending."

—Carl Bard

TABLE 8-1. Comparison of Task/Production Management (left column) and Collaborative Management (right column)

• Creates power base	• Creates trust relationship
• Identifies problem	• Defines problem solution
• Provides plan for employee	• Develops action plan together
• Threat—if you don't do it	• Supports risks taking
• Oversees—punishment/reward	• Coaches and follows-up

Adapted from Hunsaker PL, Alessandra AP. Building productive managerial relationships. In *The New Art of Managing People*, 2nd ed. Simon & Schuster, New York, NY, 2008.

Research on human personality suggests that individuals need to be treated with civility and respect. They want opportunities to feel independent and competent. They actively desire to pursue goals to which they are committed and motivated. However, most organizations manage individuals using **task/production management**. Research on production management indicates its characteristics, which are production/task-oriented, tend to create situations in which the individual feels submissive, passive, and dependent. For consistency task/production management does not encourage individuals to use the abilities they believe to be important or develop them. Activities are not aimed at the individual's needs but at the manager and organization's, thus creating frustration, resentment, and underproduction.

The **collaborative management** philosophy incorporates the belief that individuals participate in this type of management because they feel appreciated and understood. They are not being forced to comply by a mandate from their supervisor. The collaborative management process must be built around trust. Trust requires openness and honesty on the part of both the supervisor and the employee. A successful win-win relationship is built on trust. If there is trust the employee will collaborate because he or she feels understood by the supervisor and the supervisor understands the problems. The employee wants to make decisions to solve problems. Table 8-1 explains the difference between production/ task management and collaborative management.

PRINCIPLES OF COLLABORATIVE MANAGEMENT

The four basic principles of collaborative management are trust, understanding, independence, and solutions (Table 8-2). By using these principles you can (1) increase job effectiveness and improve performance and (2) create an atmosphere of growth and learning for professional development. Actions always speak louder than words. Therefore, you must be willing to trust your employees and give them opportunities for independence and collaboration. Remember you cannot succeed with these principles unless you are willing to trust your

TABLE 8-2.   Four Basic Principles of Collaborative Management

Trust	Relationship between employee and manager that requires openness and honesty.
Understanding	Individuals perform because they feel understood by the manager and understand the problem.
Independence	Individuals resent being manipulated, controlled, or persuaded into making a decision, even if that was the decision they would eventually have made. They need the right to make their own decisions.
Solutions	Management should not solve the employee's problems. They will resent this. Rather, point out problems and ask for solutions.

employees. This means you must be open and honest, and your employee must feel he or she can be open and honest with you. You can then form a trust-bond relationship. This relationship provides the foundation for collaborative management.

Five-Step Performance Development Process

To move successfully into collaborative management we recommend a five-step process to establish an effective relationship for joint problem solving. Keep in mind actions speak louder than words. If you are not willing to trust your employees and develop a partnership then you cannot be successful in our current work environment. We are in an age of four generations in today's workforce—each generation motivated by their own background and experience. Our world of constant change requires teams, collaboration, and partnership. Learning collaborative management techniques will ensure successful outcomes with many of your relationships. The 5 steps recommended to establish an effective relationship for joint problem solving are identified and described as follows:

1. *Trust:* Mutual respect and understanding is prerequisite for joint problem solving. Collaboration and teamwork cannot happen unless a firm trust relationship is developed with the employee. Employees want a supervisor who they feel understands and cares about them. They prefer a supervisor they know they can rely on. They need to know that the manager is interested in their personal needs, career goals, and continual growth and development. They need to know they can take risks, which will help in their personal and professional development.

2. *Problem solving:* The manager can promote trust by being involved in problem solving with the employee. The manager must continually review personal and task goals and provide praise as often as possible. He or she must

also guide and coach the subordinate when there is a problem to be solved or a plan correction to be made to successfully accomplish goals. The success of this activity hinges on effective information sharing and information-gathering skills.

3. *Action plans:* The major role of the manager is to listen "actively" and ask questions. Direct the action planning process toward personal and professional goals as well as business objectives. The new action plan should be mutually beneficial toward improved performance and development with clearly stated measurable outcomes.

4. *Implementation:* Subordinates become committed to plans when they are allowed to have a major role in determining goals and objectives of a plan of action.

5. *Feedback:* The supervisor must continually seek feedback from the subordinate and provide support in order to monitor the plan and desired results. The supervisor uses **feedback skills** by responding quickly with praise when results are positive and to situations needing plan corrections before they become a problem.

"Successful people are always looking for opportunities to help others. Unsuccessful people are always asking, 'What's in it for me?'"

—Brian Tracy

Understanding People

Managers cannot promote professional development unless they understand people. They need to be aware of the importance of recognizing differences both in learning and behavioral styles. Awareness can help keep tensions at a minimum. Managers can enhance their knowledge of these learning concepts.

Learn How to Learn
Successful managers are distinguished by their ability to adapt and master change within the organization. This affects their jobs and career demands. All individuals have unique ways of learning, with both strong and weak points. It is important for managers to be aware of their own and subordinates' learning styles and the alternatives made available. Personal and team development can then proceed in the most efficient and effective manner.

Keep Tension at a Minimum
Individuals have different behavioral styles and process information in different ways, which often creates tension. The collaborative manager must be able to perceive these differences and adapt to them to use employees' abilities most effectively. Trust decreases when tension increases. It is important to recognize difference in order to maintain a balance.

Interactive Communication Skills

Communication skills need continual learning. It is the single most important skill we often fail to master both personally and professionally. This section provides an overview and framework for improving communication skills that will assist managers in the evaluation and professional development process.

Questioning:

"Would you tell me, please, which way I ought to go from here?"
"That depends a good deal on where you want to get to," said the Cat.
"I don't much care where—" said Alice.
"Then it doesn't matter which way you go," said the Cat.

—Lewis Carroll, *Alice in Wonderland*

How to ask questions requires practice. To coach the employee successfully the manager must have the ability to ask the right question at the right time. This is critical for the development of collaboration and teamwork. Getting people to "open up" and discover things for themselves is an art. Questions are used to:

1. Gather information.
2. Understand perspectives and frame of reference.
3. Provide information. For example, did you know there is a training program to develop computer skills?
4. Obtain participation.
5. Clarify understanding.
6. Receive opinions and suggestions. This provides an opportunity for positive feedback and building trust.
7. Create consensus to reach agreement or discover differences.

Listening:

The supervisor must attempt to be objective to be successful at listening. Listening is not simply hearing. It requires emotional, intellectual, and physical input in search of truly hearing what is being said. The listener must concentrate and physically demonstrate sensitivity by showing various physical changes, so that the person speaking feels that he or she is being heard. Managers who are poor listeners will miss messages and opportunities, and perhaps, address the wrong problems. More important, the manager who is a poor listener will create distrust.

Barriers to effective listening are the following:

1. No motivation
2. Lack of attention
3. Poor attitude
4. Lack of awareness of good listening skills

5. Inappropriate setting
6. Emotions
7. Prejudices

"I discovered I always have choices and sometimes it's only a choice of attitude."

—Judith M. Knowlton

Image:

First impressions are lasting impressions and the most important.

How others see you often determines how you will be treated. By projecting an image that is professional, authoritative, knowledgeable, successful, and enthusiastic, managers are more likely to be trusted by those they supervise. It is important to develop an image and style that promote trust. To accomplish this goal the manager must pay attention to the following:

1. Body language. How you walk—erect and strong; shake hands—firm; eye contact—direct when appropriate (always consider culture preferences); approachable (smile or pleasant expression).
2. Clothing and accessories—neat and professional, in moderation with current business standards.
3. Demonstrate competencies with respect to knowledge, skills, and ability regarding the field of expertise.
4. Flexibility—requires recognizing differences and willingness to accommodate individual preferences when appropriate. The manager will need to sometimes negotiate and ensure that everybody wins. He or she must be understanding, reasonable, and tactful.
5. Positive/enthusiastic—look for the opportunities. Recognize and praise accomplishments frequently.

Voice Tones:

People usually choose the meaning of what is said rather than how it is said.

The exact words said with a different vocal emphasis can have significantly different meanings. To communicate effectively the manager must be aware of not only the way to say things but also of the vocal intonations of others. This is how to gather more information, meaning, and feeling from the words spoken. How the manager uses his or her voice will help or hurt the development of trust. Build trust with voice tones by:

1. Projecting in a strong and confident resonance.
2. Speaking clearly.
3. Demonstrating enthusiasm through the use of pitch, volume, and inflection.

4. Never speaking in monotones.
5. Using a natural rather than "put-on" voice.
6. Speaking slowly or rapidly depending on the subject and emphasis desired (always pay attention to facial expressions).

How to Develop Feedback Skills

Most managers, even experienced ones, dislike conducting performance evalua-tions because they wish to avoid:

- Conflict
- Taking responsibility for their evaluation of another person's performance
- Giving feedback

Few managers know how to give and receive feedback well. Nevertheless, managers must learn how to give feedback to maximize employees' performance. Managers need to think differently about giving feedback. They need to shift their focus from feedback avoidance to feedback skill development. They must practice how to:

- Establish clear and agreed to goals, expectations, and measurable outcomes.
- Meet on a regular basis to discuss progress.
- Request feedback from the employee on their support.

Key Principles

- *Feedback needs both manager and employee.* A two-way conversation must take place in which both parties speak openly and listen to each other's points of view. When we engage in conversation, we create the opportunity to build collaboration and trust.
- *Feedback must provide for individual focus.* The manager must create a pro-cess that allows both the manager and employee to share individual points of view. When each person brings his or her professional history and value system into the conversation, the results can be much richer.
- *Feedback must begin with what is working.* Managers must always begin by focusing on the positive. How can we do more of the good that is happen-ing? Always be forward focused. When the manager begins with the posi-tive, it sets the stage for good feedback. The manager will not be effective unless he or she genuinely wants to help the employee to be successful.

Managers can put these three principles into action by addressing four key elements when they prepare for performance evaluations: observe, assess, look at performance results, and develop a plan of action (Table 8-3).

TABLE 8-3. Key Elements in Preparing for Performance Evaluations

- **Observe**—Review core responsibilities, goals, and accomplishments.
- **Assess**—What are the results of established measurable outcomes?
- **Results**—Success or failure?
- **Develop**—Plan of action.

Performance Evaluation and Performance Development Approach for Diversity of Employee Workforce

The primary responsibility of all managers is mentoring and providing opportunities for growth and development of their staff. The performance evaluation is the tool for documenting collaborative plans for development. The process provides an opportunity to reflect on the past year and reward the employee for contributions to the organization. It is an opportunity to talk about strengths and what is working. It is the supervisor's responsibility to support the employee with positive feedback and encourage open communications. Employees take pride in their work and want to feel appreciated and respected. A formal process, such as a performance evaluation, offers the opportunity to show appreciation and/ or indicate which activities need improvement. One of the many supervisor responsibilities consists of helping employees contribute to the overall department and/or facility goals through accomplishing specifically defined **performance objectives**. These performance objectives should be kept in mind as the manager completes the evaluation. This evaluation is a critical part of performance development. Employees will be more motivated and much more productive, producing a higher quantity and quality of work when certain principles are followed (Table 8-4).

A well-planned performance development program should provide supervisors and employees with a tool to improve performance and enhance laboratory/institutional effectiveness. By motivating and directing employees' efforts and providing adequate resources, a performance development program can help

TABLE 8-4. Principles of Performance Development

- Clearly define objectives and clearly outline the performance assessment process.
- Clearly define how the employee's work contributes to the overall goals and subsequent success of the laboratory/institution.
- Provide timely and accurate feedback throughout the assessment period (usually a year).
- Provide direction, guidance, and support to employees throughout the assessment period.
- Conduct occasional performance review discussions with written documentation at least two to three times a year.
- Provide recognition and reward linked to excellent performance.

the laboratory and institution achieve their long-range goals and foster improved ongoing communication between supervisors and employees.

"Never become so much of an expert that you stop gaining expertise. View life as a continuous learning experience."

—Denis Waitley

PERFORMANCE EVALUATION AND PERFORMANCE DEVELOPMENT GUIDELINES

Step One: Preparation for Process

1. Ensure that a job/position description is updated and available when the self-evaluation form is submitted to the employee. Oftentimes, if the job description is over 2 years old, this could be a good time to have the employee establish an updated version as part of their annual goals.

2. Review previous goals and feedback meetings, which have taken place during the year.

3. As soon as the employee has completed the self-evaluation, compare notes from previous meetings and compare evaluation of goals.

4. Schedule a mutually agreed upon meeting date for the evaluation well in advance to provide the employee time to prepare.

Step Two: Assessment Preparation

1. Conduct the assessment in a private atmosphere. Sometimes a "neutral" site may be helpful, such as a conference room instead of the manager's office.

2. Consider personal biases and do not allow them to influence the evaluation.

3. Consider the whole period of evaluation, not just the employee's performance at the end of the period.

4. Use the feedback tools and keep the assessment an interactive two-way feedback discussion.

5. Avoid these tendencies:

   - *Consistent leniency:* Tendency to "go easy on people" to be nice to everyone.
   - *Consistent severity:* Tendency to "be too hard on people" to uphold high standards.
   - *Central tendency:* Tendency to rate almost everyone as 'average' on nearly every goal/standard/competency, instead of being more realistic in judgment.

- *Prejudice:* Tendency to allow a personal feeling toward the person being rated to influence judgment, including biases that relate to age, sex, race, nationality, or other non-job-related factors.
- *Other tendencies:* (1) Overlooking problems outside the staff member's control; (2) Blaming the person's "personality;" (3) Allowing the last evaluation to influence judgment on this evaluation; do not be trapped into thinking that you have to give a rating of 'outstanding' because you have in the past; (4) Giving high ratings to those who appear to be most active, rather than those who are most productive (Table 8-5).

"When you talk, you repeat what you already know; when you listen, you often learn something."

—Jared Sparks

An important area in the performance development program is the rating scale, which should be clearly defined and reviewed with the employee during the performance development cycle phase. Table 8-6 gives an example of a rating scale. Definitions and examples of the rating scale should be provided to the employee in clear understandable language. These definitions should serve as guidelines that can be used to measure the level of each employee's performance. Table 8-7 gives some selected examples for each level of rating, but does not represent the comprehensive list available.

TABLE 8-5.   Factors Important in Establishing Clear Performance Objectives and Expectations

- Collaborate on an updated, current, and accurate job description.
- Define reasonable and attainable expectations jointly.
- Review relevance and importance of the expectations to successful performance of the job.
- Expectations should support and relate to the unit/team, laboratory department and/or organizational or professional goals.
- Skills of the employee should match expectations (if not, an action plan should be established to acquire skills).
- Define examples of behavior/results for each performance factor.

TABLE 8-6.   Rating Scales

Outstanding
Above Standards
Meets Standards
Below Standards
Unsatisfactory

TABLE 8-7.   Rating Scale Explanation

Outstanding:

- Performance that exceeds expectations, performing duties above and beyond those of his or her regular job.
- An employee who has taken the initiative to develop new strategies that have benefited the success of the laboratory and/or institution.
- An employee who has improved the work environment by anticipating problems and planning for their solution.
- An employee who creatively designed or developed innovative approaches to achieving success in the workplace.

Above Standards:

- An employee who has shown one or more examples of having the ability to work at a level that exceeds his or her regular job-related duties.
- An employee who continues to show growth and a willingness to improve performance.
- Employee demonstrates unusual proficiency in performing difficult and complex aspects of the job competently and thoroughly, including extra and unique tasks assigned.

Meets Standards:

- Employee's performance meets the criteria and standards of job performance for practically all aspects of the job.
- Performance is steady and reliable and is maintained with a minimum of supervision.
- An employee who regularly performs his or her job functions with reliability and competence.

Below Standards:

- Performance that is in need of improvement in one or more areas related to job duties and responsibilities.
- Performance meets some requirements of the position but does not consistently meet the key, most important duties, responsibilities, requirements, and expectations of the job.
- Occasionally meets the performance expectations, but requires development.

Unsatisfactory:

- Fails to meet expectations and assignments were frequently completed at an unacceptable level of performance.
- Quality of work is poor and requires an unreasonable amount of supervision.
- Consistently fails to meet deadlines and standards of accuracy.

A more concise rating may incorporate a 3 criteria scale of: Exceeds Expectations, Meets Expectations, Below Expectations.

Step Three: Assessment Evaluation

1. A performance evaluation interview is central to the process. It is a formal discussion between the manager and staff member to evaluate how the staff

member is performing in terms of accomplishments, responsibilities, and outcomes, as well as how the staff member can perform more effectively in the future.

2. The purpose of this meeting is to (a) discuss the staff member's self-assessment, (b) give the manager's own assessment, and (c) plan for the next period. The performance evaluation meeting provides both the manager and staff member the opportunity to give and receive feedback on performance. How well the manager uses that opportunity depends in large part on excellent feedback and communication skills.

3. Here are a few tips on how to begin the interview. Make every effort to begin the interview on the right foot, putting the staff member at ease with a friendly and open introduction. The initial few minutes have a great impact on the outcome of the interview.
   - Explain the purpose of the performance evaluation.
   - Let the staff member discuss his or her self-evaluation first.
   - Ask the staff member to discuss, clarify, or elaborate on the information given on the form prepared. This is especially important if the staff member's self-evaluation is dramatically different from the evaluation.
   - Tell the staff member what you agree with first and then what you disagree with. Finally, bring up areas that the staff member has not discussed that are important.
   - Avoid criticizing personality traits.
   - Be objective: talk about measurable, observable behaviors or results.

4. Use effective communication skills:
   - Listen for emotional and logical content.
   - Listen attentively.
   - Allow time for discussion.
   - Coach rather than criticize.
   - Ask for clarification of points you do not understand.
   - Say what you think the speaker is feeling.
   - Be supportive.
   - Observe nonverbal cues.
   - Avoid defensiveness.
   - Emphasize mutual problem solving.
   - Summarize and give feedback.

5. Praise:
   - Be specific.
   - Be direct.
   - Praise often.

6. Use constructive criticism:
   - Be specific.
   - Define desired outcomes.

- Offer suggestions about how to achieve desired outcomes.
- Encourage the staff member by expressing faith that he or she can change.
- Listen attentively to the staff member's response.

7. Before closing, review the interview to make sure:
   - You have made clear the points you wanted to cover.
   - The staff member has expressed his or her ideas thoroughly.
   - You have learned about the staff member's motivations and concerns on the job.
   - The staff member understands your expectations and how you evaluated his or her overall performance.
   - Goals have been set and prioritized or activities defined.
   - An action plan has been cooperatively developed and is mutually supported.

Step Four: Feedback—Interactive and Constant

1. Follow-up with feedback. The performance appraisal process does not end with the evaluation interview. Continue to give feedback consistently throughout the next appraisal period.
2. Make feedback consistent with day-to-day information exchange that you share with the staff member. These comments are usually unplanned and spontaneous, yet should always be clearly stated.
3. To be an effective reinforcer, feedback, whether positive or negative, must occur soon after a behavior.
4. Do not defer dealing with unpleasant issues until the next performance evaluation session. They should be addressed as they occur, which requires direct confrontation.

"Remember not only to say the right thing in the right place, but far more difficult still, to leave unsaid the wrong thing at the tempting moment."

—Benjamin Franklin

Step Five: Mentoring

1. Remove roadblocks to productivity. There are a variety of ways to help support the staff member's work more efficiently and effectively. A large part of improving performance and professional development is a state of mind—a way of doing things better and emphasizing continual improvement.
2. The following are suggestions for removing roadblocks to improve performance and increase opportunities:

- Make necessary resources available.
- Open channels of communication.
- Be flexible with action plan revisions.
- Give staff members information they may need to be effective.
- Provide support for risk taking.
- Give recognition of progress on an ongoing basis.
- Acknowledge achievements departmentally.
- Provide constructive feedback when appropriate.

"Small differences in your performance can lead to large differences in your results."

—Brian Tracy

COMPETENCY MODELING

A method for performance development and evaluation is **competency modeling**. The idea for testing for competence was first proposed in the early 1970s by David McClelland, a former Harvard psychologist. McClelland was asked by the U.S. Foreign Service to find new research methods that could predict human performance and reduce the bias of traditional intelligence and aptitude testing. The definitions of competency, core competency, and competency model follow:

- **Competency:** The knowledge, skill, ability, or characteristic associated with high performance on a job, such as problem solving, analytical thinking, or leadership. Some definitions of a competency include motives, beliefs, and values.

- **Core competency:** Organizational capabilities or strengths—what an organization does best. A core competency might be product development or customer service.

- **Competency model:** A performance evaluation design that uses core competencies (organizational capabilities or strengths, that is, what an organization does best). Examples of such model formats are located later in this chapter.

To construct the appropriate competency model one of the following tools must be used for building the model:

- *Job-analysis interviews:* The interviews can be conducted in person, or in focus groups. Interviews are the best method of data collection.

- *Questionnaires:* Normally used when there are many employees to be interviewed. It is critical, however, to have appropriate questions, a sufficient sample returned, and results analyzed for accuracy.

- *Competency-model formats:* Some models use statistical data to describe the competency requirements in specific detail and use less detail in the competency descriptions. Others reverse the balance.

The competency model for a manager or supervisor might be to identify success factors (competencies), provide a behavioral description of each one, rank-order the factors by criticality, and establish a proficiency level for each factor (Table 8-8). Success factors might include managing change, setting a vision, sharing information, and supporting teams.

TABLE 8-8. Sample Competency Model for a Systems Engineer

Technical Cluster	Proficiency Ratings	
Systems Architecture		
Ability to design complex software applications, establish protocols, and create prototypes.	0-	Is not able to perform basic tasks.
	1-	Understands basic principles; can perform tasks with assistance or direction.
	2-	Performs routine tasks with reliable results; works with minimal supervision.
	3-	Performs complex and multiple tasks; can coach or teach others.
	4-	Considered an expert in this task; can describe, teach, and lead others.
Data Migration		
Ability to establish the necessary platform requirements to efficiently and completely coordinate data transfer.	0-	Is not able to perform basic tasks.
	1-	Understands basic principles; can perform tasks with assistance or direction.
	2-	Performs routine tasks with reliable results; works with minimal supervision.
	3-	Performs complex and multiple tasks; can coach or teach others.
	4-	Considered an expert in this task; can describe, teach, and lead others.
Documentation		
Ability to prepare comprehensive and complete documentation including specifications, flow diagrams, process control, and budgets.	0-	Is not able to perform basic tasks.
	1-	Understands basic principles; can perform tasks with assistance or direction.
	2-	Performs routine tasks with reliable results; works with minimal supervision.
	3-	Performs complex and multiple tasks; can coach or teach others.
	4-	Considered an expert in this task; can describe, teach and lead others.

Competency models must be governed by the collective wisdom of the people that need and build them. The decision to use a particular type of competency model should be determined by the desired applications.

If competency modeling is used, the self-appraisal form should be adjusted by replacing core responsibility with core competency or competencies. An example of a self-appraisal form is included in Appendix 8-A.

SUMMARY

The performance development program can be an excellent tool for professional development of both employees and supervisors. By using this program, employees can be introduced to the basic principles of professional development, which are built on the foundation of a commitment to learning, independent thinking, a willingness to share expertise, and the development of professional pride. Specific performance and measurable results are used to establish a common understanding of the employees' performance strengths and weaknesses. Performance discussions are based on previously agreed to, job-related factors important to the overall success on the job. Performance discussions are highly individualized and reflect employees' unique goals, abilities, and development needs.

The performance management program guides the employee in analyzing his or her own performance and with the support from the supervisor, the employee can both understand strengths and define improvement needs. The performance discussion should be based on the entire review period and not on just recent performance. All the meetings should incorporate constructive criticism and focus on how to improve performance rather than reiterating past failures or shortcomings. Using a well-planned and implemented performance development program should allow the employee to address professional issues, interpersonal skills, career planning, goal setting, and foster pride and recognition of the employees' strengths and contributions to the laboratory/institution.

SUMMARY CHART:
Important Points to Remember

➤ Performance evaluation should be based on standards detailed in the job description.

➤ Feedback on performance should be ongoing, and interlocked directly with expected actions and outcomes of the job responsibilities.

➤ A developmental action plan is goal-oriented with clearly stated measurable outcomes.

➤ A performance assessment should involve a self-evaluation with management feedback.

➤ Interactive feedback and recognition is a key to a collaborative, open and honest performance evaluation.

➤ A collaborative management process creates a trust relationship, defines problem solutions, and supports risk taking through coaching and follow-up communication.

➤ The four basic tenets of collaborative management are Trust, Understanding, Independence, and Solutions.

➤ Successful communication involves understanding, active listening, and verbal/non-verbal skill sets.

➤ Successful managers are adaptable and flexible while mastering change in their organization.

➤ Guidelines for successful performance evaluations are Preparation for the Process, Assessment Preparation, Evaluation, Interactive Feedback and Mentoring.

➤ Competency modeling is a performance evaluation design that uses core competencies needed to achieve organizational success.

➤ A rating scale based on objective criteria of the job description and responsibility is a valuable tool for specific competencies reviewed in the performance evaluation.

➤ Building a relationship of trust and openness will drive a win-win approach to effective performance and professional development.

➤ Feedback should always be forward-focused, and emphasize what is working to set the stage for improving performance and success.

➤ Diversity in background and culture of the workforce requires adaptability in both relationship building and motivation of the employee, and continuous learning by both employee and supervisor.

Suggested Problem-Based Learning Activities

Chapter 8: Performance Evaluation and Development

Instructions: Use Internet resources, books, articles, colleagues, etc., to present solutions to the problems listed below. There is no one correct solution to any problem.

Note to Instructor: Students in class may be divided into groups and given the problem-based learning activity to discuss and solve. Once the group has reached consensus as to a solution, the group may present it to the other students in the class. This activity will provide all students with information regarding solutions to the problem.

Problem #1

Suppose a minority employee feels that he or she was not promoted based on their minority status. As manager, how do you handle this situation?

Problem #2

Design a performance appraisal and supporting documents to be used in your laboratory.

Problem #3

Create a problem employee and prepare a plan of action for correcting the issues relating to this problem behavior.

BIBLIOGRAPHY

Bridges W: *Managing Transitions.* Harper Collins Publishers, New York, NY, 1991.

Butteriss M: *Re-Inventing HR Changing Roles to Create the High-Performance Organization.* John Wiley & Sons Canada Limited, Etobicoke, Ontario, 1998.

Chang RY, De Young P: *Measuring Organizational Improvement Impact.* Richard Chang Associates, Inc. Publications Division, Irvine, CA, 1995.

Citrin JM, Smith RA: *The Five Patterns of Extraordinary Careers: The Guide for Achieving Success and Satisfaction.* Crown Business, New York, NY, 2003.

Conger JA: *Learning to Lead.* Jossey-Bass Publishers, San Francisco, CA, 1992.

Covey SR: *Principle Centered Leadership.* Summit Books, New York, NY, 1991.

Dichter E: *Motivating Human Behavior.* McGraw-Hill Book Company, New York, NY, 1971.

Dotlich DL, Cairo PC: *Action Coaching.* Jossey-Bass Publishers, San Francisco, CA, 1999.

Fisher R, Ury W: *Getting to Yes.* Penguin Books, New York, NY, 1992.

Gilbert TF: *Measuring Potential for Performance Improvement.* Lakewood Publications, Minneapolis, MN, 2003.

Hunsaker PL, Alessandra AP. Building productive managerial relationships. In *The New Art of Managing People,* 2nd ed. Simon & Schuster, New York, NY, 2008.

Jones JE, Bearley WL: *360 Degree Feedback.* HRD Press & Lakewood Publications, Amherst, MA, 1996.

Kravetz DJ: *The Directory for Building Competencies.* Kravetz Associates, Bartlett, IL, 1995.

Krugg D: *Enlightened Leadership.* Enlightened Leadership International, Inc. Englewood, CO, 1998.

Neal JE: *Effective Phrases for Performance Appraisals: A Guide to Successful Evaluations,* 9th ed. Neal Publications, 2000.

Nigon DL: *Clinical Laboratory Management, Leadership Principles for the 21st Century.* McGraw-Hill Health Professions Division, New York, NY, 2000.

Rummler GA: *Performance Is The Purpose.* Lakewood Publications, Minneapolis, MN, 2002.

Simmons A: When Performance Reviews Fail. *T+D Magazine,* September 2004.

Tjosvold D: *Learning to Manage Conflict.* Lexington Books, New York, NY, 1993.

Varnadoe LA: *Medical Laboratory Management and Supervision.* F.A. Davis, Philadelphia, PA, 1996.

INTERNET RESOURCES

Employee Appraisal, SuccessFactors, Inc., 2010.
http://www.successfactors.com/topics/employee-appraisal/

Human Resources Internet Guide. HR—Guide, 2010.
http://www.hr-guide.com

Institute for Professional Development, 2004.
http://www.ipd.org

McNamara, C: Performance Management: Performance Appraisal (Generic to Performance Management). Free Management Library, © Copyright Authenticity Consulting, LLC., 2010.
http://www.managementhelp.org/perf_mng/appraisl.htm

Pam Pohly's Net Guide: Management Resources for Healthcare & Medical Professionals. Pam Pohly, 2011.
http://www.pohly.com/

Pam Pohly's Net Guide: Toolbox for Health Managers & Administrators. Pam Pohly, 2011.
http://www.pohly.com/admin.html

Powerful Tools for Positive Performance. American Productivity & Quality Center, Houston, TX, 2010.
http://www.apqc.org

Tapped In. SRI International, 2010.
http://www.tappedin.org

APPENDIX 8-A: SAMPLE/SELF-APPRAISAL

*Employee Name:*_____

Project/Location: _____*Supervisor:* _____

Period Covered: *From:* _____ *To:* _____

1. *Attached is the most recent description for your position. Does this description accurately reflect your current duties and responsibilities?*_____ *Yes* _____*No* (*if No, attached edited/updated job description*)

2. *Based on your position description, indicate your core responsibilities and what was accomplished during the year. Please include responsibilities relating to customer service, whether external or internal customers. Indicate where previous objectives were accomplished and where they were not met. Please include any special projects or assignments that were outside of your normal day-to-day responsibilities or other major accomplishments.*

Core Responsibilities	Accomplishments
Supervisor's Remarks:	

If appropriate:

Special Assignments/ Objectives from the Prior Year	Target Date	Accomplishments
Supervisor's Remarks:		

(*Continued*)

APPENDIX 8-A (*Continued*)

3. *What are the strengths of your performance? How would you improve the way you perform your responsibilities? Consider the performance factors indicated in the introduction and any others you feel appropriate in your response. These may include:*

Commitment to Excellence	*Communication*
Job Knowledge	*(Listening as well as Expressing)*
Customer Knowledge	*Initiative and Independent*
Administrative Capabilities	*Action*
Decision Making	*Managing Resources*
Teamwork	*Contributions to Stated Goals*
Problem Solving	*Professional Behavior*
Human Relations Skills	

Supervisor's Remarks:

4. *What roadblocks did you encounter in your position during the appraisal period? Include difficulties that were within and outside your control. What assistance from the organization or your supervisor would be helpful to you in meeting these challenges in the future?*

5. *What additional responsibilities would you recommend for yourself? Are there aspects of your position you would like to change or improve? What actions are you currently taking or planning to take to further develop your skills and potential in this position? What actions can your supervisor, co-workers, or company take to assist you?*

6. *In preparation for your upcoming discussion with your supervisor, list at least three possible performance objectives for yourself for the coming year. (Because each position has different responsibilities the number of objectives will vary depending on the position.) Please list them in order of priority, beginning with your highest priorities.*

These objectives should be related to the key responsibilities of your position and, as much as possible, to the mission and plans of your department and the organization. Consider the corporate objectives and the objectives of your customers, and how your objectives relate to them. Focus on long-term objectives as well as short-term. Each of us should include specific objectives relating to customer service and how to improve quality service.

Objectives should include continuous improvement and/or growth in a position rather than simply a continuation of current responsibilities and how you carry

APPENDIX 8-A (*Continued*)

them out. What can be improved? How can quality be assured? How can we assist the customer further?

If improvements are needed in particular areas of your performance, develop objectives for those improvements. Be as specific as possible.

Objectives may involve acquiring new knowledge and skills, improvements in activities in which you are already involved, and new activities and projects. Objectives should be specific, measurable in terms of quantity or quality, useful and attainable (although significant effort may be required).

Briefly describe each objective, include a timetable, and any resources or training you might need in order to achieve your objectives.

Objective 1: (Regarding Organizational Goals)

_____

Timetable: _____

Resources or Training Necessary: _____

Objective 2: (Regarding Teamwork/Departmental Goals)

_____

Timetable: _____

Resources or Training Necessary: _____

Objective 3: (Regarding Personal/Professional Development)

_____

Timetable: _____

Resources or Training Necessary: _____

Feel free to attach additional sheets as necessary.
Please feel free to include any additional comments or suggestions you care to make.

_____

Employee's Signature   ***Date***

_____

Supervisor's Signature   ***Date***   ***Date of Appraisal***
                                                    Discussion

(Continued)

APPENDIX 8-A (*Continued*)

SUPERVISOR'S SUMMARY

Provide an overall summary of the meeting with the employee. Include discussion of any areas of disagreement between yourself and the employee. You may want to describe the strengths of the employee's performance. Please indicate if any improvements are needed for satisfactory performance.

Indicate overall description of the employee's performance:
_____ *Unsatisfactory/Needs Significant Improvement*
_____ *Below Standards*
_____ *Meets Standards*
_____ *Above Standards*
_____ *Outstanding*

_____   _____

Supervisor's Signature   *Date*

_____   _____

Manager's Signature   *Date*

_____   _____

Employee's Signature   *Date*

CHAPTER 9

Education and Training: Practical Tips for Educators and Trainers

Denise M. Harmening, Phd, MT(ASCP), CLS(NCA)
Amber G. Tuten, Med, MLS(ASCP)^{CM}, DLM(ASCP)^{CM}

CHAPTER OUTLINE

Objectives
Key Terms
Case Study
Introduction
Domains and Levels of
   Learning
Application of Instructional
   Objectives as Learning
   Outcomes
Assigning Taxonomy Levels to
   Educational Objectives

Matching the Level of Instruction
   to the Needs of the Learner and
   the Task
The Clinical Preceptor
Summary
Summary Chart: Important Points
   to Remember
Suggested Problem-Based Learning
   Activities
Bibliography
Internet Resources

OBJECTIVES

Following successful completion of this chapter, the learner will be able to:

1. List and define the three domains of learning.
2. List Bloom's taxonomy levels.
3. Apply Bloom's taxonomy levels to the construction of behavioral objectives.
4. Assign taxonomy levels to the educational objectives.
5. Define learning outcomes.

KEY TERMS

Affective Domain   Learning Outcome
Cognitive Domain   Psychomotor Domain
Instructional/Educational Objectives   Taxonomy Levels

Case Study — Education and Training: Practical Tips for Educators and Trainers

You are a manager of a laboratory at a large university-based hospital in an academic health center. You have received complaints from your employees that "Mary" is not a team player. You have observed that Mary prefers to work alone and is not receptive to training student interns. At times, she can be abrasive toward others; however, she is extremely knowledgeable and her work is meticulous and accurate. She is never late and has never used sick time in her 5-year tenure with your department. Your counseling meeting with Mary reveals that she is intimidated by the prospect of training student interns because she has no background or experience in providing instruction.

Issues and Questions to Consider:

1. *Evaluate Mary's potential as an instructor in your laboratory. Assess both her strengths and weaknesses.*
2. *How would you approach facilitating Mary's participation in the clinical training of student interns?*
3. *At the most basic level, what would Mary need to know to match the level of instruction to the needs of the learner?*
4. *How would Mary develop specific learning objectives for the student interns?*
5. *What would Mary need to do to ensure that the learning outcomes were met?*

INTRODUCTION

In a teaching hospital, many individuals are required to provide instruction as part of their job without any formal training in education. One of their most difficult tasks is planning for instruction and matching the level of instruction to the needs of the learner. For example, training objectives for laboratory technicians who have two years of college education should be at a different level than technologists who have four years of college. *Training* at a specialist level would require an even higher level of complexity. Regardless of the level of instruction, it has been well established that the educational process of teaching and learning are significantly enhanced if both the teacher and learner have a clear definition

TABLE 9-1.　The Three Domains of Learning

Domain	Definition
Cognitive	Acquiring and applying knowledge
Psychomotor	Ability to perform tasks or skills
Affective	Attitudes or feelings

of the expected **learning outcome** for the instructional task; however, several differences exist in expectations for learning outcomes.

For example, in some cases the learner is expected to acquire or apply knowledge; in other situations, the learner is expected to develop a skill or demonstrate proficiency. Even still, in other instances the outcome requires the learner to acquire an appropriate attitude or work ethic toward a task. These different educational outcomes define what is commonly known as the three "domains of learning" (Table 9-1).

DOMAINS AND LEVELS OF LEARNING

This chapter provides the learner with an overview of the domains and levels of learning followed by an in-depth discussion of the design and application of instructional objectives as learning outcomes. In addition, the chapter also describes the process of assigning learning levels to instructional objectives, as well as matching the level of instruction to the needs of the learner and the task.

The different levels of learning or **taxonomy levels** describe how a learner may progress from beginner to expert in each domain of learning. The main purpose of the taxonomy levels is to aid the instructor in defining the different learning outcomes. By using taxonomy levels, specific learning objectives can be developed starting with a basic level and progressing to increasing levels of difficulty in all three domains of learning (Table 9-2).

The taxonomy level for the **cognitive domain** is probably the most recognized and well used of those currently developed. This taxonomy level was formulated in 1958 by a committee headed by Dr. Benjamin Bloom and is now commonly referred to as Bloom's taxonomy levels. Table 9-3 lists and defines the six taxonomy levels of the cognitive domain.

If objectives in the cognitive domain are well written, the intended learning outcomes should be clear and easy to measure through testing. A major problem experienced by educators in this domain is that the six levels overlap, creating some confusion related to the correct level in which to place the objective. As a result, Bloom et al. have listed a number of verbs that can be used in writing objectives. The intended purpose of this list is to facilitate the selection of the correct verb in writing the instructional objective. The taxonomy level is defined by the verb. Table 9-4 lists the verbs (behavioral terms) and instructional objectives of the various taxonomy levels of the cognitive domain.

Many educators and trainers find these verbs helpful. Irrespective of the verb used, however, one should keep in mind the intent of the objective regardless of

TABLE 9-2.   Taxonomy Levels of the Three Domains of Learning

Cognitive	Psychomotor	Affective
Levels of Understanding	*Levels of Psychomotor Development*	*Levels of Feeling*
1. Knowledge	1. Reflex movements	1. Receiving
2. Comprehension	2. Basic fundamental	2. Responding
3. Application	movements	3. Valuing
4. Analysis	3. Perceptual abilities	4. Organization
5. Synthesis	4. Physical abilities	5. Characterization
6. Evaluation	5. Skilled movements	
	6. Non-discursive movement	

TABLE 9-3.   Bloom's Taxonomy Levels

1. **KNOWLEDGE: (Recall) The remembering of previously learned material.** This may involve the recall of material ranging from specific facts to complete theories, but all that is required is the bringing to mind of the appropriate information. Knowledge is defined as the remembering of previously learned material.

2. **COMPREHENSION: (Understanding) The ability to grasp the meaning of material.** This may be shown by translating the material from one form to another (words to numbers), by interpreting material (explaining or summarizing), and by estimating future trends (predicting consequences or effects). Comprehension is defined as the ability to grasp the meaning of material. These learning outcomes go one step beyond the simple remembering of material and represent the lowest level of understanding.

3. **APPLICATION: The ability to use the learned material in new and concrete situations.** This may include such things as rules, methods, concepts, principles, laws, and theories. Application refers to the ability to use learned material in new and concrete situations. Learning outcomes in this area require a higher level of understanding than those under comprehension.

4. **ANALYSIS: The ability to break down learned material into its component parts so that its organizational structure can be understood.** This may include identification of the parts, analysis of the relationship between the parts, and recognition of the organizational principles involved. Analysis refers to the ability to break down material into its component parts so that its organizational structure may be understood. Learning outcomes here represent a higher intellectual level than comprehension and application because they require an understanding of both the content and the structural form of the material.

5. **SYNTHESIS: The ability to put parts together to form a new whole.** This area stresses creative behaviors with emphasis on formulation of *new* patterns or structures. Synthesis refers to the ability to put parts together to form a new whole. This may involve the production of a unique communication (theme or speech), a plan of operations (research proposal), or a set of abstract relations (scheme for classifying information). Learning outcomes in this area stress creative behaviors, with major emphasis on the formulation of new patterns or structures.

6. **EVALUATION: The ability to judge the value of material for a given purpose.** Judgments are based on definite criteria. These may be internal criteria (organization) or external criteria (relevance to the purpose), and the student may determine the criteria or be given them. Evaluation is concerned with the ability to judge the value of material (statement, novel, poem, research report) for a given purpose. Learning outcomes in this area are highest in the cognitive hierarchy because they contain elements of all of the other categories, plus conscious value judgments based on clearly defined criteria.

TABLE 9-4. Verbs (Behavioral Terms) and Instructional Objectives of the Taxonomy Levels of the Cognitive Domain

Taxonomy Level	Verbs (Behavioral Terms)	Instructional Objectives
Knowledge	Defines, describes, labels, identifies, matches, names, states, selects	*Know* terms, facts, methods, procedures, concepts, principles
Comprehensive	Explains, estimates, infers, distinguishes, defends, converts, generalizes, gives examples, summarizes, paraphrases, rewrites	*Understand* facts and principles, *interpret* charts and graphs, *translate* verbal to mathematical formulas, *estimate* future consequences inferred from data
Application	Changes, calculates, demonstrates, discovers, manipulates, modifies, operates, predicts, prepares, produces, relates, shows, solves, uses	*Applies* concepts and principles to new situations, *applies* laws and theories to practical situations, *solves* mathematical problems, *constructs* charts or graphs
Analysis	Breaks down, diagrams, differentiates, distinguishes, identifies, illustrates, infers, outlines, points out, relates, selects, separates, subdivides	*Recognizes* unstated assumptions, *evaluates* relevancy of the data, *distinguishes* between facts and inferences
Synthesis	Categorizes, combines, complies, composes, creates, designs, generates, modifies	*Proposes* or *plans* a new entity, *integrates* learning from different parts to solve a problem, *formulates* a new concept
Evaluation	Appraises, compares, concludes, criticizes, justifies, interprets, explains, supports, describes	*Judges* the value of written material and the value of work by use of internal criteria or external standards of excellence

experience in writing objectives. The verb used for the intended learning outcome may be interpreted differently by the learner. For example, the verb *illustrate* in an objective may be intended to have the learning outcome be a drawing or diagram of a complex structure, but the learner may interpret this verb to mean that he or she must point out something to satisfy the learning objective. The best way to learn to use Bloom's taxonomy levels is to provide some examples which are presented in the next section.

In practice, the taxonomy levels of the cognitive domain are by far the most widely used; however, the psychomotor and affective domains are not well used in educational settings.

The **psychomotor domain** can be well used in the laboratory training area to define the level of competency expected of a learner in performing a variety of tasks, for example, performing tests with a 100% accuracy or operating instrumentation. Once the objectives are written for this domain, the learning outcomes are relatively easy to measure. Measurement may require a checklist of steps to be completed for a procedure or performance of the task with 100% accuracy or within a specified time frame. Practical examinations are frequently used to assess objectives written in the psychomotor domain. A simple check or "s", "u" grading system is not sufficient to evaluate psychomotor objectives. A rubric with well defined categories should be created that assists the evaluator in determining levels of skill to make grading less subjective.

The **affective domain** can be helpful in defining learning expectations for students with respect to work ethic, initiative, interpersonal skills with co-workers, patient confidentiality of laboratory results, and professional interaction with other individuals on the healthcare team. The major problem experienced by most educators or trainers is that objectives in this domain are difficult to write and even more difficult to measure objectively and quantitatively.

The National Accrediting Agency for Clinical Laboratory Science (NAACLS) currently requires that clinical and didactic educational objectives be written in all three domains. The didactic training should involve more cognitive learning

TABLE 9-5.   Examples of Immunohematology Clinical Educational Objectives

On completion of the immunohematology rotation the student will be able to meet the following objectives within acceptable limits as determined by the clinical faculty.

1. Evaluate quality control in the immunohematology laboratory and formulate a logical course of action when reagent controls fall outside normal limits.
2. Perform ABO and Rh grouping including weak D (formerly Du) status on designated patients and donor units.
3. Describe the principle and applications of direct antiglobulin testing and include the follow-up testing of positive direct antiglobulin tests.
4. Perform antibody screening and identification procedures and select any of the following special techniques that may be useful for investigating antibody problems:

   - Elution
   - Enzyme treatment
   - Enhancement media
   - Adsorption
   - Temperature manipulation
   - Neutralization (optional)

5. List the federal, state, and peer review agencies and committees that monitor blood banks and transfusion services.
6. Compare and contrast the following adverse reactions to transfusion in regard to cause, classic signs and symptoms, recommendations for future transfusion, and serologic investigation (if applicable).

   - Immediate hemolytic
   - Delayed hemolytic
   - Febrile nonhemolytic
   - Urticarial
   - Anaphylactic
   - Bacterial

7. Formulate a strategy for troubleshooting basic problems in technique and procedure.
8. Exhibit professional attributes and attitudes and maintain professional standards when interacting with professionals within the laboratory and the healthcare facility.

objectives and the clinical setting more psychomotor. Table 9-5 lists examples of clinical educational objectives for the blood bank laboratory rotations of the University of Maryland School of Medicine's Medical Technology program. The reader should quickly review this list and classify the domain of learning for each objective.

APPLICATION OF INSTRUCTIONAL OBJECTIVES AS LEARNING OUTCOMES

Instructional/educational objectives may be written in many different formats. It is important to use instructional objectives to balance the level of instruction with the needs of the learner. Achieving this balance with clearly written objectives will provide the basis for the measurable outcome assessment. One of the most common errors in writing objectives is to state the objective in a manner that focuses attention on the teaching activity rather than the learning outcome, for example, to demonstrate to students how to use a cell washer. Can this be measured as a learning outcome for the student? Actually, the educator has achieved this objective once the demonstration is completed. A better way to write this objective is in terms of the type of learning outcomes we expect. After the teacher's demonstration, the objectives may be written as follows: After observing the demonstration, the learner will be able to:

(Cognitive)   1. Describe the steps of proper operation of the blood bank cell washer.

(Cognitive)   2. List the precautions necessary when using the cell washer.

(Cognitive)   3. List the steps for calibration of the cell washer.

(Psychomotor)   4. Demonstrate skill by using the cell washer with acceptable motor performance for five patient samples.

Instructional objectives written in this format place the focus on the student and the type of knowledge and proficiency required as a result of the learning experience. A shift in focus from the learning process to the learning outcomes clarifies the intent of the instruction and sets the stage for evaluation of that instruction. The verbs *describe, list,* and *demonstrate* are specific types of behavior that indicate how the student shows that he or she has learned. Furthermore, these objectives are easily measured. It is important to be able to distinguish between stating objectives in terms of what will be taught and learning outcomes expected from students.

Read the following two objectives and decide which one is stated as an expected learning outcome.

The learner will be able to:

1. Instill an appreciation for the different types of transfusion reactions.

2. List and define the different types of transfusion reactions.

Clearly, the second objective specifies how a student will demonstrate learning after the instructional period. Note the second objective begins with a verb that implies an activity (which can be measured) on the part of the student.

An educational objective should clearly indicate the intent of the instruction in terms of the type of behavior ("list and define") that the student is expected to demonstrate.

The verb in the first objective, *instills*, implies that the *teacher*, not the student, is engaged in the activity, and the objective cannot be appropriately measured. Stating educational or instructional objectives as learning outcomes contributes to the instructional process by:

1. Providing direction for the educator/trainer.
2. Conveying clearly the instructional intent to others.
3. Providing a guide for instructional content, teaching methods, and materials to be used during instruction.
4. Providing a guide for constructing tests and other methods of evaluation of student competency.

A common error made in teaching is neglecting to use the educational objectives to construct tests. As a result the student does not know what is important and is not guided or focused in the learning process; consequently, the test may not be a valid measure of the student's knowledge or proficiency.

Another common error in writing objectives is stating the objective in terms of the learning process instead of the learning outcome. Which of the following objectives is stated as an instructional/learning outcome?

The learner will be able to:

1. Gain knowledge of antigen-antibody reactions
2. Apply the basic principles of antigen-antibody reactions in performing ABO typing

The second objective clearly indicates what the student can do at the end of instruction. The first objective focuses on the "gaining of knowledge" (the learning process) rather than the type of behavior that provides evidence of the expected outcome of the learning experience.

These errors of stating objectives in terms of the teacher's performance and the learning process can be avoided by focusing on the type of student performance expected (learning outcome) at the end of instruction. To summarize, instructional/educational objectives should be concise, clear statements that define instructional intent in terms of the desired learning outcomes.

ASSIGNING TAXONOMY LEVELS TO EDUCATIONAL OBJECTIVES

One of the most difficult tasks is selecting the proper taxonomy level for the objective in the domain of learning. NAACLS requires, as a part of their accreditation process, that Medical Technology/Clinical Laboratory Science programs use objectives in various taxonomy levels and that examination questions assign taxonomy levels. The reader should refer to Table 9-3, which lists and defines Bloom's taxonomy levels, before working through the following examples:

Level 1, *knowledge,* involves recall, the remembering of previously learned material. This simplest level of learning requires basic memorization of information that may range from simple facts to complex principles or theories.

Example

The student will be able to list the hemoglobin/hematocrit required for the donation of blood.

Level 2, *comprehension,* is the ability to grasp the meaning of the material or information. This usually requires interpretation of information to indicate learning.

Example

The student will be able to interpret the ABO group from the serologic reactions listed for each patient.

Level 3, *application,* requires the ability to use the learned material in new and defined situations.

Example

The student will be able to calculate the number of platelet units needed to increase a patient's platelet count from 10,000 to 50,000.

Level 4, *analysis,* requires using the first three levels of knowledge, comprehension, and application previously described. It represents the ability to break down learned material into component parts so that the overall structure or organization can be understood. The level requires the learner to demonstrate insight in selecting the most significant parts of the material, identifying important components, and understanding relationships. The learner must be able to distinguish relevant from irrelevant information, distinguish facts from assumptions, and identify the underlying principles of the concepts.

Example

The student will be able to select the appropriate product for transfusion after review and interpretation of the patient's clinical history and laboratory results.

Level 5, *synthesis*, is the ability to put parts or components together to form a new whole. This level requires the learner to combine elements to form something new through some creative or intuitive process. The learner is expected to develop an original application of the material learned.

Example

The student will be able to design a protocol for the investigation of hemolytic transfusion reactions in a 350-bed community hospital.

Level 6, *evaluation*, is the ability to judge the value of material for a given purpose. This is the highest level of understanding and requires the learner to use all five taxonomy levels in forming an assessment or judgment. This level usually involves the use of values and value judgments. Evaluation implies the determination of the value or quality of information in making a judgment that is usually based on appropriate established criteria. Evaluation involves making judgments based on factual information or values.

Example

Using the criteria for "ruling-out," the student will determine the appropriate "selective cells" to identify the patient's antibody(ies).

By now, it is apparent that trying to use all six taxonomy levels, which greatly overlap, for writing educational objectives is not only burdensome, but impractical for our field. As a result, most educators use the abbreviated version of taxonomy levels published by the American Society for Clinical Pathology (ASCP) (Table 9-6). In practice, these three levels are used to assign taxonomy levels for test questions used for the certifying examinations given by the ASCP Board of Registry. In addition, Standard 22 of the NAACLS self-study process also requires assignment of taxonomy levels for test questions used in Clinical Laboratory science programs.

In the cognitive domain of learning, the Bloom's taxonomy levels can be correlated with the ASCP levels by arbitrarily assigning: knowledge as taxonomy level 1; comprehension and application as level 2; and analysis, synthesis, and evaluation as level 3.

TABLE 9-6.   ASCP Taxonomy Levels

TAXONOMY 1 — *Recall:* Ability to recall or recognize previously learned (memorized) knowledge ranging from specific facts to complete theories.

TAXONOMY 2 — *Interpretive Skills:* Ability to use recalled knowledge to interpret or apply verbal, numeric, or visual data.

TAXONOMY 3 — *Problem Solving:* Ability to use recalled knowledge and the interpretation/application of distinct criteria to resolve a problem or situation and/or make an appropriate decision.

MATCHING THE LEVEL OF INSTRUCTION TO THE NEEDS OF THE LEARNER AND THE TASK

The final component in planning for clinical instruction is to match the level of instruction to the needs of the learner. Clinical laboratory instructors must possess the ability to train individuals at several different levels of education and to ensure that the training received at each is appropriate to the tasks. Clinical rotational training is especially difficult for both the student and the clinical instructor because of variations that exist among laboratories. Numerous factors affect the student's clinical rotation experience, including the type and size of the laboratory, geographic region, urban versus rural setting, patient population, and knowledge and expertise of laboratory clinical instructors. Too often, clinical training is tied to the resources available within the laboratory rather than to the knowledge and proficiency needs of the learner. Furthermore, the clinical instructor is faced with the ongoing debate regarding which tasks should be associated with technologists at the various levels of education. For example, a clinical laboratory instructor employed in a large, urban, teaching hospital affiliated with a School of Medicine presented a student with a patient sample containing four unknown antibodies, one of which was anti-G. If one were to match the needs of the learner with this antibody exercise, what would be the appropriate educational level of the student, MLT, MLS, or Specialist? Believe it or not, this sample was presented to an undergraduate MLS student, and the clinical instructor firmly believed that MLSs should be proficient in performing specialized antibody techniques. The confusion with regard to matching the level of instruction to the needs of the learner is understandable when clinical educators lack appropriate information on which to base their clinical instruction.

An excellent resource for clinical instructors is the report from the ASCLS position paper dated July 25, 2009. Entitled, *Practice Levels and Educational Needs for Clinical Laboratory Personnel,* the report delineates the knowledge and abilities expected of career-entry graduates.

Table 9-7 further summarizes the knowledge and ability associated with immunohematology/blood bank procedures and tests as required at various learner levels. The ability to perform specialized high-frequency/low-frequency antibody techniques is not considered appropriate at the medical laboratory scientist level, but rather should be an integral part of the training at the specialist level.

THE CLINICAL PRECEPTOR

One of the greatest ways to contribute to the profession of medical laboratory science is to serve as a clinical preceptor assisting in the training of new medical laboratory scientists and medical laboratory technicians during their clinical rotations. In the case study at the beginning of this chapter, Mary did not feel comfortable serving

TABLE 9-7.   Examples of Consensus Results: Immunohematology/Blood Bank

Knowledge	Ability
A—Specimen collection, labeling, storage, and preparation	A—None required
B—Immunologic genetic theory	B—Has observed
C—Principles of methods including recognition and resolution of common problems	C—Has performed satisfactorily on practice specimens; may require additional experience
D—Disease manifestation/clinical correlations	D—Proficient; able to perform in job setting after usual employee orientation
E—Differentiates/resolves technical, instrument, physiologic causes of problems or unexpected test results	

	Knowledge		Ability	
Competencies	MLS	MLT	MLS	MLT
ABO blood typing	A, B, C, D, E	A, B, C, D, E	D	D
Rh blood grouping	A, B, C, D, E	A, B, C, D, E	D	D
Kell/Kidd Duffy systems	A, B, C, D, E	A, C, D	C	C
Miscellaneous blood group systems	None	None	A	A
Antibody screen	A, B, C, D, E	A, B, C, D	D	D
Antibody identification	A, B, C, D, E	A, B, C, D	D	C
Antibody titering	A, B, C, D, E	A, C	C	B
Elutions	A, B, C, D, E	A, C	C	B
Cold antibody workup using IgG AHG	A, B, C, D, E	C	C	A
Antibody removal by ZZAP	A, C	None	A	A
HLA testing	B, C, D	None	A	A

as a clinical preceptor. To be a good clinical preceptor, one must not feel intimidated by teaching. Students will ask questions that the preceptor may not readily be able to answer, but may be seen as a learning opportunity for both the student and the preceptor. It is perfectly acceptable to say, "I do not know, but let's find out."

When teaching a student or a new employee a test procedure, be sure to use a method similar to the following:

1. **Discuss:** Have the student read the procedure and discuss the individual steps to be sure he understands how the test is performed.

2. **Demonstrate:** Demonstrate a procedure, explaining each step, while the student follows along with the written procedure.

3. **Guided practice:** Let the student perform the procedure under your guidance, allowing him to ask questions along the way, while following the written procedure.

4. **Independent practice:** Have the student perform the test without asking questions while you watch.

5. **Evaluate:** After the student has practiced the test independently several times, evaluate the skill level achieved.

In evaluating students, be cognizant of the "halo" effect, where preceptors tend to assign better grades to students with personalities similar to theirs regardless of skill level, or tend to give all students high or low grades. Creating grading rubrics will assist in making the evaluation of all students less biased than standard check-off forms. An example of a simple rubric for the evaluation of the basic cross-match is included in Table 9-8.

Above all, enjoy sharing your knowledge and expertise. By serving as a clinical preceptor you are contributing to the future of the profession and to a standard of excellence in healthcare.

TABLE 9-8. Immunohematology Competency

Cross-Match
Immunohematology Clinical Practicum

In order to meet the cross-match competency, the student must perform a cross-match, using proper procedure and technique, with 100% accuracy within a 20-minute time limit.
Student Name: _____

Total Scores:

95 - 100%

Technique is <u>good</u> with proper procedure, steps and technique. Student interpreted result accurately and <u>required no assistance or prompting.</u>

80 - 94%

Technique is <u>adequate</u> with proper procedure, steps and technique. Student <u>required minimal prompting or assistance.</u>

70 - 79%

Technique is <u>minimally adequate</u> with proper procedure steps, and technique. Student <u>required prompting or assistance</u> with several steps.

Failure to meet competency

Technique is <u>inadequate</u> with failure to follow proper procedure steps, and technique. Student cannot perform this task without <u>constant assistance or prompting.</u>
Evaluator should use the following point system to evaluate each step in the procedure:

(Continued)

TABLE 9-8.   Immunohematology Competency (*Continued*)

10 points	8 points	6 points	4 points	2 points	0 points
Performs task using proper procedure and technique with <u>no</u> <u>prompting.</u>	Performs task, but <u>needs a little</u> <u>improvement</u> on this step.	Performs task, but <u>needs a</u> <u>lot more</u> <u>practice</u> on this step.	Performs task but demonstrates <u>very poor</u> <u>skill</u> in this step.	Performs task, but performs this step in an <u>unacceptable</u> manner.	<u>Totally</u> <u>eliminated</u> this step.

Evaluation Sheet

Student Name: _____

10 points	8 points	6 points	4 points	2 points	0 points
Performs task using proper procedure and technique with <u>no prompting.</u>	Performs task, but <u>needs a little</u> <u>improvement</u> on this step.	Performs task, but <u>needs a</u> <u>lot more</u> <u>practice</u> on this step.	Performs task but demonstrates <u>very poor</u> <u>skill</u> in this step.	Performs task, but performs this step in an <u>unacceptable</u> manner.	<u>Totally</u> <u>eliminated</u> this step.

Objectives		Scores				
1. Bring reagents to room temperature.	10	8	6	4	2	0
2. Put on gloves.	10	8	6	4	2	0
3. Properly identify specimen.	10	8	6	4	2	0
4. Check records for patient history.	10	8	6	4	2	0
5. Perform ABO and Rh following facility procedure.	10	8	6	4	2	0
6. Perform antibody screen following facility procedure.	10	8	6	4	2	0
7. Perform cross-match following facility procedure.	10	8	6	4	2	0
8. Read and record all results following facility procedure.	10	8	6	4	2	0
9. Label RBC unit properly.	10	8	6	4	2	0
10. Place unit and sample in refrigerator and clean work area.	10	8	6	4	2	0
Totals						

Total Score: _____ Evaluator Signature: _____

Date Completed: _____

SUMMARY

Clinical training is a vital component of the student's total educational experience. Armed with the resources and knowledge of what to teach, how to construct behavioral objectives and measurable learning outcomes, as well as how to match the level of instruction to the needs of the learner, the clinical laboratory instructor becomes a highly effective partner in training and mentoring the next generation of clinical laboratory science professionals.

SUMMARY CHART:
Important Points to Remember

➤ The three domains of learning are: cognitive domain (knowledge), psychomotor domain (performance), affective domain (attitude/ behavior).

➤ The taxonomy levels are: Knowledge, Comprehension, Application, Analysis, Synthesis, and Evaluation. A mnemonic to use to remember taxonomy levels: Killing Cats Almost Always Seems Evil (or Easy depending on how you feel about cats).

➤ ASCP Taxonomy levels: Level 1 = Recall; Level 2 = Interpretive skills; Level 3 = Problem solving.

➤ Objectives must be written so that they describe the method of evaluation. A student should be able to determine from the written objective what he has to do to successfully achieve this task. If the objective says "the student will explain Bloom's taxonomy", the evaluation should have the student explain Bloom's taxonomy.

➤ Objectives must be measurable. Do not use verbs like "understand" or "know" because you cannot measure whether the student has achieved that objective.

➤ When writing objectives, start with the end in mind. Determine what it is you want the student to be able to do (psychomotor) or know (cognitive), or how you want them to do it (affective). Determine how you plan to evaluate the student, and then create the objectives that match that evaluation.

SUGGESTED PROBLEM-BASED LEARNING ACTIVITIES

Chapter 9: Education and Training: Practical Tips for Educators and Trainers

Instructions: Use Internet resources, books, articles, colleagues, etc., to present solutions to the problems listed below. There is no one correct solution to any problem.

Note to Instructor: Students in class may be divided into groups and given the problem-based learning activity to discuss and solve. Once the group has reached consensus as to a solution, the group may present it to the other students in the class. This activity will provide all students with information regarding solutions to the problem.

Problem #1

Develop a training program for employees/students.

Problem #2

How do you, as a laboratory scientist, develop skills to train students or new employees?

Problem #3

Develop a tool to assess annual employee competence.

Problem #4

Design an objective and a rubric for evaluating a psychomotor skill.

Problem # 5

Role playing: Have one student play the role of the preceptor and another student play the role of the student. Practice teaching a new procedure using the method given in this chapter.

BIBLIOGRAPHY

American Society for Clinical Laboratory Science. *Practice Levels and Educational Needs for Clinical Laboratory Personnel,* position paper, 25 July 2009.

Anderson LW, Krathwohl DR: *A taxonomy for learning, teaching, and assessing: A revision of Bloom's taxonomy of educational objectives.* New York, NY: Longman, 2001.

Bloom BS, et al: *Taxonomy of Educational Objectives, The Classification of Educational Goals, Handbook I: Cognitive Domain,* David McKray Company, Inc, New York, NY, 1956.

Bransford JD, Brown AL, Cocking RR (Ed.): How People Learn: Brain, Mind, Experience, and School: Expanded Edition. Commission on Behavioral and Social Sciences and Education, 2000. Copyright 2000 by the National Academy of Sciences, Washington, D.C.

Henderson T: "Classroom Assessment Techniques in Asynchronous Learning Networks." *The Technology Source,* September/October 2001. Available online at http://ts.mivu.org/default.asp?show=article&id=1034.

Olson VD: Instruction of Competent Psychomotor Skill, *College Teaching Methods and Styles Journal,* 2008; 4(9).

Orey M (Ed.): *Emerging perspectives on learning, teaching, and technology.* Association for Educational Communications and Technology, 2001.

Panzarella KJ, Manyon ATJ: *A model for integrated assessment of clinical competence.* Allied Health 2007; 36(3):157–64. PMID: 17941410

Pohl M: *Learning to Think, Thinking to Learn: Models and Strategies to Develop a Classroom Culture of Thinking.* Cheltenham, Vic.: Hawker Brownlow, 2000.

Shepherd C, Mullane AM: Rubrics: The Key to Fairness in Performance Based Assessments. *Journal of College Teaching and Learning,* 2008; 5(9).

Spearman LR: *The Rotation Manual for Clinical Laboratory Science.* Williams & Wilkins, 1995.

Suskie L: What are good assessment practices? In *Assessing Student Learning: A Common Sense Guide.* Bolton, MA: Anker, 2004.

Wass V, Van der Vleuten C, Shatzer J, Jones R: "Assessment of clinical competence." *The Lancet* - 2001; 357 (9260): 945-9. DOI: 10.1016/S0140-6736(00)04221-5

Wiggins G, McTighe J: *Understanding by Design,* 2nd ed. Association for Supervision and Curriculum Development, Alexandria, VA, 2005.

INTERNET RESOURCES

American Psychological Association (APA), *The Assessment Cyberguide for Learning Goals & Outcomes in the Undergraduate Psychology Major.* Washington, DC, 2010. http://www.apa.org/ed/new_blooms.html

American Society for Clinical Pathology (ASCP). http://www.ascp.org/

Bloom's Taxonomy. University of Victoria, 2004. http://www.coun.uvic.ca/learn/program/hndouts/bloom.html

Enerson D, Plank K, Johnson N: *An Introduction to Classroom Assessment Techniques.* Schreyer Institute for Teaching Excellence, Penn State, University Park, PA, 2007.

http://www.schreyerinstitute.psu.edu/pdf/Classroom_Assessment_Techniques_Intro.pdf

FIPSE project group, Office of Educational Development, University of North Carolina School of Medicine. The Expert Preceptor Interactive Curriculum, 1998. Accessed Sept. 2010. http://www.med.unc.edu/epic/

Kruse K: *How to Write Great Learning Objectives.* http://www.e-learningguru.com/articles/art3_4.htm

Major Categories in the Taxonomy of Educational Objectives. Bloom, 1956.

http://faculty.washington.edu/krumme/
guides/bloom.html

National Accrediting Agency for Clinical Laboratory Sciences (NAACLS).
http://www.naacls.org/

Waller K: *Writing Instructional Objectives.* NAACLS Board of Directors.
http://www.naacls.org/PDFviewer.asp?
mainUrl=/docs/announcement/writing-objectives.pdf

Financial Management

For any business to remain successful, it must maintain sound business and management practices. Clinical laboratories must be mindful of these requirements and maintain proper procedures and practices to assure continued profitability and adequate solvency. This is especially important in times of volatile swings in activity and dramatic changes in volume. Laboratory managers must focus on the business aspects of their activities to safeguard their operations and assure continued success.

Section III includes five chapters designed to provide a basic introduction to the financial aspects of management. Business and financial terms are discussed as appropriate for the topic. Some are covered in more than one chapter. Brief descriptions of these terms and concepts are intended to assist the learner in understanding basic financial management and its interrelationships.

Section III Contents:

CHAPTER 10

Fundamentals of Financial Management

Jan R. Heier, DBA, CPA
Joseph J. Collins, MS, CPA

CHAPTER OUTLINE

OBJECTIVES

Following successful completion of this chapter, the learner will be able to:

1. Discuss the importance of financial management in the healthcare industry.
2. Identify the different types of organizational business operations.
3. Identify and interpret basic financial statements.
4. Compare and contrast financial and managerial accounting.
5. Recognize revenues and expenses involved with laboratory operations.
6. Explain basic performance tools and ratios used by management in forecasting performance and in the decision making process.
7. Briefly discuss budgeting and the way it relates to revenue and expense management.
8. Explain how to use a Cost-Volume-Profit Analysis.
9. Understand the behavior of laboratory costs.
10. Explain the costs associated with laboratory testing.
11. Explain how to analyze laboratory costs.
12. Explain how to derive and use Cost-per-Test Analysis.

KEY TERMS

Assets
Balance Sheet
Break-Even Analysis
Budget-Performance Report
Cash Flow Statement
Contribution Margin
Cost-Benefit Analysis
Cost-per-Test
Cost-Volume-Profit (CVP) Analysis
Debt Ratios
Economies of Scale
Financial Accounting
Financial Ratios
Fixed Costs

High-Low Analysis
Income Statement
Liabilities
Liquidity Ratios
Managerial Cost Accounting
Mixed/Semi-Variable Costs
Owner's Equity
Profitability Ratios
Retained Earnings
Return on Investment (ROI)
SWOT Analysis
Unit Costs
Variable Costs

Case Study   Fundamentals of Financial Management

You are the manager of a "for-profit" laboratory associated with a community-based teaching hospital. Your lab is housed in a building adjacent to the main facility. You have been notified by the hospital administration that reimbursements from both private pay insurance and government sources have been reduced due to the process of capitation. The hospital is negotiating with the insurance companies and agencies to increase reimbursements based on the organization's overall cost structure and related costs for specific services. As laboratory manager, you have been asked to determine the cost of your operations in total, and pretest as well as analyze, the behavior of the costs incurred.

Issues and Questions to Consider:
1. *How do you read and understand Financial Statements?*
2. *Discuss the financial tools and ratios that may be used in analyzing the financial performance of the laboratory.*
3. *How do you plan for the financial future of the laboratory using budgets?*
4. *How do you determine the total costs of the lab operations?*
5. *How do you determine the costs of individual laboratory tests?*
6. *What is driving the costs of the laboratory tests?*

INTRODUCTION

With the introduction of the Health Care Reform Act in 2010, and its stated objective to reign in costs, the importance of understanding the unit cost structure and efficiencies of the average *for profit* clinical laboratory becomes a critical necessity. Efficient operations help to provide a basis for the allocation of financial, human, and technological resources. The first steps in understanding laboratory financial management are rooted in the issues of both micro- and macroeconomics associated with the healthcare industry. Healthcare providers today are continuingly challenged to provide high standards of quality care and easy access to services while maintaining low costs. In today's managed care environment with ever-increasing governmental regulation, the laboratory manager must have an understanding of the complex relationships between and among costs, productivity, and revenues. An understanding of the financial and economic environment of healthcare is a critical component in the decision-making processes of the laboratory manager.

Regardless of whether the clinical laboratory is managed by a hospital or acts as an independent contractor, the manager must be able to understand the cost structure of the organization. In addition, the manager must view this cost structure in relationship to the complex external healthcare environment of regulations, third party payers, capitation and service reimbursements based on a set fee or rate regardless of the laboratory's costs. To properly manage a laboratory in this environment, the manager must understand the sources of cost information that are used to analyze the laboratory's structure. Second, the manager should use these sources to determine the lab's base costs of services and what causes these costs to occur. Next, the manager must understand the tools necessary to analyze the magnitude of the costs (both total and per unit) and compare these with past performance. Finally, the manager should be able to use the data to negotiate a more favorable reimbursement rate. He can also use the data to prepare budgets for future operations.

This chapter introduces the reader to the aspects of the fiscal and organizational environment of the healthcare industry as they relate to laboratory managers. This background information provides the framework for a detailed discussion of financial management, an essential portion of a laboratory manager's job. The discussion begins with a review of accounting terminology and reporting. Next, the chapter will cover the concepts of revenue management, budgeting, and ratio analysis to assist managers in financial decision-making. Finally, the chapter will focus on the types of costs used in determining the aggregate cost of services provided and other productivity measures.

THE HEALTHCARE INDUSTRY AND ITS ORGANIZATIONAL ENVIRONMENT

Health care facilities operate in a variety of business environments. Many are public sector activities, maintained by local, county, state, or federal entities. Others function as private sector activities, and are owned or managed by persons or organizations in non-governmental organizations. While these operations may generate a substantial portion of their income from government sources, they remain private activities.

Private operations may take different forms and may operate as proprietary operations, also referred to as "for-profit" organizations or as social associations, more commonly known as "not-for-profit" entities. A proprietary organization can be developed along a number of different lines. These are basic business formations that are common throughout the economic world.

It can be created as: (1) a proprietorship, meaning that it is owned and operated by a single individual; (2) a partnership, an entity owned by two or more individuals with joint and several responsibilities for debts and obligations of the organization, and a defined expression of the manner in which gains and or losses are to be shared; or (3) a corporation (may also be a professional association which has a more limited latitude of a corporate structure). A corporation is a legal entity and has an existence of its own, apart from its stockholders. A corporation is created by application to a state or federal agency requesting that a charter be granted. This application will define the original capital structure and officers of the organization. It may further be defined as a stock company, a "for-profit" company with a certain number of shares authorized and number of shares issued, or it may be a social association, a "not-for-profit" organization with no shareholders and no stock issued. Such an organization is viewed under the law as being owned by the community, meaning that no private individual or institution has an equity (ownership) interest in the company.

A not-for-profit company is not automatically immune from a responsibility for paying federal and state income tax. To be considered exempt from tax liability, it must file a request with the Department of the Treasury for an exemption based on the type of social benefit activity in which it operates. While an exemption will ordinarily be granted by the Treasury Department, a not-for-profit organization will continue to be liable for state and federal income tax on earnings it may earn, which are outside of the scope of its not-for-profit status.

REVIEW OF FINANCIAL ACCOUNTING CONCEPTS

A primary goal of financial management is to ensure the profitability and the survival of the organization. The manager must have sources of information from which to plan and later evaluate the outcome of operations. The primary source of information is the organization's **financial accounting system**. This reflects the necessary data on revenues, expenses, assets, and liabilities, and can provide reports for the manager to both review and control operations. In contrast to the financial accounting system, managerial accounting analyzes the information to make it useful for budgeting, decision-making, and organizational evaluation. The **periodic financial statements** provide the framework for financial accounting, and reflect the structure of the business as a whole.

The nature of the Balance Sheet and other vital financial and accounting report terms are defined below.

Balance Sheet (Table 10-1) is a document that represents the financial position of an organization at a particular point, typically the end of an accounting period. The Balance Sheet reflects an organization's assets, liabilities, and equity.

Assets represent the resources of the organization. These assets can have a physical form, such as a building, or may be intangible and have economic value.

Liabilities are the obligations that an organization has to creditors. These may be short-term, due in one year or less; or long-term, greater than one year.

Owners' Equity represents the "book value" of the organization. In a *for-profit* organization, the Owner's Equity is usually made up of Capital Stock, representing the ownership in the company, and **Retained Earnings** representing the company's earnings over time less any dividends distributed. In a not-for profit organization, the equity will be represented by either

TABLE 10-1.   Sample Balance Sheet

For-Profit Labs Balance Sheet as of December 31, 2011			
Assets		**Liabilities**	
Cash	15,936	Short-Term Debt	1,999
Accounts Receivable	54,962	Accounts Payable	21,874
Restricted Funds	6,467	Accrued Salaried and Expenses	39,436
Accrued Income	7,212	Other Current Liabilities	18,448
Inventory	10,722	Advances from Third Party Payers[1]	20,397
Prepaid Expenses	4,896	Unearned Revenue	2,642
Total Current Assets	**100,195**	**Total Current Liabilities**	**104,796**
Property and Equipment	567,877	Pension and Related Costs	783
Less: Accumulated Depreciation	(160,075)	Long-Term Debt	175,309
Net Property & Equipment[2]	**407,802**	**Total Liabilities**	**280,888**
		Stockholder's Equity	
Total Other Assets[3]	**115,186**	Common Stock	100,000
		Retained Earnings[4]	242,295
		Total Equity	**342,295**
Total Assets[5]	**$623,183**	**Total Liabilities and Equity**[6]	**$623,183**

Notes:

[1] In the cases of accruals noted above, an Asset would represent accruals from insurance carriers that related to tests completed but not yet billed for, the liability side represents funds dispersed to the company for which the tests are yet to be completed.

[2] Depreciation is the systematic allocation of long-term cost to expense over the estimated life of the asset and Net PP&E represents the accounting or book value of the fixed assets after depreciation accumulated over a number of years has been recognized.

[3] Other assets encompass a number of accounting transactions that do not fit the primary classifications noted above. These items usually the accounting investments and intangible assets such as patents and trademarks.

[4] Total Assets Calculation = Total Current Assets + Net PP&E + Total Other Assets

[5] Retained Earnings represent earnings (not cash) held for future investment in the business. It is calculated by Beginning Retained Earnings + Net Income − Dividend Distribution = Beginning Retained Earnings

[6] Total Liabilities and Equity Calculation = Total Liabilities + Total Equity.

the terms "Net Assets" or the "Excess of Assets over Liabilities" because such an organization has no capital shareholders.

Income Statement (Table 10-2) presents the financial results of an organization over a stated period of time. In a *for-profit* organization this will be referred to as "Net Income"; in a *not-for-profit* organization the net gain is referred to as "Excess Revenues over Expenses."

TABLE 10-2. Sample Income Statement

For- Profit Labs Income Statement for the Year Ended December 31, 2011		
Sales	$240,000	
Cost of Goods and Services	168,000	
Gross Margin (Sales – Cost of Goods Sold)		72,000
Less: Operating Expenses		
Wages and Salaries	46,000	
Miscellaneous Expenses	8,000	
Depreciation	2,000	
Insurance	800	
Total Operating Expenses	56,800	
Total Operating Income (Gross Margin – Total Operating Expenses)		15,200
Less: Interest Expense	1,220	
Earnings Before Taxes		13,980
Less: Provision for Income Taxes	4,560	
Net Income		$9,420

Accrual Accounting—In accrual accounting systems, revenues are recognized or reflected in an income statement when they are earned, not when they are collected. Expenses are recognized or reflected in the income statement when they are incurred, not when they are paid.

Cash Basis Accounting—In a cash basis accounting system, revenues are not reflected until the cash payment is received and expenses are not reflected until payment is made for the purchase. The cash basis system may not reflect an accurate picture of actual operations, since it is heavily skewed based on payments received or paid. It is not considered a valid representation of an organization's financial position.

Revenue—Revenues reflect the earnings of the organization, both billed and unbilled, and collected or yet to be collected.

Expense—Expenses or costs are recognized as charges to the income statement as they are incurred.

Inventories—Inventory represents the value of merchandise that has been purchased for resale or for inclusion in the value of merchandise that is to be sold, but is at the date of the financial report, as yet unsold.

Property, Plant and Equipment—Property, plant and equipment (PP&E) represents assets that have been purchased that are to be used in the revenue producing activities of the organization. Additionally they will have a value of some stated minimum, usually $500, and an estimated useful life of three years or greater. When purchased, they are capitalized rather than expensed, meaning that their cost is assigned to the balance sheet rather than the income statement. Their cost is then recaptured or charged off by periodic charges of depreciation, which allows for their cost to be absorbed in the income statement over a period of years, usually consistent with their estimated useful life span.

Accrued Liabilities—Accrued liabilities represent the accumulation of costs which have been incurred in operations, but which are not yet due for payment, and thus have not been reflected as accounts payable or cash disbursements.

Depreciation—Depreciation represents the periodic charges of costs to recapture the value of property, plant and equipment items that have been purchased and assigned to the balance sheet as long-term assets. The cost assigned in each period is proportionate to the useful life of the asset, and represents a reflection of the absorption of cost over a period of time rather than as a cost incurred in only the period purchased. Depreciation over a period of time, consistent with the estimated useful life of the item, reflects a better matching of the revenues attributable to the use of the equipment, with the cost of the equipment over time.

Accumulated Depreciation—As depreciation is charged as a periodic cost, an offset is necessary to absorb this expense. Logically, it would seem appropriate to charge this cost off against the PP&E accounts. Doing so, however, might cause an organization to lose track of the true full cost of the item or its remaining unabsorbed cost. To resolve this problem, charges for periodic depreciation costs are offset by credits to an Accumulated Depreciation account. This account serves to act as an offset against the PP&E accounts, and thus reflects both a gross cost and a net cost of capital assets shown on a balance sheet.

Tax Issues—While accounting requirements require that equipment costs be recovered over a periodic basis, current tax regulations allow for the cost of equipment to be absorbed in the year of purchase. This will result in a difference between the cost and net profit shown on the income statement and the net profit shown on the tax return.

Cash Flow Statement—Financial statements produced for a for-profit company are required to include a Cash Flow Statement. This statement reflects the flow of cash through an organization over the period and is segmented in three distinct categories: cash flow from operating activities, cash flow from investing activities, and cash flow from financing activities. Since this statement deals with cash, it is essentially a reconciliation of the net gain or loss shown on the income statement, with the net change in the cash balances reflected on the balance sheet between the beginning and the end of the period.

Notes to Financial Statements—To allow for a broader understanding of items included in a company's financial reports, the notes to financial statements are presented as an addendum to define and qualify items that may need further clarification. Typically, they will specify that the reports have been prepared on an accrual basis, a modified accrual basis or a cash basis. (Statements not on an accrual basis will usually have a disclaimer in an accountant's opinion statement, stating that he cannot certify to the accuracy of the information presented.) This statement will also delineate information relative to items such as: long-term lease requirements, debt amortization, capital structures and similar information that is deemed relevant. Information relative to subsequent events, such as actions taking place subsequent to the date of the reports that might have a significant impact on the organization, are also to be included.

Annual Audit—An annual audit may or may not be required. If the company has significant loan indebtedness, the bank or others holding the debt may require a certified audited financial report. If the company has publicly traded stock, the Securities and Exchange Commission (SEC) will require such an audit. Whether a formal audit is mandated or not, the company should develop and maintain a system of adequate and effective internal controls, to assure that its accounting systems are functioning properly. An audit does not attempt to report that everything is precisely accurate. Much of financial accounting depends on reasonable estimates and good judgment. Audits are completed to obtain reasonable assurance that financial statements presented are free from material misstatement, and that effective internal control has been maintained. In an unqualified opinion as to the company's reports, the auditor will state that in his judgment, the statements reflected are free from material defect. The auditor's report which will be attached to the financial statement after an audit has been completed, and will include a statement as to the scope of the audit, and a statement as to the accountant's opinion regarding the material accuracy of the information presented.

Internal Control Systems—Internal controls are systems and procedures that are designed to maintain a proper flow of information; reduce opportunities for mistakes; and preclude deliberate acts of fraud, theft or defalcation. Proper internal control systems define responsibility for different tasks, and separate individual efforts in such a manner as to preclude theft or abuse. As an example of proper internal control, a person who is responsible for purchasing should not be the same person who prepares checks, or who reconciles the bank statement with the company's records.

EVALUATION OF LABORATORY OPERATIONS: REVENUES AND EXPENSES

Operating managers depend on a variety of sources to keep abreast of the performance of their activities. Among these are periodic financial reports, typically generated monthly or quarterly. These will usually include an income statement, a statement of assets, liabilities, and equity; budget projections and comparisons to actual; and various statistical performance reports which help to analyze the information and to make informed judgments going forward.

Revenues

Gross revenues or charges represent the total billings generated from service efforts provided by the operation, and also from the sale of any product or merchandise sold. These include all charges generated, both billed and unbilled, and all funds as yet uncollected. Charges generated are recorded at a standard gross price level for each product or service. Often, discounts are provided to customers on selected or varied basis which reflect a reduction of the level of gross charges. Additionally, particularly in the healthcare environment, price reductions are offered to large customers, or to clients that have entered into contractual agreements that specify a variation in the price agreed upon for specific items. These are referred to in the income statements as "contractual allowances," and are reflected in the income statement as a reduction from gross income. These allowances reflect a difference between the standard gross charge levied for a product or a service rendered, and the amount that is actually being billed to the customer and expected to be received as payment. The aggregation of gross charges will be reflected as the lead item in the income statement, followed by the accumulation of discounts granted, contractual allowances awarded, and any other credits that are recorded as a reduction in revenues. (Other items such as billing adjustments or the correction of errors, will be reflected as adjustments in gross revenues. Additionally, accounts written off as bad debts, or charged against bad debt allowances, will be reflected as an expense and not as a reduction of income.) The income statement will then show a "Gross revenue" accumulation, an additional line for "Total Contractual Allowances, Discounts, etc.," and a third line for the difference between the above, designated "Net Sales." It is important to keep in mind that while initial charges levied will result in gross sales at one level, contractual agreements and preferred customer agreements previously agreed upon with customers will result in a net sales income level which is lower. This will be the level that must be referred to when planning for expense or cost provisions.

Balance Sheet and Ratio Analysis

The laboratory manager should monitor the financial operations of the laboratory on an ongoing basis. Periodic financial reports contain valuable information and reflect trends that should be followed closely. A widely used tool to analyze financial statements is the use of ratio analysis. **Financial ratios** can be categorized in three distinct groups: Liquidity ratios, Debt-Equity ratios, and Profitability Indicators. **Liquidity ratios**, such as the current ratio or times interest earned ratio, is used to determine the organization's ability to meet short-term debt obligations. **Debt ratios** are used to determine an organization's ability to meet long-term debt. **Profitability ratios**, such as the **Return on Investment (ROI)** ratio demonstrate the organization's efficiency of operations. A rate of return ratio is used to evaluate the operation of the organization as a whole, by comparing net income with the organization's total equity. As an example, a net income of $13,980 compared with a total equity of $342,295 results in a 4.08% return on investment.

Return on Investment
Table 10-3 provides a sample of ratios commonly used in financial analysis.

Internal Ratios
In addition to financial ratios, the laboratory manager can also develop internal statistics that can help to control costs and evaluate operations. Much of the data needed to develop these internal ratios can be derived from the accounting system. Certain non-financial data such as testing time can be correlated with the financial data to provide a more informed analysis. Ratios developed from internal

TABLE 10-3. List of Common Financial Ratios Used in Financial Analysis

Name	Common Formula	Purpose
Current Ratio	Current Assets ÷ Current Liabilities	Ability to pay current debts
Accounts Receivable Turnover	Sales ÷ Average Receivables	Measure of collection efficiency
Days Receivable	365 ÷ Accounts Receivable Turnover	The time it takes to collect accounts receivable
Asset Turnover	Sales ÷ Total Assets	Measure of sales developed from assets
Times Interest Earned	Operating Income ÷ Interest	Test on income available to pay interest expenses
Liabilities to Assets	Total Liabilities Debt ÷ Total Assets	Measure of assets funded by debt rather than equity
Gross Margin	Gross Profit ÷ Sales	Measure of profitability
Operating Margin	Operating Profit ÷ Sales	Measure of profitability
Net Margin	Net Profit ÷ Sales	Measure of profitability
Return on Assets	Net Income + Interest ÷ Average Total Assets	Measure of profitability
Return on Investment	Net Income ÷ Average Equity	Measure of profitability

operating data can typically highlight individual elements of a laboratory's financial operating activities, and present a clearer picture of both the efficiency of the laboratory and financial impact of the individual tests performed. Examples of ratios important to the laboratory manager are:

- Cost-per-test (procedure)
- Total cost per billable test
- Direct cost per billable test
- Technical labor cost per billable test
- Billable tests per labor cost
- Billable tests per patient admission
- Revenue per billable test
- Profit margin per billable test

REVIEW OF PLANNING AND MANAGEMENT ACCOUNTING

Financial Management

Financial management is the process of planning, controlling and evaluating available fiscal, material and personnel resources of an organization. The goal of sound financial management is the proper and efficient allocation of these resources within the laboratory, and the application of ongoing improvements to ensure quality, efficiency, and cost-effectiveness within the laboratory. Managers should be familiar with the basic accounting, economic, and financial principles, and their relationship to laboratory operations to achieve and maintain success. Equally important is the manager's involvement in the planning process and control of operations through sound internal planning and proper budgeting. Figure 10-1 depicts the relationship between management and accounting functions.

The manager must be familiar with the full range costs incurred, or associated with all the efforts required to perform testing and provide services in the laboratory. He should be able to evaluate these costs both at an overall level, and also on a per-unit or individual test case level. Having a clear picture of how revenues are generated and how these relate to costs on both an aggregate and a per-unit basis is vital to the effective operation of the larger organization. Net revenues, that is gross charges less all contractual adjustments, discounts, and other price or rate adjustments, must be sufficient to provide for the full range of costs, both direct and indirect, that are associated with the activity. While a not-for-profit activity has the provision of service as its principal goal, it must nevertheless generate sufficient revenues to provide an amount equal to its cost or a modest surplus. A proprietary, for-profit organization must also allow enough earnings to provide for a return on equity for its shareholders or investors and an ample provision for applicable federal and state taxes.

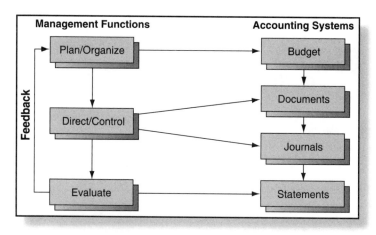

FIGURE 10-1.   Relationship Between Management and Accounting Functions

Budget Planning

A universal tool that is used in business to guide an activity and plan/provide for the needs of the activity is a well formulated and comprehensive budget.

Budgeting is a system for formalizing in writing a quantitative financial plan, supportive of the institution's financial mission, for a given time period.

Budget—Performance Report

Tables 10-4a and 10-4b are examples of budget comparison documents. Projections for a given time period are compared with actual performance. The variances (actual performance minus budgeted performance) and related percentages allow the manager to track both the actual and relative magnitude of the laboratory's performance against the budgeted amounts. Comparison of actual expenses with projected budgeted expenses provides important information to the laboratory manager, and helps to evaluate the original projection of available resources for a given period. The manager must pay close attention to and scrutinize the variances between budget and actual expenditures. This variance analysis should provide information in a timely fashion so that the manager can adjust operations to correct for any inefficiency. As a side note, when developing the variance report, consistency is important with the calculation traditionally made on an actual vs. budgeted basis. In addition, terminology related to the variance effects are reversed between revenues and expenses. A negative variance on a revenue account indicates an unfavorable variance because the revenue was less than expected. By contrast, a negative variance on an expense account indicates a favorable variance because the cost was lower than expected. The opposite effect is also true. The difference between Tables 10-4a and 10-4b are in the level of detail. In the first case, the document represents a report for only one month of operations. In the second case, Table 10-4b provides the manager a quarterly analysis of the lab's operations. The monthly and quarterly reports are often combined.

TABLE 10-4a. For-Profit Labs

Budget and Performance Report: March 2011					
		March Actual	March Budget	Variance	Variance %
Wages and Salaries					
Technical Salaries		26,680	25,000	1,680 U	6.72%
Non-Technical Wages					
Regular		6,900	6,700	200 U	2.99%
Overtime		800	500	300 U	60.00%
TOTAL SALARIES AND WAGES		34,380	32,200	2,180 U	6.77%
Benefits					
Retirement	10% TS&W	3,438	3,220	218 U	6.77%
Health	15% TS&W	5,157	4,830	327 U	6.77%
Total Benefits		8,595	8,050	545 U	6.77%
TOTAL EMPLOYMENT		42,975	40,250	2,725 U	6.77%
OPERATING EXPENSES					
Reagents		20,700	19,900	800 U	4.02%
Supplies		16,500	17,200	−700 F	−4.07%
Maintenance and Repairs		950	1,100	−150 F	−13.64%
Equipment Leases		650	650	0	0.00%
Utilities		1,100	1,000	100 U	10.00%
TOTAL OPERATING EXPENSES		39,900	39,850	50 U	0.13%
TOTAL EXPENSES		82,875	80,100	2,775 U	3.46%
ESTIMATED REVENUES		95,000	90,000	5,000 F	5.56%
ESTIMATED INCOME		12,125	9,900	2,225 F	22.47%

Notes: U = Unfavorable; F = Favorable

Cash Flow Projection

While the operating budget is necessary to maintain the activities of the organization on an ongoing basis (consistent with the larger goals of remaining profitable and assuring that revenues are sufficient to provide for operations), an organization must also plan for proper cash flow to assure that ample sources of cash are available to meet obligations (See Table 10-5). While these goals may seem to be very similar, the cash flow projection report will take into account any timing differences or disparities between when revenues are generated and when

TABLE 10-4b. For-Profit Labs

Budget and Performance Report: Year-to-Date March 2011

	March Actual	February Actual	January Actual	March YTD	Budget YTD	Variance		Variance %
Wages and Salaries								
Technical Salaries	26,680	25,100	26,200	77,980	75,000	2,980	U	3.97%
Non-Technical Wages								
Regular	6,900	7,500	6,300	20,700	20,000	700	U	3.50%
Overtime	800	900	500	2,200	500	1,700	U	340.00%
TOTAL SALARIES AND WAGES	34,380	33,500	33,000	100,880	95,500	5,380	U	5.63%
Benefits								
Retirement 10% of TS&W	3,438	3,350	3,300	10,088	9,550	538	U	5.63%
Health 15% of TS&W	5,157	5,025	4,950	15,132	14,325	807	U	5.63%
Total Benefits	8,595	8,375	8,250	25,220	23,875	1,345	U	5.63%
TOTAL EMPLOYMENT	42,975	41,875	41,250	126,100	119,375	6,725	U	5.63%
OPERATING EXPENSES								
Reagents	20,700	18,700	19,700	59,100	55,500	3,600	U	6.49%
Supplies	16,500	15,900	15,600	48,000	44,500	3,500	U	7.87%
Maintenance and Repairs	950	3,200	6,100	10,250	12,000	(1,750)	F	–14.58%
Equipment Leases	650	650	650	1,950	2,000	(50)	F	–2.50%
Utilities	1,100	950	1,000	3,050	3,000	50	U	1.67%
TOTAL OPERATING EXPENSES	39,900	39,400	43,050	122,350	117,000	5,350	U	4.57%
TOTAL EXPENSES	82,875	81,275	84,300	248,450	236,375	12,075	U	5.11%
ESTIMATED REVENUES	95,000	94,000	92,000	281,000	270,000	(11,000)	F	–4.07%
ESTIMATED INCOME	12,125	12,725	7,700	32,550	33,625	1,075	F	3.20%

253

TABLE 10-5.   For-Profit Labs – Sample Cash Budget

	9/30/2011	10/31/2011	11/30/2011	12/31/2011
Beginning Cash Balance	$10,000	$10,480	$10,860	$10,195
Cash Receipts Collections	46,000	68,000	68,000	54,000
Total Cash Available	56,000	78,480	78,860	64,195
Cash Disbursements				
Purchases	42,700	48,300	40,600	32,900
Wages and Commissions	9,250	12,250	13,000	10,750
Miscellaneous Expenses	2,500	4,000	3,000	2,500
Equipment Purchases	3,000			
Lease Payments per Month	2,000	2,000	2,000	2,000
Total Disbursements	59,450	66,550	58,600	48,150
Minimum Cash Balance Desired	10,000	10,000	10,000	10,000
Total Cash Needed	69,450	76,550	68,600	58,150
Excess (Deficit) Cash	−13,450	1,930	10,260	6,045
Financing				
Borrowings (at Beginning)	14,000			
Repayments (at End)		1,000	10,000	3,000
Interest (@ 6% Annually)[1]	70	70	65	15
Total Effect of Financing	14,000	1,070	10,065	3,015
Ending Cash Balance[2]	$10,480	$10,860	$10,195	$13,030
Loan Balance	$14,000	$13,000	$3,000	$0

Notes:

1 Assuming interest is accrued for the entire month, September Interest Calculation = 1/12 × .06 × $14,000 = 70; October Interest Calculation = 1/12 × .06 × $14,000 = 70; November Interest Calculation = 1/12 × .06 × $13,000 = 65; December Interest Calculation = 1/12 × .06 × $3,000 = 15

2 September Ending Balance Calculation = $56,000 − $59,450 + $14,000 − $70 = $10,480; October Ending Balance Calculation = $78,480 − $66,550 − $1,070 = $10,860; November Ending Balance Calculation = $78,860 − $58,600 − $10,065 = $10,195; December Ending Balance Calculation = $64,195 − $48,150 − $3,015 = $13,030

collections are received. Similarly, differences in the timing of when expenses are incurred and when those obligations are paid may also be different than that shown in the budget. For these reasons, a laboratory operating as an independent entity may have a need to project its cash flow over a period of time as a projection apart from its financial budget. There are a number of reasons why cash flow may differ from revenue and expense on an accrual basis.

Certain obligations for operating leases or rental contracts may call for asymmetrical schedules of payment. Debt instruments may be required to be paid quarterly or semi-annually. Some purchases of major equipment may be capitalized and thus will not be included as expenses. Rather, the cost of these

TABLE 10-6. Example of SWOT Analysis

Strengths	Weaknesses
Leading market position in the U.S. diagnostics industry. Operational effectiveness increasing shareholders confidence. Focus on product development providing competitive advantage.	Low bargaining power affecting company's revenues and profitability.

Opportunities	Threats
Acquisition of Monogram Biosciences to solidify LabCorp's position in the personalized medicine market. Growth in genomic and esoteric testing represents significant revenue growth opportunities. Aging population boosting demand for clinical laboratory services.	High competition could put downward pressure on the market share. Legal proceedings could affect company's brand image. Prolonging global economic crisis could restrict the company's growth.

DATAMONITOR. *Laboratory Corporation of America Holdings Company Profile* 26 Nov. 2009, p. 5.

items will be reflected as depreciation over a greater length of time, usually consistent with their estimated useful lifespan of the item. Certain revenues may be forthcoming from large bulk purchasers of service who may pay in bulk at designates dates. Any or all of these anomalies will create a disparity between an operating budget and a parallel cash flow projection.

SWOT

Although subjective in nature, an analysis to determine the **S**trengths, **W**eaknesses, **O**pportunities and **T**hreats facing the organization may give a different view from that presented in the budget process. Managers must plan for alternative strategies and possible problems or events that may appear on the horizon. This analysis, commonly referred to as a **SWOT analysis**, is the result of comprehensive planning, including brainstorming sessions among managers and employees, to anticipate future events that may have an impact on the organization.

ANALYZING THE COST OF SERVICE

Cost Behavior

Managerial Cost accounting is a system for providing an analysis of cost information used in decision-making. In today's health care environment, correct cost

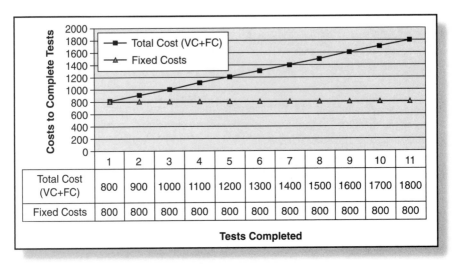

FIGURE 10-2. **Cost Behavior Graph**
VC = Variable Cost; FC = Fixed Cost

information is critical to ensure that future participation in third party contracts maintains adequate operations, and assures profitability for the lab. To accomplish this, the manager must identify the total costs associated with services and assign responsibility for those costs. The costs of adhering to requirements mandated by accreditation and certification agencies must also be considered along with traditional costs such as labor, materials, and depreciation. The laboratory manager must be effective in defining and itemizing all costs associated with the testing and other services provided by the lab.

For an effective analysis of both unit costs and total costs, the laboratory must address both fixed and variable components of cost behaviors (Figure 10-2). Cost behaviors will vary in relationship to the laboratory's testing volume.

> **Fixed costs** are those that do not change because they are not related to volume; examples of fixed costs are administrative salaries, rent, and lease commitments. Since fixed costs are not increased or decreased by volume the "per test fixed cost" will change in an inverse proportion to volume, and thus represents a measure for the laboratory's "**economies of scale.**" For example, if the lab has $10,000 in fixed costs and performs 1,000 tests, the fixed cost-per-test is $10.00. If however, the lab completes 10,000 tests, the fixed cost-per-test drops dramatically to $1.00 per test, making the lab more cost competitive.

> **Variable costs** are those that move in relationship to the laboratory's testing volume and change in a direct relationship to that volume. Supplies required to perform a specific test are variable costs. Managing variable costs require

an understanding of both the type and cost the inputs used to conduct a test, as well as the "normal" usage of the materials. For example, if a certain test requires two ounces of liquid reagent, then normal (or standard) volume of 20,000 ounces is used to complete 10,000 tests. If, however, an inventory reveals that 21,000 ounces were used, then an unfavorable quantity of 1,000 ounces has occurred and the manager should investigate this problem. By contrast, a favorable variance of 1,000 ounces would indicate that less material than normal actually was used, leading the manager to have possible concerns about problems related to service quality. The same analysis can be applied to areas such as labor hours and prices of supplies using the following two formulas:

Price Variance = Actual Unit Quantity Purchased × [Actual Price/Unit – Budgeted Price/Unit]

Quantity Variance = Budgeted Price/Unit × [Actual Quantity Used/Test – Budgeted Quantity Used per Test]

Semi-variable costs or **mixed costs**: Some expenses incurred in the laboratory will vary, but only incrementally. These costs are termed **semi-variable costs** or **mixed costs** and change in increments based on workload or volume change. An example of a semi-variable cost may be a laboratory's utilities cost. In this case, there is a flat fee paid for a minimum amount of kilowatt hours used. As the number of tests performed grows, the amount of electricity used will increase as well, with greater total costs.

Table 10-7 presents a simple **high-low analysis** that shows how to determine the relationship between two related variables and derive a cost formula or function that determines the levels of fixed and variable costs. As noted in the table, the function can then be used to estimate or budget future costs. The related graph (Figure 10-3) shows a graphical relationship between the two variables (the long line is the high-low relationship that shows the slope of the line and its fixed position of the Y-axis).

Cost-Volume-Profit (CVP) Analysis

Understanding the cost behavior of the laboratory allows the manager the opportunity to analyze the position of the lab with respect to profitability, and to determine what measures are needed to control costs (or increase revenues if that is possible). One of the primary tools for completing this analysis is **Cost-Volume-Profit (CVP) Analysis**, more commonly called **Breakeven**. To complete a CVP analysis it is important to determine behavior of the laboratory's costs.

To illustrate CVP, (Table 10-8), assume a lab had fixed costs to cover of $300,000; if the lab charges $15 per test when the incremental cost is $9.00 per test, how many tests need to be completed to cover the lab's fixed costs? As the table indicates, 50,000 tests allow the lab to breakeven.

TABLE 10-7.   High-Low Example—Estimated Relationship Between Two Variables

| EXAMPLE: Lab Tests Performed Compared to Utility Costs per Month | | |
Month	Lab Tests Performed	Utility Cost per Month
January	75,000	5,100
February	78,000	5,300
March	80,000	5,650
April	92,000	6,300
May	98,000	6,400
June	108,000	6,700
July	118,000	7,035
August	112,000	7,000
September	95,000	6,200
October	90,000	6,100
November	85,000	5,600
December	90,000	5,900
	X or Independent Data	Y or Dependent Data

$$\frac{(\text{High Cost} - \text{Low Cost})}{(\text{High Activity} - \text{Low Activity})} = \text{Est. Variable Rate/Test}$$

$$\frac{(\$7,035 - \$5,100)}{(118,000 - 75,000)} = \frac{\$1,935}{43,000} = \$0.045 \text{ per Test}$$

Use the slope of the line to find the best average relationship between the high and low data points.

High Cost – (High Activity × Variable Rate) = Est. Fixed Cost
[$7,035 – (118,000 × $0.45)] = ($7,035 – 5,310) = $1,725
Note: The Est. Fixed Cost can be calculated using the low data point.
Low Cost – (Low Activity × Variable rate) = Est. Fixed Cost
[$5100 – (75,000 × $0.045)] = ($5100 – 3,375) = $1,725

A Cost Formula or Function for the data enables the manager to make estimates of future cash needs.

Cost Formula: Fixed + (Variable Rate × Number of Tests) = Y

Budget Use: In January of the following year, it is projected that test volume will be at 100,000 units. What will be the month's estimated costs for utilities?

$1,725 + ($0.045 × 100,000) = $6,225

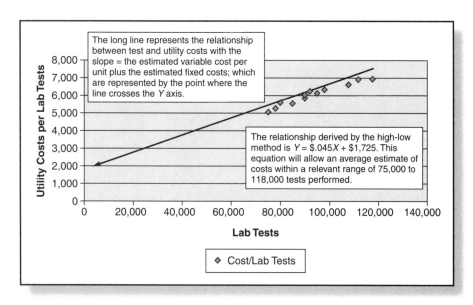

The long line represents the relationship between test and utility costs with the slope = the estimated variable cost per unit plus the estimated fixed costs; which are represented by the point where the line crosses the *Y* axis.

The relationship derived by the high-low method is *Y* = $.045*X* + $1,725. This equation will allow an average estimate of costs within a relevant range of 75,000 to 118,000 tests performed.

FIGURE 10-3. High-Low Graph

For simplicity sake, the lab can determine the amount of tests it needs to perform to break even using the following formula.

$$\frac{\text{TOTAL FIXED COST}}{\text{CONTRIBUTION MARGIN/TEST}} = \frac{\$300,000}{\$15.00 - \$9.00} = 50,000 \text{ Tests}$$

(CONTRIBUTION MARGIN/TEST = SALES PRICE minus VARIABLE COST PER TEST)

In the above example, the $15.00 — $9.00 or $6.00 represents **Contribution Margin** per test, first towards covering fixed costs, and then income. The result can also be shown by the use of the graph in Figure 10-4.

Cost-Volume-Profit Analysis as illustrated above, allows for the projection of costs and revenues at a given change in volume and pricing, and provides the necessary information to make decisions regarding potential service contracts with payers (insurers, managed care, or other third-party organizations). In addition, such analysis allows for planning purchases of materials and staffing as volume changes. In order to complete a CVP analysis, it may be necessary to identify and allocate the various costs to the services being rendered to determine **cost-per-test**. The process of determining fixed versus variable costs is covered in more detail in the next section of this chapter.

Cost per test data is extremely useful for decision-making. Pricing decisions related to alternative contracts to offer in response to a managed care group or a request for bids are critical. In addition, decisions on whether to provide testing in-house, or contracting out to an affiliated lab or reference laboratory, may be made by comparing costs of the alternative service methods.

TABLE 10-8.   Cost-Volume-Profit (Breakeven Analysis)

Tests Performed	Revenue $15/test	Variable Cost $9.00/test	Contribution Margin (Revenue – VC)	Fixed Costs	Total Costs	Operating Income (CM – FC)	Total Test Cost (FC + VC)/Tests
0	0	0	0	300,000	300,000	(300,000)	0.00
10,000	150,000	90,000	60,000	300,000	390,000	(240,000)	39.00
20,000	300,000	180,000	120,000	300,000	480,000	(180,000)	24.00
30,000	450,000	270,000	180,000	300,000	570,000	(120,000)	19.00
40,000	600,000	360,000	240,000	300,000	660,000	(60,000)	16.50
50,000	750,000	450,000	300,000	300,000	750,000	0	15.00
60,000	900,000	540,000	360,000	300,000	840,000	60,000	14.00
70,000	1,050,000	630,000	420,000	300,000	930,000	120,000	13.29
80,000	1,200,000	720,000	480,000	300,000	1,020,000	180,000	12.75

Note: Test cost decrease is due to Fixed Costs that are spread more thinly over an ever-increasing amount of Tests Performed.

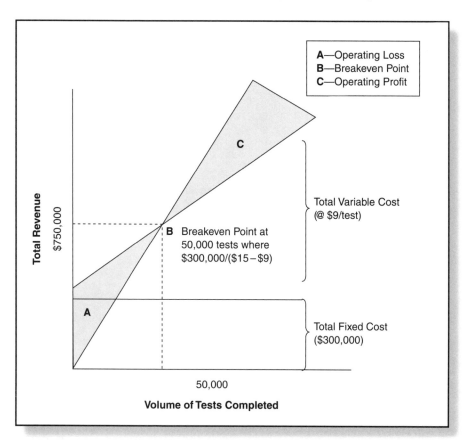

FIGURE 10-4. **CVP Graph**

A **cost-benefit analysis** can be performed using costing information to determine which alternative is the most financially beneficial for the organization (Refer to Chapter 11).

PRODUCTIVITY AND MEASURING THE COST-PER-TEST

Cost-per-test analysis is a means of identifying the productivity of a laboratory. Within the obvious guidelines of quality and efficacy, the lower the cost-per-test, the more efficient the laboratory is in providing its services. A laboratory with high productivity should yield a lower cost-per-test compared to a less productive counterpart. A cost-per-test analysis begins with the identification and allocation of component costs and their identification and relationship to the service provided. As previously discussed, the laboratory manager must first identify the lab's

TABLE 10-9.   Cost Analysis Checklist

Fixed Costs	Labor Costs	
__ Rent	__ Base Wages	
__ Utilities	__ Taxes	
__ Compliance cost	__ Insurance	
__ PT Subscription	__ Retirement	
__ Leases	__ Other Benefits	
__ Management		

Variable Costs		
Test-Specific Costs:	**Test-System Costs:**	
__ Reagent	__ Sample Cups	
__ Calibration	__ Sample Tips	
__ Control	__ Reagent Kit	
__ Other	__ Cuvettes	
	__ Multi-Analyte Calibrators/Controls	
	__ Printing Supplies	

fixed costs (i.e., those costs that remain constant regardless of volume). Examples of fixed costs are administrative salaries, rent, and lease payments. In addition, the variable costs, those that vary proportionally with the volume of testing, must then be identified. Examples are supplies and reagents needed to perform a test. Labor costs may fall into either fixed or variable costs, and sometimes both categories, depending on how various staff members are compensated (hourly versus salaried). All testing services in the laboratory will inevitably consist of both fixed and variable components.

Cost-per-test (or more generically — unit costs) are the sum of both fixed and variable costs divided by the number of unit tests. The unit cost-per-test is used to measure the laboratory's productivity and demonstrate the laboratory's economies compared with other comparable laboratories. One of the primary objectives of the process is to identify the costs associated with the testing process, both direct and indirect, and efficiently attach or allocate all of the costs related to the test to determine the actual cost of that particular test. In the case of indirect costs, they must be allocated using a particular unit of production such as, in this case, the glucose assay. Table 10-9 can serve as a template to determine the costs associated with testing.

Test-specific (variable) costs are the simplest to identify and allocate. For example, the cost of both glucose reagents and calibration and/or control materials specific for the glucose assay test are known from previous purchases and usage. Costs of consumable supplies, such as sample cups (cuvettes) and pipette tips needed to perform the assay, are also be identified and allocated appropriately. Consumable supplies may be shared among other assays being performed on the same analyzer, and thus the portion of the purchase cost that can be attributed only to the glucose assays performed must be determined. Finally, fixed costs associated with the laboratory services must be identified and allocated. To illustrate the cost allocation and the determination of cost-per-test in more detail, the example of a glucose assay test performed on an automated analyzer will be the illustrated using the following data:

Total tests per month	50,000
Glucose tests per month	3,120
Runs per month	40
Tests per run	78
Test repeats	3
Patient dilutions	6
Controls per run	2
Control repeats	2
Failed runs per month	1
Calibrators (per 6 months)	12
Reagent cost per month	$400
Control cost per month	$60
Calibrator cost per month	$60
Cuvettes per month	3,405
Cost per Cuvettes	$0.05
Technologist time per run in minutes	20
Fixed OVERHEAD cost per month	$500

Analysis of Cost-per-Test

Variable Costs

1. Cost of one Cuvette per test $0.0500
2. Cost of reagents, controls, and calibrators (allocated based on cuvette usage) per month:

   Reagents $400
   Controls $60
   + Calibrators $60
   Total $520 $520/3405   = $0.1527
   Number of Cuvettes per month: 3405*

*The total number of patients per run is 78, and 3 patient samples per run require dilution, adding 3 additional. The 2 controls per run are analyzed and there are 6 calibrators run in duplicate, once per each 6 months; therefore 2 calibrators are allocated per month. In all, 83 (78 + 3 + 2) are needed per run, which equates to 3320 (83 × 40 runs per month). The one failed run per month and the additional control repeat increases the total to 3405 (3320 + 83 + 2) per month.

Labor Costs

(Depending on the situation, these may be variable, fixed, or semi-variable)

$24.00 per hr. × 20 minutes (tech time) $= \dfrac{\$8.00 \text{ per run}}{78 \text{ tests per run}} =$ $0.1026

Fixed Costs

(The allocation rate is based on the number of tests)
Fixed costs/Total tests per month = Fixed cost per test
$500/50, 000 = $0.0100
Total cost per test = $0.3153
Total glucose tests performed: 3,120
Total cost for completing glucose assay test: 3,120 × $0.3153 = $983.74

As the analysis indicates, all costs need to be considered including both fixed and variable costs. Costs are often shared with other tests, and thus will need to be allocated by some standard measure. In this case, the fixed costs are allocated or applied to each test based on the number of tests performed by the lab; whereas, variable costs of reagent, control, and calibrator reagents are allocated based on the usage of cuvettes. This analysis allows for a proper understanding of the laboratory's costs of operations per test and total costs, as well as the charges to the patient necessary to cover the costs. This type of analysis will also help in negotiating reimbursements from third-party payers, by giving them a base estimate or budget for the laboratory's actual per unit costs.

SUMMARY

Making decisions that ensure future financial performance is an important aspect for any laboratory manager. Financial management provides a variety of benefits. First, for the patients, it provides for better quality services at a reduced cost. Next, for the healthcare administrator, it provides information for strategic planning and the best use of available funds. Finally, for the laboratory manager, it provides financial information for effective cost reductions, appropriate test utilization, equipment utilization, staffing utilization, and material usage.

SUMMARY CHART:
Important Points to Remember

➤ Knowledge of financial accounting terminology and application is necessary to properly run a medical laboratory and make decisions.

➤ Budgets should be prepared annually to chart the future financial course of the laboratory.

➤ Financial statements containing current operating results should be obtained and analyzed through ratio analysis or historical comparisons

➤ Current operating results should be compared with budgeted expectations and any variances analyzed and dealt with to enhance the laboratory's efficiency.

➤ Determine the cost behaviors associated with the laboratory activities and conduct a breakeven analysis to determine the current profitability position of the laboratory.

➤ Determine the "cost-per-test" of the laboratory.

➤ Use the "cost-per-test" as a standard to compare the laboratory's operating efficiency over time.

➤ The "cost-per-test" can also be used to negotiate reimbursement with third party payers.

➤ A non-financial SWOT analysis is useful in determining the future direction of the company.

SUGGESTED PROBLEM-BASED LEARNING ACTIVITIES

Chapter 10: Fundamentals of Financial Management

Instructions: Use Internet resources, books, articles, colleagues, etc., to present solutions to the problems listed below. There is no one correct solution to any problem.

Note to Instructor: Students in class may be divided into groups and given the problem-based learning activity to discuss and solve. Once the group has reached consensus as to a solution, the group may present it to the other students in the class. This activity will provide all students with information regarding solutions to the problem.

Problem #1

Go to the Internet and download a copy of the **annual report** of a publicly held clinical laboratory such as *Laboratory Corporation of America (LAB-CORP)* and review the financial statements for the definitions used in the chapter. Read through the Balance Sheet, Income Statement, and Cash Flow Statement for the financial definitions covered in this chapter. Peruse the notes to the financial statements to understand the expanded information provided about the materials presented in the financial statements.

Problem #2

Develop a plan to evaluate your department's financial productivity and illustrate this process using financial ratios and productivity measures.

Problem #3

Prioritize and discuss the financial and productivity issues that may be affected by the HealthCare Reform Legislations.

Problem #4

Develop a plan to evaluate your lab's productivity and cost structure using managerial accounting measures and unit cost performance.

Problem #5

Develop a hypothetical SWOT analysis of your laboratory company.

BIBLIOGRAPHY

Baker JJ, Baker RW: *Health Care Finance, Basic Tools for Nonfinancial Managers.* Aspen Publications, Gaithersburg, MD, 2000.

Brigham EF, Houston SC: *Fundamentals of Financial Management,* ed 10. South-Western College Publications, Cincinnati, OH, 2004.

Datamonitor. *Laboratory Corporation of America Holdings Company Profile.* 26 Nov. 2009, p 5; 35.

Fields E: *Essentials of Finance and Accounting for Non-Financial Managers.* AMACOM, New York, NY, 2002.

Horngren CT, Sundum GL, Elliot JA: *Introduction to Financial Accounting,* ed 9. Pearson Prentice Hall and Company, Upper Saddle River, NJ, 2006.

Horngren CT, Sundum GL, Stratton WO: *Introduction to Management Accounting,* ed 13. Pearson Prentice Hall and Company, Upper Saddle River, NJ, 2005.

Ives M, Razak JA, Hosch GA: *Introduction to Governmental and Not-for-Profit Accounting.* Pearson Prentice Hall and Company, Upper Saddle River, NJ, 2004.

Snyder JR, Wilkinson D: *Management in Laboratory Medicine,* ed 3. Lippincott, Philadelphia, PA, 1998.

INTERNET RESOURCES

American Association for Clinical Chemistry (AACC)
http://www.AACC.org

American Society for Clinical Pathology (ASCP)
http://www.ASCP.org

Center for Disease Control (CDC), FastStats, Health Expenditures.
http://www.cdc.gov/nchs/fastats/hexpense.htm

Clinical Laboratory Management Association (CLMA)
http://www.CLMA.org

"Cost-Volume-Profit (CVP) Analysis." Business Glossary, Allbusiness.com, 2010.
http://www.allbusiness.com/glossaries/cost-volume-profit-cvp-analysis/4950439-1.html

Organization for Economic Cooperation and Development (OECD)
http://www.oecd.org/

Cost/Benefit Analysis

Joseph J. Wawrzynski, Jr., MBA, MT(ASCP)BB,
DLM^{CM}, CQA(ASQ)CQIA
Janet S. Hall, MS, CC(NRCC)

CHAPTER OUTLINE

OBJECTIVES

Following successful completion of this chapter, the learner will be able to:

1. Define and manipulate the key elements of managerial cost accounting.
2. Identify and discuss the five types of expenses (costs).
3. Identify and describe the information required to calculate expected revenue.
4. List potential intangible factors that should be assessed when performing a make versus buy analysis.
5. Perform a break-even analysis for a proposed new test.
6. Price a new test.
7. Evaluate the special considerations for capital equipment acquisition.
8. Summarize the relationship between micro, departmental, and institutional financial analysis and planning.

KEY TERMS

Billable Procedure
Break-Even Point
Charge Description Master (CDM)
Cost Per Reportable
Current Value of Money
Depreciation
Direct Expense (Cost)
Expense
Financial Accounting
For-Profit Entity
Indirect Expense (Cost)
Lease

Management Accounting
Microcosting
Non-Billable Procedure
Not-For-Profit Entity
Overhead
Payback Period
Private Accounting
Public Accounting
Reagent Rental
Return on Investment (ROI)
Surcharge/Cost Plus Method

Cost/Benefit Analysis

You are the laboratory manager. The hospital administration wants to penetrate the market and expand the business by performing Parathyroid Surgeries (reimbursement $15,000). They have enticed a prominent surgeon to join the staff. He plans on scheduling four surgeries per week – two on Tuesday and two on Thursdays. Every case will need an intact Parathyroid Hormone (PTH) performed STAT during surgery. You currently send this test to your reference laboratory with a minimum 24-hour TAT. None of the analyzers currently in your lab are capable of running this test. The best pricing you obtain is from Siemens Diagnostics for an Immulite 1000. The price of the analyzer is $75,000. The price of the test kit is $800 for 100 tests. The test requires three levels of controls run per 24 hours. The stability of the test kit once opened is eight weeks. Reimbursement for the test is $20. You realize that you will only be able to run on average 32 tests (patient reportable results) before discarding the reagent ($25 per test for reagent alone).

Issues and Questions to Consider:
1. *Would you bring the test in-house as per the physician's request?*
2. *What other departments need to be involved in developing this service?*
3. *What assumptions should be made modifying the Chemistry operating budget?*
4. *What financial tools would be useful in justifying the addition of this test?*
5. *Would further explanation be needed in justifying the addition of this test as addition does not appear to be warranted on its own merits?*

INTRODUCTION

One of the most important tasks of a laboratory manager is assessing and comparing expense (cost) with associated revenue (benefit), a process known as a cost/benefit analysis. This chapter provides the reader with a global perspective on using financial information followed by details on the nuts and bolts of cost/benefit analysis including evaluation of expenses, evaluation of revenues, and pricing formulas. Two related topics—making business decisions and capital purchases—are also discussed. Finally, the chapter includes suggested resources to assist laboratory managers in evaluating the financial position of their institutions, as well as to compare their findings to financial situations of other comparable institutions.

USING FINANCIAL INFORMATION: THE BIG PICTURE

Healthcare is a huge business (expenditures surpassed $2.3 trillion in 2008, was expected to have reached $2.5 trillion in 2009 and is projected to reach $4.5 trillion and comprise 19.3 percent of GDP by 2019) in the United States that is composed of a complex system of providers and payers.[1,2] The providers perform healthcare services and attempt to maximize the reimbursement received. The payers, conversely, pay out only what they deem necessary. This was not always the case.

The healthcare market before 1982 was based on fee-for-service reimbursement. A healthcare provider performed a service (e.g., a laboratory test) and a payer paid for that service. Cost was not an issue. When the cost of performing a test increased, the provider increased the price to the payer, and the payer paid the increased rate. This system eventually began to burden payers. In 1982, laboratories came to realize that they needed to act like businesses when the federal government instituted a payment system for Medicare patients that was based on DRGs (diagnostic-related groups). Under that system, all services provided for hospital in-patients were grouped together, and a single payment amount was made based on the DRG assigned to the case. Whether the laboratory charged $5.00 or $50.00 for a test, the amount received to cover the test plus all other services performed was the same. It suddenly became important for laboratories to contain costs. In August 2000, Medicare instituted the hospital outpatient prospective payment system (OPPS), commonly known as the ambulatory payment classification system (APC), a similar system to the in-patient DRG system. Payment under the APC system is determined by the services provided during the outpatient visit.[3]

In 1983 TEFRA (Tax Equity and Fiscal Responsibility Act) was passed. TEFRA set limits of reimbursement (the section 223 limits on routine per diem costs were extended to cover total costs per discharge) and established a system to monitor and adjust reimbursement to providers.[4] Most recently the Balanced Budget Amendment of 1997 set more limitations on Medicare payment schedules and defined a systematic scheme for decreasing payments over time.[5] Healthcare providers, including laboratory managers, have been forced to take a hard look at expenses and revenues, and to modify operations to control expense.

Entities providing healthcare in the United States are divided into two categories: for-profit and not-for-profit. A **for-profit entity** is privately held (e.g., a corporation). Its profits are distributed to the owners (individuals or shareholders) and its primary purpose is to generate revenue. Any profits it is able to generate are taxed. Examples of for-profit healthcare entities include the large commercial laboratories and some large hospital systems such as Columbia HCA or Community Health Systems. A **not-for-profit entity** (e.g., most community based hospitals) is one whose profits are held by the entity to further its cause. These entities usually exist to provide a service, such as healthcare. In these entities the "profits" are not taxed and are retained by the entity and used for purchase of capital equipment or other goods and services required to sustain the business entity. The objectives of for-profit and not-for-profit businesses are different, but the bottom line is that both must balance expense and revenue to remain solvent.

Further, in the business world there are two levels of oversight of the financial side of a business. The first, **management accounting**, is the analysis of cost and revenue data that provides information on operations and budgeting for managers. Managerial accounting is also called *cost accounting*. In the laboratory, managerial accounting includes activities such as **microcosting** (the process of determining the actual cost of performing a billable procedure), performing analyses of services and equipment in order to evaluate their profitability, and budgeting (the compilation of expected expenses and revenue into a financial plan).

Information generated through management accounting in all departments of a hospital is then collated and evaluated by the Department of Finance, which generates financial records, and forecasts and performs strategic planning for the entire entity. These activities are called **financial accounting**.

The activities performed in the laboratory and other departments which are evaluated and reported by the Department of Finance are facets of **private accounting** (i.e., they are performed by an entity for its own managerial activities). Once done, however, they are made available to regulatory, government, and private accounting firms for both informational purposes and to meet regulatory requirements. This activity is called **public accounting**. Table 11-1 shows the relationships between private and public accounting and between management and financial accounting.

All entities, whether for-profit or not-for-profit, go through the same general accounting processes, although the information may be distributed differently outside the entity based on applicable regulations.

EVALUATING EXPENSES

It is important for managers to know what it costs to operate a laboratory section or department. It is the only side of the cost/revenue equation over which they

TABLE 11-1.   Accounting Relationships

Public Accounting	Governments	
	Outside Accountants (Auditors)	
	Stockholders	
	Regulatory Agencies	
	Income Tax Services	
Private Accounting	Strategic Planning ⎫	
	Forecasting ⎬ ◄——— Financial Accounting	
	Department Audits ⎭	
	Budgets ⎫	
	Line Item Analysis ⎬ ◄——— Management Accounting	
	Microcosting ⎭	

have direct control. In order to perform the evaluations, the manager must have accurate records, including, but not limited to, test counts, vendor contracts, staff salary and benefit information and consumable costs.

For this discussion, **expense** is defined as the *cost* of providing a billable procedure. In the laboratory, a **billable procedure** is a test that is billed to a payer. The payer may be an individual or a private or government insurance. The charge for a billable procedure includes all the expenses (costs) incurred in generating the test result, including the cost of collecting and processing the specimen, performing the test (reagents, consumables, labor, laboratory and equipment costs), and numerous other costs plus some measure of profit. A **non-billable procedure** contributes to the generation of a billable test result, but which is not directly reimbursable. Examples of non-billable procedures include standards, quality control specimens, and repeats. Some non-reimbursable procedures are occasionally performed in the laboratory, but should not be billed because payment is unlikely. These include tests considered to be experimental and tests for which appropriate medical necessity or diagnosis information has not been gathered. Obviously the volume of such tests should be kept to a minimum, if allowed at all.

The most effective method for determining the actual cost to perform a billable procedure is to perform a microcost analysis. Microcosting accounts for all expenses associated with performing a given test including reagents, consumables, laboratory costs, and reporting costs and includes pre-analytical, analytical, and post-analytical expenses. It is a structured approach that, when built into a template, can be used to price any new test being considered or to be an ongoing evaluation tool for tests currently being performed.

There are two types of expenses to consider when performing a microcosting evaluation. **Direct expense (cost)** includes all costs directly related to performing a test. It includes the reagents, consumables, labor and benefits, etc. Examples of direct costs are shown in Table 11-2.

Indirect expense (cost) includes expenses that are part of doing business, but that are not directly related to the cost of the test being evaluated. Indirect costs are also called **overhead**. Examples of indirect costs are shown in Table 11-3.

Direct costs are relatively easy to determine and should be calculated using a line-by-line approach. For example, the cost of consumables needed to collect a blood specimen is straightforward:

Alcohol swab	$ 0.13
Needle	0.34
Vacutainer tube(s)	0.60
Tourniquet	0.05
Adapter	0.21
Gauze pad	0.13
Band-Aid	0.05
Total cost	$ 1.51

TABLE 11-2.   Examples of Direct Costs

Specimen Collection Consumables (preps, Vacutainers, needles, etc.)
Processing Consumables (tubes, caps, transfer pipets, labels, etc.)
Reagents

    Calibrators
    Controls
    Reagents, stains, etc.

Analytical Consumables (sample cups, tips, media plates, etc.)
Proficiency Testing Materials
Labor

    Collections
    Accessioning
    Analysis
    QC
    Reporting
    Other

Equipment Costs

    Monthly Lease/Rental Cost
    Depreciation (purchases only)
    Maintenance

        Ongoing/in-house/daily/weekly/monthly
        Contracted

Office Supplies
Reporting Costs (fax, paper, printheads, etc.)

If more than one test is performed per collection, the cost of the collection expendables can be spread over multiple tests, thereby decreasing the cost per test. The same can be done for processing costs. Pricing information for the consumables used is available from the purchasing department and from utilization reports generated monthly by the finance department.

When calculating reagent costs, the cost of the reagent actually used to run a single test is easy to calculate based on the known volume of reagent used and the cost per volume. These numbers are readily available from contracting information generated by vendors or from records in the purchasing department. The cost of calibrators and controls is also available. The actual cost of these per test can be determined by dividing the total amount used, by the total number of tests performed, using a particular calibration and/or control schedule. For example, if three levels of controls are run once per shift, and the instrument uses 0.2 ml of control, the cost of 0.2 ml of control can be divided by the total number of tests run on that shift to determine the actual cost of the control per reportable result.

TABLE 11-3.   Examples of Indirect Costs

Licenses
Marketing
   Labor
   Materials
Information Systems Requirements
   Programming (Ongoing)
   Maintenance Fees
   Training
      Initial
      Ongoing
Supervisory and Administrative Salaries
Secretarial Support
Other Facility Overhead (as determined by the facility)
Intangibles
   Signatures – ABN (Advanced Beneficiary Notice) risk, F/U (Failure/Unable) to obtain
   Liability Costs (Insurance)
   Public Relations
   Involvement in Product Line
      Physician Relations
      Markets
      Network Requirements
      Long-Term Survival
      Medical Involvement

An alternative option that has found favor lately is **cost per reportable** contracts directly from the vendor. In a cost per reportable contract, the cost of the reagents and the equipment used to run the test is a set, pre-determined amount contracted with the vendor for each test *reported*. For example, each potassium reportable test may result in the laboratory being charged $0.11 by the vendor. As in the traditional method of calculating test cost, the cost of calibrators and controls also needs to be considered and added to the cost per reportable to determine the total cost for each test. In either case, a large sample size should be used to determine accurate average volumes of tests, controls, repeats, proficiency tests, etc. Sometimes, when these numbers are very small, they can be included as a factor and not evaluated directly.

Laboratory labor cost calculations are generally done using the number of minutes required to perform the test, multiplied by an average hourly rate plus 35% of the rate to cover benefits. For example, if a test takes 3 minutes of a medical technologist's/clinical laboratory scientist's time to perform and report a laboratory test and the hourly rate of the medical technologist is $33.75

($25.00 per hour salary + $8.75 (35%) for benefits), the tech labor cost of the test would be $1.69 ($0.5625 per minute × 3 minutes = $1.6875). The cost of labor for collections, accessioning/processing, etc. can be calculated in the same way using the hourly rates of the personnel who perform these tasks. See Table 11-4 for two examples. Remember to include the benefits when determining the total cost.

Equipment costs per test can be determined in a similar fashion. Reports of monthly rental costs for rented or leased equipment and any additional ongoing maintenance costs are specified in the vendor contract. Generally, calculating the part of those costs that apply to a single analysis of a single analyte can be performed by dividing the total cost over a given period by the total number of tests performed on the equipment during the same time period. Depreciation cost for owned capital equipment should be calculated as a direct cost, but it will not vary with the number of tests performed. Each analyzer should be evaluated independently based on how it is used. A detailed discussion of advantages/disadvantages of purchase/lease/rental will occur later in this chapter under Capital Acquisition.

Indirect costs may be calculated in two ways. The first is to do a line-by-line analysis of all indirect costs. This method can be time consuming, and sometimes the information is not readily available. The second method is to multiply the direct cost by a factor that is a reasonable assumption of the total indirect cost. Many not-for-profit laboratories use a factor of 1.3, but the factor for any given entity may vary greatly, depending on the type of entity and the overall overhead costs. The finance department is the best source for determining the factor for your institution.

When costing out a test that will be added to the menu of a current piece of equipment, it is sometimes valuable to consider only the direct variable costs involved, as the indirect costs will not change. In that case, the true indirect cost per analysis is not performed, but only the additional direct cost is of significance.

Costs may also be fixed, variable, or semi-variable. A fixed cost remains constant despite any change in the volume of tests performed. Examples of fixed costs include salaries and benefits for supervisors and administrators, the cost of a courier, and depreciation on a piece of equipment. Variable costs, however, vary proportionately to the change in test volume. Examples of variable costs include reagent costs and consumables (e.g., pipette tips, cups). Semi-variable costs

TABLE 11-4.   Labor Cost Calculations

	Average Salary (includes benefits)	Per Minute Cost
Tech Time (@ $25 per Hour)	$33.75/60 min.	= $0.5625 (Tech)
Lab Assistant/Phleb Time (@ $15 per Hour)	$20.25/60 min.	= $0.34 (Phleb)

vary with the volume, but not in direct proportion. Technologist labor is a good example. If a 5% increase in test volume occurs, and the work can be covered by current staffing, the total labor cost does not increase and the labor cost per billable actually decreases. If a 30% increase occurs, additional technical staff is required and the total cost will increase. The cost per laboratory may remain the same or increase.

Knowing the total costs of each laboratory is an important first step in determining profitability. Unfortunately, not enough laboratories have done a microcosting analysis within the recent past, but rely instead on historical data generated during the budget process and calculate a small percentage increase for increased labor costs (annual raises). Consequently, many actually have little or no idea of their true costs. A microcosting analysis should be performed whenever there are major changes, for example vendor or equipment changes, market adjustments for salaries or laboratory renovations.

EVALUATING REVENUE

Revenue is defined as the price of services rendered. It is the amount charged for a test or service. Do not confuse revenue with reimbursement, which will be discussed later (in Chapter 14).

In medical laboratories, the charges billed for a test are attached to a specific CPT (current procedural terminology) code. The CPT coding system is maintained by the CPT Editorial Board of the American Medical Association (AMA) and is considered the standard for healthcare billing practices in the United States.[6] Codes are assigned for all healthcare procedures, including operating room, imaging, respiratory therapy and others, and are updated annually. Codes for laboratory tests are in the range of 80000 to 89999. The following are examples of current laboratory CPT codes:

CPT codes may refer to a single test (total cholesterol) or to specific panels of tests (basic metabolic profile) that are constructed by the AMA and approved for reimbursement by Medicare. Only tests that have CPT codes are reimbursed.

80162   Digoxin

82465   Cholesterol, serum or whole blood, total

85025   Complete (CBC) automated (Hgb, Hct, RBC, WBC and platelet count) and automated differential WBC count

87040   Culture bacterial; blood, aerobic with isolation and presumptive identification of isolates (includes anaerobic culture, if appropriate)

86900   Blood typing; ABO

80048   Basic metabolic panel (Calcium, total)

This panel must include the following:

Calcium, total (82310)

Carbon dioxide (82374)

Chloride (82435)

Creatinine (82565)

Glucose (82947)

Potassium (84132)

Sodium (84295)

Urea nitrogen (BUN)(84520)

Generally the hospital has a list of all billable services, their associated CPT code, and the price charged to the patient or insurance carrier. This list is called a **Charge Description Master** or **CDM**. As a manager, you should be closely involved in updating and validating the information in the CDM that applies to your area of responsibility, in order to maximize revenue and avoid Medicare fraud and abuse issues. The CDM is used to price in-patient and on-campus outpatient or regulated visits. A separate CDM may be in place for unregulated visits for patients not admitted to the hospital, which include laboratory outreach programs. This CDM is used for outreach business, which may be brought in to expand the hospital laboratory's revenue base. Although the CPTs are the same for the tests rendered, the charges usually differ. Both taxable and nontaxable entities may have one CDM, but may offer discounted pricing to other entities to which they provide services. This is possible because they are not billing the patient directly (or Medicare), but are billing the institution or organization, who is purchasing the tests. The institution, in turn, bills the patient or other responsible party.

Revenue projections for the laboratory are compiled using a number of means including the following:

1. Historical data
2. Patient day forecasts
3. Regulatory changes
4. Growth projections based on new markets and changing technologies

Historical data are gathered from the statistics of the previous fiscal (financial) year and then modified based on expected or actual regulatory changes, growth projections related to strategic planning initiatives and other factors that could have a decrease in volume. These factors may include increased competition or reduced demand due to economic changes. Revenue based on patient day forecasts is based on the expected DRG reimbursement rate multiplied by the number of patient days expected to fall into each DRG. In many organizations, most of these calculations are performed by the finance department, but input by laboratory management, especially that related to outreach initiatives, is important. In theory, all billed charges are reimbursed. However, there are several caveats that can affect whether a billed charge is actually paid. Most of these apply to Medicare and Medicaid (state-run programs), and many of the commercial insurances are following Medicare's lead and not reimbursing without having secured the appropriate information. In any event, in order to ensure proper cash flow for the organization, the documentation must be complete and accurate. The patient's entire bill may be denied if there is a single error, resulting in correcting the error and resubmitting the bill.

First, all work reimbursed by Medicare must be authenticated as "medically necessary" by the person ordering the test. To do that, there must be a physician signature with the order (many Medicare programs accept other providers) or an indication in the patient's chart that a physician ordered the test. Second, there must be a valid ICD-9CM code, which is a numerical code indicating a specific diagnosis for which the test is ordered. A narrative description of symptoms or diagnosis is generally not acceptable. If the ICD-9CM code does not match criteria developed by Medicare for tests it considers to be medically necessary for that ICD-9CM code, the test will not be reimbursed. Laboratories have the option of having a Medicare patient sign an ABN (advanced beneficiary notice), which certifies that the patient accepts financial responsibility for tests not covered by Medicare. Accomplishing this task on in-patients can be difficult; even on outpatients and outreach patients, it is a complex and tedious procedure. Medicare holds laboratories responsible for obtaining ABN signatures and also for educating their users about the necessity of providing this information. It is a difficult task for laboratories and a cause of ongoing concern.

The type of insurance held by the patient is also a factor in determining what is paid. Medical assistance programs (Medicaid), which are governed at the state level but partially funded by the federal government, have many of the same rules as Medicare. In addition, many patients are enrolled in managed care insurance plans that do not pay fee-for-service, but instead pay the institution a flat per-member-per-month rate. These contracts are becoming more common and involve the shared risk by healthcare providers and insurance companies to keep utilization low. If the laboratory bills most HMOs (Health Maintenance Organizations) for fee-for-service, it will not be reimbursed. The laboratory test fees are all included in the flat rate.

Although budgeted revenue is carefully calculated and based on in-patient rates, actual revenues collected may differ. Actual reimbursement, however, is constantly monitored, and changes noted are included in the next year's revenue projections.

PRICING FORMULAS

Pricing for in-patient and outpatient procedures (tests) may be done using several methods (Table 11-5).

Using the **surcharge/cost plus method**, the actual cost of performing the test is determined using the microcosting method. The total cost is then multiplied by a factor (e.g., 1.5 times cost) or a dollar amount is added to the cost (surcharge) to arrive at the final price. See Table 11-6 for an example.

Note that in the example in Table 11-6, the contract is a cost per reportable and includes the cost of the analyzer, the cost of the reagents, and the cost of service. If the laboratory has purchased analyzers, the cost of reagents, service, and depreciation of the analyzer should be included and utilized for the cost per test.

TABLE 11-5.   Pricing Formulas

Surcharge/Cost Plus
Weighted Value/RVU
Historical Data

TABLE 11-6.   Surcharge/Cost Plus Method

Laboratory Charge for a CBC Using Surcharge/Cost Plus Method (Cost per reportable contract with vendor)		
Direct Costs		
Supplies Phlebotomy (from earlier example)		$1.51
Labor: Phlebotomy (6 minutes @ rate)		$2.03
Cost per Test (includes supplies, reagents, analyzer)		$1.51
Labor: Medical Technologist (5 minutes @ rate)		$2.81
Indirect Costs		
Hospital Overhead		$8.75
Laboratory Overhead		$7.25
Total Cost		$23.86
Upcharge Factor 150%		
Charge for CBC on CDM	= 23.86 × 150%	= **$35.79**

Pricing based on *weighted value/RVUs* (relative value units) is performed by assigning an RVU to the test. RVUs are generally based on the complexity and time required to perform the test, although other factors such as reagent cost for more esoteric tests may be included. The RVU so determined is then multiplied by a fixed dollar amount to determine the pricing for the test. For example, if cholesterol is weighted at 4 RVUs and the fixed dollar amount per RVU is $1.50, the price for a cholesterol test would be 4 x $1.50 or $6.00.

Pricing may also be determined based on historical data, which may be modified to reflect current market trends and expected adjustments.

Reimbursement issues (see chapter 14 for more details) are key in evaluating real revenue, as where a test is priced and what the expected reimbursement is, determine how much revenue is actually generated. For in-patients, the need to control utilization is more important so that unnecessary tests are not performed for which the laboratory incurs expense, but is not reimbursed.

MAKING BUSINESS DECISIONS

For *most* laboratory tests, the evaluation process for bringing in a new test or deciding to continue to perform a test should include a break-even analysis. The **break-even point** is the point at which there is no profit or loss from performing a test, but that the total of all fixed and variable costs equals the amount of revenue generated by the test. The reasons for performing a break-even analysis are: (1) to determine where to price the test and (2) to determine the volume of tests required to meet the break-even point.

The break-even point is determined by dividing the fixed costs plus the dollar amount of the profit expected per test by the revenues generated minus the total variable expense. Figure 11-1 shows the relationships among the factors used to calculate the break-even point.

The **break-even point** may be expressed by the following:

Where V = the volume of tests needed to break even, R = the expected revenue generated by the test, VC = the total variable cost per test, FC = the fixed cost per test, and I = the net income (revenue — total cost).

$$V = (FC + I) / (R - VC)$$

Comparing the expected number of tests to the number of tests required to balance the equation will indicate whether the test will be profitable. Adjusting the price of the test will also change the volume required to break even.

The break-even analysis formula is based on several assumptions.

1. When costs increase, profits decrease.
2. When costs decrease, profits increase.
3. When volumes increase, costs and profits increase.
4. When volumes decrease, costs and profits decrease.

Although the increases and decreases may not be linear, it is prudent to keep in mind that these relationships do exist. Quantifying their relationships is generally possible, given the availability of appropriate information.

The astute manager also needs to remember that many things other than volumes can affect costs. Those include, but are not limited to, changes in method, changes in equipment, changes from manual to automated methods or vice versa, changes in test mix, changes in unit prices for laboratory, consumables or purchased services, and changes in regulations. The best defense in monitoring these potential changes is to become fast friends with the purchasing department, the human resources department, and the group purchasing organization, if the facility belongs to one. In addition, it is desirable to keep abreast of regulatory issues and information via Internet access, publications, and professional associations.

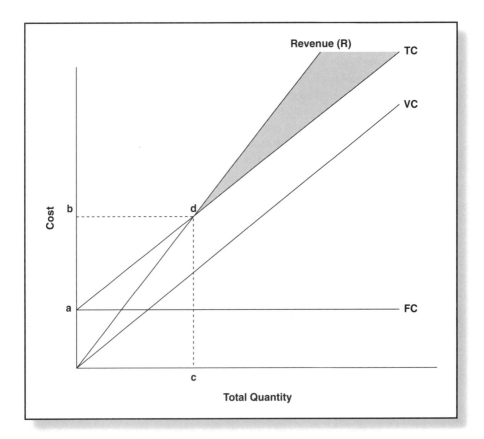

FIGURE 11-1.   **Break-Even Point**

Notes: TC = Total Cost, VC = Variable Cost, FC = Fixed Cost, R = Revenue, I = Income (represented by shaded area). TC = FC + VC. Point "d" is the break-even point (the revenues are equal to the costs). Point "c" is the quantity of tests we need to perform, point "a" is the fixed cost and point "b" is the total cost of the revenue we need to break even.

Source: Dr. Luka Powanga, *Managerial Economics in Effective Business Decisions*.[7]

The degree of profitability should also be evaluated in light of a number of "intangibles." These may include the following:

1. Will this give us a foothold in a not-yet-developed market?
2. Is this necessary for a new service or program being developed by ours or another department?
3. Is this required to keep us competitive in the outreach market?
4. Is there a particular high profile physician who requires this test?
5. Will providing this test shorten the length of stay?
6. Will providing this test decrease downstream costs by not having to perform expensive interventional procedures that might otherwise be ordered?

In some cases it is better to break even while managing to accommodate an intangible, than to make a large profit for profit's sake alone. Particularly in the community-based hospital, not all testing will be profitable. These hospitals do not have the luxury enjoyed by the commercial laboratories of accepting only "good" business or those which are most profitable. Instead, they provide the continuum of care and the support services required in the community setting, while having to work harder on at least breaking even on their overall business volume.

Taking all of these factors into account, the make-versus-buy decision can be made with some certainty. If it is determined that it is more profitable to perform the test than to send it elsewhere and incur the additional cost, the test should be brought in. In not-for-profit institutions, it may even be logical to bring in a test if doing so saves expense downstream, even if the expense to the laboratory is slightly higher. If, on the other hand, there are either financial or intangible reasons not to perform the test, it should continue to be referred out. In many instances, the laboratory manager must provide this information to senior management and they will ultimately decide where the test will be performed.

CAPITAL ACQUISITIONS

Today, there are many payment options a laboratory manager may consider when selecting a new piece of equipment including capital purchase, leasing and reagent rental. The cost of renting (most organizations will place this cost in the operating budget) or leasing the equipment, should be compared with the cost of interest and depreciation of purchase (capital budget). Most equipment companies will perform these analyses for the laboratory, but the finance department will likely want to perform the same analyses themselves. Keep in mind that you may be "competing" against project or equipment requests submitted by other departments and the financial predictions that you submit (return on investment, payback, etc.) may be determining factors in approving your request.

Generally speaking, the industry (laboratory managers and hospital finance and administration) expects a 5–7 year life expectancy for diagnostic medical laboratory equipment. Specific life expectancies can be researched in more detail in references such as the American Hospital Association's *Estimated Useful Lives of Depreciable Hospital Assets.*[8]

As the procurement of new equipment can take a great deal of time and due diligence (determining need for new equipment, capital submission, capital approval process, Request for Purchase process, site visits, contract proposal with funding options, legal review, etc.), it is important to begin the process early (at least one year prior). As stated earlier, based on available resources, it must be determined whether equipment should be purchased, leased, or re-agent rented.

The issue of capital equipment lies in the **current value of money**. The outlay of a sum of money that has a current value, but will increase in value over time, and if not spent today, will be more valuable in purchasing goods or services at a future date, is the center of discussion. Once spent, that money is no longer available and must be written off over the life of the equipment. If that money is spent in increments over a period of time, it has a greater total value over that time.

The evaluation of **depreciation** of capital equipment is key. The amount of depreciation is determined by the number of years over which the equipment is accounted for on the general ledger. Most hospitals use a straight-line depreciation formula, where the dollar value of the equipment is "written off" at the same rate over the useful lifetime of the instrument. That period of time is determined by the hospital's general accounting practices but is typically the expected life-cycle of the analyzer (5–7 years).

The calculation of the **return on investment (ROI)** is another common practice when evaluating the cost-versus-rent or lease option. The return on investment can be expressed in many ways, but generally ROI = profit margin × asset turnover. Profit margin and asset turnover, therefore, work in opposite directions. For the profit margin to increase, the turnover in assets (money) must decrease. Several factors increase profit margins, including automation, decreasing discretionary costs, eliminating obsolete and redundant services or testing, increasing collections of billed revenue, and decreasing direct costs. If a direct cost of a piece of equipment increases, the profitability of the testing scenario decreases. The goal is to at least break even on the return.

A **payback period** calculation should also be made. The payback period indicates the time it will take to generate the incoming revenue to compensate for the money paid out for the equipment (outgoing assets). For example, if an instrument costs $100,000 and it generates $25,000 annually in incremental cash, the payback period would be $100,000 divided by $25,000 or 4 years. The goal is to keep the payback period as short as possible, so that funds are not tied up. This is critically important when cash flow is tight and capital funds are at a premium.

When lump sum capital dollars are not available, a hospital can choose to **lease** an instrument. In a lease agreement, monthly payments are spread over a specified period of time (60 months) and are based on the purchase price plus interest and taxes, insurance, and maintenance. Seeing that lease expenses can be depreciated, leasing can represent an advantage over purchasing when cash availability is an issue for the institution. Leasing also offers 100% financing at fixed rates, no money down, and protection for the laboratory against inflation. A second advantage to leasing is the equipment in the laboratory is more likely to remain current. The disadvantages of leasing include: locking the laboratory into a long-term relationship with one vendor; lack of ownership; and higher reagent and consumables prices, in most cases.

There are two advantages to a **reagent rental** agreement, the cost of the instrument is included in the reagent cost charged by the vendor, and as with leasing, the equipment in the laboratory is more likely to remain current. The laboratory signs an agreement, which usually commits it to a minimum volume of reagent, purchased over a specified period at a set price. Again, the advantage is that there are no capital costs for the laboratory. Whereas direct purchase requires a large amount of money up front, and leasing requires capital money spread over time, reagent rental requires no capital money. If the allocated resources do not allow for lease or purchase, reagent rental can be used for the first year and the equipment leased or purchased later working with the financial services of the institution and appropriate vendor(s). If the choice is for a capital purchase of an instrument, it is important to realize the concept of the payback period. The payback is the number of years it will take to pay back the original instrument purchase cost. A projected payback period for capital equipment is presented in Table 11-7. The financial services department can help with various financial calculations presented by vendors.

Getting What You Need

Most organizations define a capital acquisition (capital purchase) as an acquisition of a major piece of equipment, or infrastructure improvement greater than a specific dollar amount that has a useful life measured in years. Each department throughout the organization is responsible for compiling a list of major equipment required or desired to improve their department. Capital acquisitions for the laboratory typically include items such as analyzers, refrigerators, centrifuges, microscopes and other equipment.

TABLE 11-7. Example of a Projected Payback Period for Capital Equipment

- Instrument costs = $150,000
- Estimated annual cash flow = $30,000/year
- Payback period for the instrument = 5 years ($150,000/$30,000)

Today there are many financing options for the acquisition of capital equipment. These options include purchasing, leasing, and renting. The following five areas are the financial considerations in capital acquisition[9]:

Cash Flow—Amount of money and schedule of when it is paid. Purchase requires large outlay of cash; lease and rental spread payments over time.

Commitment—Buy-in of the company to the capital equipment with purchase being the most committed and rental the least committed.

Cost—Time value of money must be factored in to determine final cost.

Tax Impact—Depreciable or deductible expense.

Obsolescence Risk—Expected life cycle of product versus newer equipment with advances in technology.

The following is an example of justification for switching from traditional test tube blood bank testing to column agglutination testing, better known as Ortho's Gel system. Much of the information on the following pages are excerpts from a justification presentation developed by Don Strable, laboratory manager and Joseph Wawrzynski, Jr., to assist in simplifying this process.

Format and Process

The format and process for submitting capital requests differs from organization to organization. Some organizations may require electronic submission of data to a centralized database or application. This is a convenient way to track the submission as people in the process log in, access, provide comments and their approval/disapproval. As one person "rubber stamps" their approval via electronic signature, the next person in the approval process is notified the capital request is ready for their review and so forth until a capital committee or board meet and approve the requests. Keep in mind that not all requests may be approved as capital funds are limited. In this case, providing proper justification is paramount to having your request approved while another department's would not be.

In some organizations the same process occurs on paper forms. Success with this model requires the submission packet make its way to each appropriate party and not be lost along the way. It may be prudent to make copies of paperwork submitted so that in the event any paperwork is misplaced, duplicate paperwork can be submitted promptly.

In either case, the capital submission format can be generically described as follows:

Summary
Benefits
Data
Financials and Interpretation

Summary

- Outline your key points
- Keep it simple
- Make it accurate
- Minimize the length of your justification

The summary is a brief paragraph of no more than 3 or 4 sentences clearly specifying your request. The summary is used to outline your key reasons for obtaining the piece of equipment or infrastructure improvement. It should be short, sweet and to the point.

For example:

- In 2000, the automation of the Blood Bank processes began with the implementation of the Ortho Gel Card methodology for blood bank patient testing. In 2004, to continue the process with the acquisition of the Ortho ProVue technology, an integrated gel card reader and pipetting system was added, which is interfaceable with the LIS.

Benefits

The next step is to explain the important benefits that justify the acquisition of the equipment or improvement to infrastructure. Key areas of benefits include:

- Meeting Regulatory Requirement
- Patient Safety
- Improved Quality and Service
- Financial Strength
- Leadership and Market Strength
- Infrastructure Improvements

The manager is able to justify acquisition of the equipment or improvement to infrastructure by detailing as many of the areas of benefits listed above that the product will influence. Keep in mind that each manager will have capital acquisition requests and there will be a limited supply of money. Using the key areas of benefit will aid in prioritizing the needs of the organization. Obviously, equipment or infrastructure improvements needed to meet regulatory requirements have to be approved, and, in some cases, are approved on an emergency basis.

Capital acquisitions and infrastructure improvements designed to address patient safety issues also tend to be higher priorities. Patient safety improvements are measures implemented to ensure the safety of patients by providing the intended treatment to the intended recipient. Organizations can spend decades building a reputation of quality and service. It only takes one or two incidents to tarnish that reputation. This is further advanced by the number of avenues available for the media and the general population to transmit information (TV, radio, Internet, Blogs, etc.).

Capital acquisitions to improve the quality of patient care and services are also highly prioritized. "Quality" can be both real (better outcomes based on core measures that are statistically measured in venues such as the Hospital Consumer Assessment of Health Providers and Systems Surveys (HCAHPS)) and perceived (Press Ganey patient surveys asking the patient to rate the quality of care received). As each healthcare organization's "grades" or ratings are available to consumers via the Internet, healthcare consumers are becoming more educated with regard to the quality (both real and perceived) of care each organization delivers. This available information has brought a "transparency" to the healthcare industry, such that healthcare consumers are able to research and compare the quality received at specific healthcare institutions. Many institutions realize that consumers are taking advantage of this information and are scrutinizing the industry before choosing a healthcare provider. As a result, many organizations are turning to operational improvement strategies such as LEAN, Six Sigma, infrastructure and technology advances to improve quality, gain efficiencies and thereby improve service.

As reimbursement rates shrink and pay-for-performance (P4P) initiatives are adopted, including no reimbursements for hospital acquired conditions, maintaining profitability has become imperative for organizations to remain viable. Without profit, capital does not exist as the funds are used for paying operational expenses. Capital increases as the profit margin increases, allowing the organization to re-invest in itself.

Leadership and market strength are also, albeit, less, important than some of the other key benefits. Maintaining and improving market share (growth) is important for an organization to compete against other healthcare organizations. Acquisition of state-of-the-art equipment is also important in attracting quality employees and physicians.

Infrastructure improvements, while not glamorous, are often the backbone of the organization. For example, Information Technology improvements such as a network switch or wireless access point are not glamorous or may not even be apparent. They do, however, allow equipment such as wireless PDA blood collection devices to perform the following: scan a patient's bar-coded wristband, wirelessly connect to the LIS, query the LIS for patient orders, print out the specimen labels at the patient bedside, and reconfirm the patient ID by rescanning the patient's barcode.

For example:

BENEFITS OF IMPLEMENTING THE ORTHO PROVUE INCLUDE: PATIENT SAFETY

- Improved patient safety using barcode tracking
- Utilize gel reproducibility and stability
- Gel facilitates supervisory review, technical competency and training
- Reduces human clerical activity (label two gel cards vs. multiple test tubes)

IMPROVED QUALITY AND SERVICE

- Automated test processing and interpretation
- LIS bi-directional interface obtains patient demographics and sends results to LIS
- Automatic QC monitoring for reagents, test cards and QC results
- Random access for enhanced productivity and stat response
- Utilization of same reagent system as manual method
- 45 day implementation plan
- Small equipment footprint
- Expansion of current testing capability

FINANCIAL STRENGTH

- Cost avoidance by not hiring additional FTE
- Payback within life of analyzer

LEADERSHIP AND MARKET STRENGTH

Employee Satisfaction

- Nonvalue-added processing steps
- Reduces clerical activities
- State-of-the-art technology

Physician Satisfaction

- Better, more consistent results
- Better response time

DATA

- Create a capsule summary of your workload
- Review a minimum of 2 years to a maximum of 5 years
- Highlight trends
- Be able to explain the trends
- Do not forget non-revenue items

Table 11-8 outlines the key data that justify either an additional FTE or the automated analyzer. From the data given, we know that the institution implemented immediate spin crossmatches sometime after 2000. In addition, we can also see that the volume for Types, Screens and Crossmatches have increased significantly. The organization's senior administration can correlate the rise in these tests to the expansions in two programs: Maternity and Oncology & Infusion.

TABLE 11-8.   Workload Volume 2000–2004

Workload (Revenue Generators)	Year 2000	Projected Year 2004	% Change 2004/2000
Type & Screen	2643	5406	105%
ABO & Rh	65	318	489%
DAT	60	120	200%
Cord Blood ABO & Rh	828	1226	48%
Cord Blood DAT	828	1226	48%
Crossmatch IS	0	2651	
Crossmatch IgG	1656	1107	
Crossmatch IS & IgG	1656	3758	120%

Workload (Non-Revenue Generators)	Year 2000	Projected Year 2004	% Change 2004/2000
Unit Retype	1985	4000	105%
Patient Retype	550	1803	328%

Note: If data is to be submitted in a paper packet, a chart or graph may be useful in conveying the data, as a pictorial representation can make a dramatic impact. See Figure 11-2.

TRENDS: 2000 thru 2004

- Type and screens increased 105%
- Blood types increased 489% due to maternity screening
- Crossmatches increased 120%; Decreased IgG Crossmatch by switching to IS Crossmatch
- Component retypes increased 105% due to transfusion growth

Financials & Interpretation

As stated in Chapter 10, investment decisions (capital expenditures, growth into new service lines, etc.) in healthcare involve many factors including returns on investment, comparing the return on investment between different projects and intangibles such as despite a negative return on an investment, the investment will be needed to support another larger project that will provide a positive return. To aid in these decisions, three useful financial tools are:

- Payback Period
- Net Present Value (NPV)
- Internal Rate of Return (IRR)

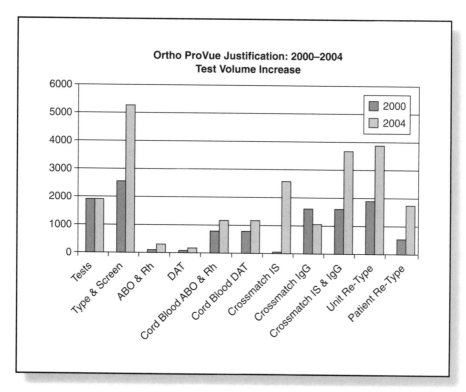

FIGURE 11-2. **Graphical Representation of Workload Comparison 2000–2004**
Source: Don Strable, MS, MT(ASCP)DLM[10]

The first step in evaluating the decision to purchase the ProVue is to outline the estimated revenue and expenses for the first five years and apportion for each year individually. In this case, revenue can also be defined as dollars being spent on an additional FTE (cost avoidance). Expenses will still mean the money being spent on the ProVue. We also needed to include the additional expense of the LIS interface (at purchase) and the yearly maintenance fees associated with this as well as the ProVue maintenance contract for years 2–5. Refer to Table 11-9.

Interpretations

- **NPV: $15,356.21** value of our $49,076 return on the project at a 10% interest rate (obtained from the CFO).

  NOTES: NPV calculated using *Microsoft Office 2003 Excel* NPV function by entering NPV(0.1, −103000, 26000, 35560, 37167, 38822, 40527). The NPV function is used to determine the net present value using cash flows that occur at regular intervals, such as monthly or annually. Each cash flow, specified as a *value*, occurs at the end of a period (*Microsoft, 2007*).

TABLE 11-9.   Projected Revenues, Expenses and Total for the First Five Years of the Automated ProVue Analyzer

Year	Revenues (Cost Avoidance)	Expenses	Expense Comments	Revenue – Expenses
Year 1	$26,000 (0.5 FTE)	$110,000	Equipment	–$103,000
		$14,000	LIS Interface	
		$0	Maintenance included	
		$5,000	Renovations	
		$129,000		
Year 2	$53,560 (1.0 FTE)	$4,000	LIS Interface maintenance	$35,560
		$14,000	ProVue maintenance	
		$18,000		
Year 3	$55,167 (1.0 FTE)	$4,000	LIS Interface maintenance	$37,167
		$14,000	ProVue maintenance	
		$18,000		
Year 4	$56,822 (1.0 FTE)	$4,000	LIS Interface maintenance	$38,822
		$14,000	ProVue maintenance	
		$18,000		
Year 5	$58,527 (1.0 FTE)	$4,000	LIS Interface maintenance	$40,527
		$14,000	ProVue maintenance	
		$18,000		
Overall	$250,076	$201,000		**$49,076**

- **IRR: 17%** return on our invested dollar

  NOTES: IRR calculated using *Microsoft Office 2003 Excel* IRR function {IRR(values, guess)} by entering our values into a table (–103000, 35560, 37167, 38822, 40527) and then using these numbers as the "values" portion of the function. We entered the Microsoft default of 0.10 for 10%.

- **PAYBACK PERIOD: 45 months**

  NOTES: Payback period is calculated as the amount of the investment/annual cash flows. As our cash flows are not equal, but are relatively the same amount, we used the average of 38,019 for the last 4 years. Dividing 103,000/38019 = 2.7 years. Adding the first year in results in a payback term of 3.7 years or approximately 45 months. As this payback period is less than the minimum 60 month expected life of the analyzer, this would be a good investment.

Final Thoughts

As a lab manager, you will be responsible for capital procurement, budgeting and the justification process. You may have to compete against other projects as capital funds are limited. As such, the more compelling an argument you can state utilizing the key benefit areas, the better your chances will be of having your capital requests approved. Listed below are a few simple rules to ensure you develop the strongest argument possible to gain approval.

- Seek input from the finance professionals; it will make a stronger case.
- Do not try to outthink the finance people; this is their sandbox (area of expertise).
- Do not overstate your case; you will have to live with it. Once an FTE is retracted, it is harder to justify reinstatement.
- Threats, failures, mistakes, and errors make a better case to replace you rather than equipment.

RESOURCES

Many resources are available to assist laboratory managers in evaluating their own profitability and in comparing that to the profitability and practices of other institutions. Information on cost accounting is available both in hard copy and online and is provided not only by financial institutions, but by government agencies and professional associations affiliated with the healthcare field. The College of American Pathologists, the Clinical Laboratory Management Association, and the Centers for Medicare and Medicaid Services (formerly the Health Care Financing Administration) are but a few. The attached bibliography and Internet resources are only a starting point for locating additional information.

SUMMARY

This chapter has presented a basic overview of the interrelationships of financial and managerial accounting, methods to evaluate expenses and revenues, issues surrounding reimbursement, methods for pricing tests, factors related to capital acquisitions, and a short list of resources available to laboratory managers. In an industry where competition is brutal and change is rapid and extensive, it becomes critical for the manager to understand and constantly evaluate the financial status of the laboratory. A strong knowledge of financial methods and practices will allow the manager to do that and to remain financially strong and competitive.

SUMMARY CHART:
Important Points to Remember

➤ The laboratory produces revenue (patient testing) and has expenses (cost of equipment, reagent, supplies, building, etc.). Expenses are the only part in which the laboratory manager has direct control.

➤ In medical laboratories, the charges billed for a test are attached to a specific CPT (current procedural terminology) code. The CPT coding system is maintained by the CPT Editorial Board of the American Medical Association.

➤ The Charge Description Master is a list of all billable services, their associated CPT code, and the price charged to the patient or insurance carrier.

➤ The cost of each laboratory test includes direct and indirect expenses; all must be accounted for to determine the true cost.

➤ Direct costs are costs directly related to performing a test including reagents, consumables, labor and benefits.

➤ Indirect costs (overhead) include expenses that are part of doing business, but that are not directly related to the cost of the test being evaluated. Examples include licenses, fees, administrative staff and the building.

➤ Fixed costs remain constant despite any change in the volume of tests performed. Examples of fixed costs include salaries and benefits for supervisors and administrators, the cost of a courier, and depreciation on a piece of equipment.

➤ Variable costs, however, vary proportionately to the change in test volume. Examples of variable costs include reagent costs and consumables (e.g., pipette tips, cups).

➤ Semi-variable costs vary with the volume, but not in direct proportion. Technologist labor is a good example. If a 5% increase in test volume occurs, and the work can be covered by current staffing, the total labor cost does not increase and the labor cost per billable actually decreases. If a 30% increase occurs, additional technical staff is required and the total cost will increase.

➤ A microcosting analysis determines the cost of a test by totaling all expenses associated with performing a given test including reagents, consumables, laboratory costs, and reporting costs and includes pre-analytical, analytical, and post-analytical expenses.

➤ A break-even analysis determines the number of tests needed to be performed to generate enough revenue to cover the expenses incurred ("break-even").

➤ In most cases, the benefit (laboratory revenue) should justify the additional direct expense when expanding the test menu and/or the cost of capital acquisitions on its own merits.

➤ There are many financing options available to procure capital equipment including purchase, lease and renting.

➤ Utilize financial analyses such as Payback, NPV, IRR, etc. to justify your request and aid your case.

➤ Utilize the key areas of benefit to build your case and justify the capital equipment you are requesting. Key areas of benefit are: Meeting Regulatory Requirement, Patient Safety, Improved Quality and Service, Financial Strength, Leadership and Market Strength and Infrastructure Improvements.

Suggested Problem-Based Learning Activities

Chapter 11: Cost/Benefit Analysis

Instructions: Use Internet resources, books, articles, colleagues, etc., to present solutions to the problems listed below. There is no one correct solution to any problem.

Note to Instructor: Students in class may be divided into groups and given the problem-based learning activity to discuss and solve. Once the group has reached consensus as to a solution, the group may present it to the other students in the class. This activity will provide all students with information regarding solutions to the problem.

Problem #1

Suppose you have just been given a project to provide new laboratory services. Project revenue and costs for this new service.

Problem #2

You have just purchased a piece of new equipment and must determine what testing to perform in-house and what testing to send to a reference laboratory.

Problem #3

Suppose your institution just received notification that the reimbursement for your inpatient laboratory testing will be reduced by 6%. What alternative do you have to maintain your current profit level?

REFERENCES

1. Centers for Medicaid & Medicare Services. *National Health Expenditure Data: NHE Fact Sheet.* 26 June 2010. Retrieved 11 July 2010, from: http://www.cms.gov/NationalHealthExpendData/25_NHE_Fact_Sheet.asp#TopOfPage

2. Centers for Medicaid & Medicare Services. *National Health Expenditure Projections 2009–2019,* Forecast Summary NHE Fact Sheet. 29 June 2010. Retrieved 22 Aug 2010, from: http://www.cms.gov/NationalHealthExpendData/downloads/proj2009.pdf

3. Centers for Medicaid & Medicare Services. *Hospital Outpatient Prospective Payment System.* Jan 2010. Retrieved 22 Aug 2010, from: https://www.cms.gov/MLNProducts/downloads/HospitalOutpaysysfctsht.pdf

4. Staff of the Human Resources and Community Development Division, Congressional Budget Office. *Analysis of Medicare Hospital Reimbursement Changes in the Tax Equity and Fiscal Responsibility Act of 1982.* March 1983. Retrieved 11 July 2010, from: http://www.cbo.gov/ftpdocs/50xx/doc5059/doc09a.pdf

5. Wilensky GR: *The Balanced Budget Act of 1997: a current look at its impact on patients and providers.* Statement (Testimony) before the Medicare Payment Advisory Commission. 19 July 2000. Retrieved 11 July 2010, from: http://pages.stern.nyu.edu/~jasker/BBA1.pdf

6. American Medical Association. *About CPT.* Retrieved 22 Aug 2010, from: http://www.ama-assn.org/ama/pub/physician-resources/solutions-managing-your-practice/coding-billing-insurance/cpt/about-cpt.shtml

7. Powanga, M, McManus, V, Donnelly, P: *Effective Business Decisions.* McGraw-Hill Primis Custom Publishing, New York, NY, 2001, p. 50.

8. American Hospital Association Health Data Management Group: *Estimated Useful Lives of Depreciable Hospital Assets.* American Hospital Association, Chicago, IL, 2008.

9. Sobel M: *MBA in a Nutshell.* McGraw-Hill Professional, New York, NY, 2010. pp. 91-92.

10. Strable D: Ortho ProVue Justification. PowerPoint presentation, 2004.

BIBLIOGRAPHY

American Medical Association: *CPT 2010 Professional Edition (Current Procedural Terminology, Professional Ed. (Spiral)).* American Medical Association, Chicago, IL, 2010.

Andersen RM, Rice TH, Kominski GF: *Changing the U.S. Health Care System: Key Issues in Health Services Policy and Management.* Jossey-Bass, A Wiley Company, San Francisco, CA, 2001.

Bozo P, ed.: *Cost-Effective Laboratory Management.* Lippincott, Williams & Wilkins Publishers, Philadelphia, PA, 1998.

Brock HR, Herrington LA: *Cost Accounting: Principles and Applications.* Glencoe McGraw-Hill, 1998.

Cooper R, Kaplan RS: *Design of Cost Management Systems.* Prentice Hall, Upper Saddle River, 1998.

Drucker P: *Management Challenges for the 21st Century.* HarperCollins Publishers, New York, NY, 1999.

Groppelli A, Nikbakht E: *Finance (Barron's Business Review Series).* Barron's Educational Series, Hauppauge, NY, 2006.

Horngren CT, Foster G, Datar SM: *Cost Accounting: A Managerial Emphasis.* Prentice Hall, Upper Saddle River, NJ, 1999.

Kimmel P, Weygandt J, Kieso D: *Financial Accounting: Tools for Business Decision Making.* John Wiley & Sons, Danvers, 2005.

Kimmel P, Weygandt J, Kieso D: *Accounting and Finance: Managerial Use and Analysis.* John Wiley & Sons, New York, NY, 2000.

Kirschner CG, et al: *Current Procedural Terminology 2010.* American Medical Association, Chicago, IL, 2009.

Label W: *Accounting for Non-Accountants.* Sourcebooks, Naperville, IL, 2010.

Schultz D: *ICD-9CM Code Book for Hospitals.* St. Anthony Publishing, Reston, VA, 2000.

Travers EM: *Clinical Laboratory Management.* Williams & Wilkins, Philadelphia, PA, 1997.

Wallace MA, Kosinski DD: *Clinical Laboratory Science Education and Management.* WB Saunders, Philadelphia, PA, 1998.

Williams J, Haka S, Bettner M: *Financial and Managerial Accounting: The Basis of Business Decisions.* McGraw-Hill/Irwin, New York, NY, 2004.

Zelman WM, McCue MJ, Millikan AR, Glick ND. *Financial Management of Health Care Organizations: An Introduction to Fundamental Tools, Concepts, and Applications.* Blackwell Publishing, Malden, MA, 2004.

INTERNET RESOURCES

American Association for Clinical Chemistry (AACC)
http://www.aacc.org

American Hospital Association (AHA)
http://www.aha.org

American Medical Association (AMA)
http://www.ama-assn.org

Centers for Medicare and Medicaid Services (CMS)
http://www.cms.gov

The Clinical Laboratory Management Association (CLMA)
http://www.clma.org

The Joint Commission. Quality Check™
http://www.qualitycheck.org/consumer/searchQCR.aspx

The Maryland Hospital Association
http://www.mdhospitals.org,
http://www.mhaonline.org

Thomson Reuters
http://www.thomsonreuters.com

U.S. Department of Health & Human Services. Hospital Compare
http://www.hospitalcompare.hhs.gov/hospital-search.aspx

12

Effective Budgeting in the Laboratory: Practical Tips

Joseph J. Wawrzynski, Jr., MBA, MT(ASCP)BB, DLM^{CM}, CQA(ASQ)CQIA
Irina Lutinger, MPH, H(ASCP)DLM

CHAPTER OUTLINE

Objectives
Key Terms
Case Study
Introduction
Types of Operating Budgets
The Successful Budget Process
Common Budget Problems and
    Possible Solutions
Surviving Budget Justification

Summary
Summary Chart: Important Points
    to Remember
Suggested Problem-Based Learning
    Activities
References
Bibliography
Internet Resources

OBJECTIVES

Following successful completion of this chapter, the learner will be able to:

1. Describe the operating budget types.
2. Explain the steps for preparation of a successful budget process.
3. Identify common budgetary problems and recommend possible solutions.
4. Describe how to write proper budget justifications.

KEY TERMS

Appropriation Budget
Budget Justification

Fixed or Static Budget
Flexible or Variable Budget

Case Study   Planning to Open an Outpatient Infusion Center

You are the manager of the clinical laboratory in the hospital. The hospital administration wants to penetrate the market and expand the business by opening an Oncology Outpatient Infusion Center. It will complement the existing Radiation Oncology Department and will be dedicated to the treatment and support of patients receiving Outpatient chemotherapy infusions and blood transfusions. The center will provide services in two settings: 1) a contemporary indoor "hospital" atmosphere, in comfortable reclining lounges with amenities such as choices for music, television, DVD movies, reading material, and Internet access. Ample comfortable seating for family members persuades them to remain with their loved one during treatment and 2) a tranquil nature setting for patients to receive infusions in an outdoor shaded garden complete with bamboo shoots and a cascading waterfall that empties into a reflection pond populated with Japanese Koi fish. Outdoor landscaping will also include stunning horticultural displays that are visually pleasing with reduced fragrance. Chairs and benches in shaded areas encourage family members to stay with loved ones during the treatment period. Consideration was given for a standalone laboratory; however, as space is at a premium, administration has requested the testing be absorbed by your existing laboratory with specimens transported to your location. Test turn-around-time (TAT) will be an important factor, as patients need to be on schedule. Administration has informed you that test volumes will increase 10% (30 CBCs) in Hematology and 25% (10 Type & Screens) in Blood Bank. Hematology and Blood Bank are currently staffed with two technologists. Construction will take approximately six months to complete (completed within the existing fiscal year) as renovations will occur to an existing space.

Issues and Questions to Consider:
1. *What effect will this have on the existing budgets?*
2. *What other areas of the laboratory will be impacted?*
3. *What assumptions should be made in modifying the current operating budget?*
4. *Will any additional laboratory personnel be required for the additional test volumes and rapid TAT expectations?*
5. *Which are the major aspects of concern in proposing the new facility?*

INTRODUCTION

Why is budgeting in the Healthcare Industry, and the laboratory in particular, important?

Consider the following facts:

In a recent article entitled *"Number of uninsured Americans could grow by 10M in 5 years,"* associate editor Chelsey Ledue cited a Robert Wood Johnson Foundation report as projecting that by 2015, there could be as many as 59.7 million people uninsured.[1] In addition, the report indicated that number could swell to 67.6 million by 2020. An estimated 49.4 million individuals were without health coverage in 2010, yet these individuals are required to be seen in Emergency Departments of most hospitals when they present for treatment.[1]

In 2008, there was $36.4 billion (5.8% of total expenses) in charity or uncompensated care delivered.[2] Furthermore, there was a decline in the number of registered community hospitals with 5,828 in 1980, and 5,010 in 2008, a 14% decrease.[2]

Total spending on health care in the economy has doubled over the last 30 years to a level of about 16% of Gross Domestic Product (GDP) which was $13.7 trillion in 2007, and $14.10 trillion in 2008.[3,4] The Congressional Budget Office predicts that this percentage will approach 31% of GDP over the next 25 years, almost doubling.[5] On average the United States spends $7,290 annually per person on health care.[3] Compare this to the $2,964 average among all OECD countries (Organisation for Economic Co-operation and Development).[3] Even Norway, the nation with the second most expensive healthcare system on a per capita basis, places a distant second, spending only $4,763 ($2,527 less or almost 35% less per year than the United States).[3]

Seeking to radically change the current healthcare system, in March 2010, President Barack Obama signed into law a health care reform bill (American Affordable Care Act) that looks to rein in costs and provide coverage to most Americans. Key points of the bill are [6]:

1. Expanding health coverage to all Americans
2. Making healthcare more affordable by lowering costs
3. Increased accountability of health insurers
4. Creates a new competitive market for health care insurance
5. Ends discrimination for people with pre-existing conditions

Lastly, the Centers for Medicare and Medicaid Services (CMS) has developed "pay-for-performance" (P4P) initiatives to encourage high quality care to be delivered to Medicare beneficiaries.[7] Higher performing hospitals (top 10%) as measured against quality and clinical measures, will have the opportunity to be reimbursed a 2% bonus payment in addition to the standard diagnosis related group (DRG) payment.[7]

What do all of these statistics and pending changes mean for the laboratory? In order to remain viable, hospitals will need to become even more business-oriented, placing an increased emphasis on quality, the cost of non-quality and the bottom line. There will be fewer reimbursement dollars (cost control) to provide health care to more Americans (increased access). CMS (and other insurance companies) have begun to recognize the cost saving advantage of providing quality healthcare to their beneficiaries and will reward those organizations that excel and penalize those that fall short. Budgeting and variances will be scrutinized more closely in an effort to track and control costs.

The budget process is demanding and stressful. Within reason, the laboratory manager must be able to accurately forecast expenses for anticipated patient and test volumes and to a lesser extent, revenues. As most, if not all, inpatient testing is bundled into the DRG reimbursement rate received by the hospital, revenue projections may not be that significant for inpatients; however, they may still remain for outpatients or for contract clients. Keep in mind the budget is just that—a forecast; a best guess estimate of anticipated volumes, revenues and expenses. Many outside factors that cannot be anticipated may influence revenues or expenses. A recent example would include lower patient volumes due to the postponement of elective procedures due to many Americans' loss of jobs (and the loss of healthcare insurance) caused by the current recession. However, most test volumes, revenues and expenses should be able to be reasonably estimated by tracking past expenses, reviewing vendor contracts and accurately projecting growth.

A variance is the difference between the actual and projected (budgeted) volume, revenue or expense. Variances can be positive or negative. Variances will occur. Some variances will be obvious; others will require substantial investigation. Variances are not always problems. On the contrary, they present opportunities to correct problems. In any event, the laboratory manager must be able to justify any variance from the forecasted budget. Investigation would yield an explanation and proper justification in our decreased patient volume example above. To properly prepare a budget, the laboratory manager/supervisor should be able to respond to the following questions:

- What are the projected test volumes for the upcoming budget period?
- How much did the laboratory spend on reagents, consumables, proficiency testing, licensing fees, maintenance contracts, etc., last year? Are there any changes such as changes to the test menu, increased fees, purchase of additional proficiency tests, etc.?
- Do increased expenditures for the send-out tests to the reference laboratory warrant investigation of bringing testing in-house?
- If any tests are brought in-house, is there an increase in the testing section's budget (reagents, personnel, consumables, etc.) and a corresponding decrease in the sendout account?

An understanding of the planning, budgeting, and managing process is vital in allocation of available resources not only to meet anticipated needs but also to control actual use. The laboratory must be viewed as a business. Once this fact is recognized, considerations of long-term and short-term planning should be included, with emphasis on operating requirements; clear goals and objectives must be identified; and monitoring and control of ongoing operations must be implemented. The budget is a business tool to be used for effective resource management.

Resource management is different from **resource allocation** because it includes accountability for results. Managers are asked to justify resources needed in terms of expected results; therefore cost accounting is an important tool to accomplish this objective on an on-going basis. Cost accounting identifies, defines, measures, reports, and analyzes the elements of costs associated with providing a unit of output (test) and appropriately assigns and allocates costs to that test. For example, operating costs require daily review including but not limited to payroll, reagents, and consumable utilization. Constant justification for variances is required to explain why better/less expensive results can't be obtained by using fewer resources. Payers, patients, and the community ask questions about prices and charges, which increases pressure on the budgeting process and hospital resources. In this climate of high demands and low resources, sufficient information provided during the year from the hospital to the laboratory manager is imperative for successful budgetary planning. The challenge of budgeting and resource management is to improve existing resources, to identify realistic expectations, and to communicate these effectively to all appropriate parties.

The **operating budget** is a tool for laboratory managers to use throughout the year. Simply put, it is the calculated best-guess estimate of revenue and expenditures the laboratory is expected to realize for a 12 month period of time, the fiscal year. The budget is the overall plan for projections, identification and coordination of resources and a means to track expenditures. Today's budget must evaluate appropriate use of resources in relation to results, instead of being used as a projection and monitoring tool. Furthermore, the operating budget is a communication tool to be used with internal and external customers, but it is not a crystal ball.

When reviewing a budget, it is important not to focus on numbers only, but to understand the objectives of the department and organization behind the numbers. The laboratory manager should be able to objectively assess the needs of the organization, the resources available and appropriately allocate the resources to accomplish the established goal(s). The budgetary package should explain the objectives regarding future growth, and then the manager will be able to objectively estimate and identify the realistic expectations. The budget should be used not only to comply with the annual process but also to improve the financial aspects of one's job and the department to solve problems as they arise.

Most organizations' operating plan or budgeting cycle is based on a period of one year and is goal oriented. The goal to remain under the projected budget or have appropriate justification for surpassing the budget. This period of time is known as a fiscal year. The fiscal year may or may not coincide with the calendar year. For example, a fiscal year could run from July 1st through June 30th just as easily as from January 1st to December 31st. The fiscal year is further broken down into four quarters and further into 12 individual months.

Typically, the organization has a financial system capable of providing the laboratory and other departments with various financial report(s). The reports function as tools in identifying how well the department is achieving its identified goals and objectives. The type and format of the operating budget selected depend on the organization's requirements. The reports most likely will display the budgeted and actual revenue, test volumes, and expenses (salaries and nonsalaries). The reports may also display the percentage variance between budgeted and actual. This chapter defines the types of operating budgets, offers guidelines for the budgetary process, identifies the most common budget problems, and provides tips on surviving budget justification.

TYPES OF OPERATING BUDGETS

Among budget types are the following: fixed, flexible, program, appropriation, rolling, incremental, and zero-based budgets. Capital budgeting (purchases) was previously discussed in Chapter 11, and will not be addressed in this chapter.

A **fixed or static budget** assumes a single level of activity, and the entire budget is built around that level. If the laboratory is confident that its expenditures won't change during the budget cycle, there will be no new tests brought in and no new equipment purchased, then this type of budget can be used. A fixed budget is not a tool to monitor and control resources during changes, and thus would not be a good choice for this scenario.

A **flexible or variable budget** differs from the fixed budget in a number of ways. The flexible budget can be geared to a *range* of activity, useful if any change in services (addition or subtraction) is anticipated. The flexible budget compares actual results to the new level of activity instead of comparing against the originally budgeted level of activity. The flexible budget recognizes the difficulty of establishing a single level of achievement and provides a tool for controlling costs. It can also point out the priority expenses and its variances.

A **program budget** is created based on a specific program matrix. Included in this matrix are all proposed services and the resources required. A proposed program can include a set of activities, services, staffing, and equipment related to the program. This type of budget can be used for short-term planning.

An **appropriation budget** is usually found in governmental organizations that depend on an outside source of funds. During the review process the outside agency reviews the budget in detail and authorizes specific dollar amounts. If expenses exceed the appropriated amount, the responsible party must obtain the supplemental appropriation from the granting agency.

A **rolling budget** is a continuous budget that is updated periodically in preparation for the next budget cycle. A rolling budget for a 12-month period is reviewed and revised every quarter. The past quarter becomes history and the new quarter is added to the projection to move ahead. This type of budget is used for cash projections and therefore frequently updated.

An **incremental budget** addresses only changes like new equipment, new positions, and new programs. It assumes that all current operations are essential to the process and working at its peak performance. The advantage is the minimal time commitment for incremental budget preparation and the disadvantage is assumption that all existing operations are essential for business.

In a **zero-based budget,** management annually reevaluates all activities to decide whether they should be eliminated or funded. Projects are approved based on funds availability and funding levels are determined by priorities. A zero-based budget helps to determine levels of resource requirements within a service or program and the possible expenditure level within each responsibility center. Each department manager is required to justify the entire unit budget annually as if all of its activities were totally new. It is extremely important to have accurate records of how much cost is incurred for every resource used to produce test results.

Based on the preceding discussion in our case study, the new Outpatient Infusion Center that the hospital is planning to open, what budget should we use? While we don't know the exact volumes, but based on past history, we can develop an estimated increase to our existing test volumes, reagents, consumables and determine if our existing staff has the capacity to perform the increased workload. To be successful, we need to carefully account for all the services required including the additional test volumes and what sections will be impacted (courier, accessioning and testing) in this venture.

The budget will be based on various components of costs such as direct, indirect, variable, and fixed. The direct costs can be easily tied to a laboratory test, but the indirect costs are not involved in the production of the test. For example, direct costs include consumables and supplies, labor, and equipment to do the test. In contrast, the major component of indirect costs is the cost of time in which personnel are doing things other than producing reportable laboratory results. Supervisory personnel not doing testing, secretarial support, phlebotomist

TABLE 12-1. Example of Variable Costs for Reagents and Supplies

Number of Tests	Costs of Reagents and Supplies	Total Variable Costs
1	$0.25	$0.25
10	$0.25	$2.50
100	$0.25	$25.00

time, photocopying, utilities, employee benefits, computing services, and space are examples of indirect costs. Costs can behave as fixed or as variable. Fixed expenses do not vary with the test volume for a given period when variable expenses change proportionately with changes in volume of tests performed. Variable costs increase or decrease proportionally as activity changes. Table 12-1 provides an example of variable costs for reagents and supplies.

$$\text{Total costs} = \text{Fixed costs} + \text{Variable costs}$$
$$\text{Average cost per test} = \text{Total costs}/\# \text{ tests}$$

The average cost per test decreases as volume increases (up to a certain volume at which point additional staff will need to be hired as the volume will reach a point that exceeds the capacity of the existing staff).

Labor expenses are important to accurately estimate the budgetary needs. An example of direct variable costs is presented in Table 12-2.

Because the Outpatient Infusion Center in our example will not be performing testing, compliance with regulatory agencies should not be a problem. The Information Systems personnel will need to install appropriate devices such as computer terminals, phones and faxes and ensure their functionality in order for the laboratory test results to be communicated to the clinicians. The information services staff would be responsible for connecting laboratory information, clinical information, and registration systems operations. Failure of any of these systems could lead, for example, to the inability of the laboratory information system to retrieve, transmit, or compile results for clients or their patients leading to a loss of both revenue and future business. In addition, we will also need to educate and familiarize the Outpatient Infusion Center physicians and nursing staffs to the established normal ranges, critical values, reporting cascade, etc.

If testing were to be performed at the new facility, we would need to make sure that all the regulatory requirements are met appropriately, the appropriate paperwork is filed and licenses obtained, a Medical Director is appointed to oversee the Center and is involved with selecting the equipment, reviewing the validation paperwork and the staff training on the new equipment is completed in addition to the steps mentioned in our project. For a review of capital acquisition, including various options (purchase, leasing, reagent rental), please refer to Chapter 11.

TABLE 12-2.   Example of Direct Variable Costs

- Labor: Tech time $25/hr./60 min = $0.417/min
- Time to perform test 13 minutes: 13 minutes × $0.417/min = $5.42
- Benefits @ 35% of time to perform test = $1.90
- Consumables expense is $1.50
- Therefore our cost is $8.82

THE SUCCESSFUL BUDGET PROCESS

The success of the budget process depends on the following elements:

1. Clear goals and objectives that can guide the resource allocation.
2. Project volumes or obtain projections from senior administration.
3. Convert volumes into revenue (mostly for outpatients).
4. Convert volumes into expense requirements.
5. Detailed statistical data, economic trends, and accurate information about existing and potential clients.
6. A defined budget period and procedures for development of the budget.
7. Reports to identify actual financial and statistical information for comparison with the budget and for variance analysis.

There are three important segments for the complete budget: **income forecasting, expense budget,** and **cash flow projections.** Income forecasting estimates future revenues and should be used to set goals. In our example, what is the projected volume of testing planned for the Outpatient Infusion Center? As the Outpatient Infusion Center is a new facility, the existing laboratory operating budget will need to be modified based on the additional forecasted volume. If one knows the number of physicians re-locating to the Outpatient Infusion Center from an existing practice, the test volume history can be reviewed and used as a baseline for the additional operating expenses. Consultation with the Outpatient Infusion Center physicians is also recommended to confirm their practices and ordering habits. Once the above is determined, convert volumes into revenue. What number should the price per test be? Many charges will already be calculated and can be found in the hospitals charge description master (CDM), which should be reviewed and updated periodically. If the test is not included in the CDM, the laboratory manager will need to calculate the variable and the fixed costs for a particular test and then it can be multiplied by a specific number of tests projected. The laboratory manager will then be able to convert volumes into expense requirements: Labor expense with benefits, non-labor expense, and overhead expense. Consultation with a member of the finance department is highly recommended in establishing pricing and making any additions or modifications to the CDM.

In an effort to control labor expenses, the laboratory manager can hire part-time and/or temporary employees instead of only full-time employees, if possible. Part-time employees receive benefits in proportion to the number of hours worked. The temporary workers receive only benefits required by law. In addition, many organizations have implemented flexible scheduling, reducing staff whenever a decrease in test volumes is noticed. Staff are encouraged to use vacation time or can take time off without pay. In many cases this is well received with staff "taking turns" taking afternoons off for final winter holiday preparations or leaving early on a Friday afternoon in the summer. Obviously, the laboratory manager will need to ensure adequate staff remain to perform the reduced workload of patient testing. Expense budget should also include upcoming cost-of-living raises, if any.

The non-labor expense will be based on projected volume of testing. Theoretically managers can reduce these expenses by using generic supplies wherever possible in the laboratory. In reality, it is almost impossible to use generic materials because the main bulk of its reagents and consumables must come from a specific vendor to be used on their analyzers. The non-labor expenses also should include an estimate of anticipated increases in supplies and service contracts. Overhead expenses such as depreciation, heating, cooling, insurance premiums, etc. are assigned to each department as a specific percent.

A realistic estimate of future growth can demonstrate to management the need for additional staff to meet future revenue standards. Many organizations now subscribe to benchmarking services which attempt to compare laboratories similar in size and scope. The benchmarking service collects data submitted by subscribers and calculates an average and different percentiles based on their calculations. Data in the laboratory manager's favor from the benchmarking service makes a compelling argument for the justification of additional resources.

The expense budget can also forecast expense categories. For example, a growth in an outreach services area will require a greater commitment to travel, administrative support, and telephone and other expenses. The cash flow projections are just as important for future planning and are based on the accuracy of projected volumes and expenses. Several factors can adversely affect cash flow, including excessive investments or a too high level of debt. All of these components must be interrelated and coordinated for successful budget planning.

For our laboratory budget we need to perform a careful analysis based not only on the costs of our existing laboratory but also on the additional test volumes contributed by the new Outpatient Infusion Center. As stated earlier, we need to assess the potential volume of specimens and tests based on clinicians' projected patient population, evaluation of existing services and the forecast of clients relocating to this new facility. We may need additional staffing to process specimens efficiently and timely. A full-time phlebotomist will collect, label, and send specimens to the accessioner in the laboratory. Physicians and clients in this high quality oncology operation are expecting rapid and accurate results. In addition, by meeting with various services that will be involved in the Outpatient Infusion Center operation, one can realistically project assumptions of future growth. Once operations begin, unless the existing budget is modified, the monthly operating reports will reflect the additional volumes in the actual revenue and expenses, creating variances when compared with the budgeted. The **variance analysis** will capture changes and trends in the marketplace that affect the operation. Analyzing variances will improve the quality of the original forecasts, point out changes in operation, and offer a means of asking why goals were not met. Proper budgeting and forecasting cannot entirely eliminate problems. We can't predict the future accurately, but we can make proper distinctions.

Practical Tips to Ensure a Successful Operating Budget Process

The budgeting process should vaguely resemble the following:
The laboratory manager is tasked with developing an operating budget for a period of time, typically one fiscal year. Statistics such as test volumes, revenues and expenses have been compiled and tracked for the previous year(s). The actual run rates are tracked against the projected categories and analyzed for variance. Significant variances from budgeted volumes, revenues or expenses (positive or negative) will need to be explained or justified. Senior management or the laboratory manager will then estimate variables for the proposed budget such as growth, inflation, new programs, test menu changes, etc. The manager will utilize these projections and statistics as a basis for developing the new budget.

The seven tips outlined below should prove useful in preparing a budget:

1. Start early
2. Recognize and utilize resources
3. Review financial reports
4. Predict or obtain predictions of future test volumes
5. Predict or obtain expense increases
6. Provide documentation
7. Compare the proposed budget to the existing

Start Early

Starting early is a bit of a misnomer as the budgeting process does not "end," per se, as expenses are tracked and variances are analyzed on a continual basis. The organization will usually set deadlines as to when the drafted budget is due to be submitted for review. You need to keep two things in mind: 1) there may be many levels of reviews and approvals that will be necessary and 2) the laboratory is not the only department that will be submitting a budget for review. At a minimum, the laboratory manager will prepare the budget and submit to senior management for approval. In health care systems, the process may be convoluted and begin with section supervisors preparing the initial budget with reviews and approvals required from the laboratory manager, a local finance committee, the chief financial officer, the chief operating officer or chief executive officer, the system finance committee and finally the board. Each level may require the budget for a week or more due to the volumes they will need to review and approve.

Recognize and Utilize Resources

In most instances, the laboratory manager will not need to develop a budget "from scratch." There should be past budgets the laboratory manager can use as a guide, as most laboratories have been operating for a number of years. If there are changes to the budgeting process, the finance department may provide templates to be used. Most laboratory managers will also have access to computer applications such as spreadsheets that will be useful in preparing a budget and tracking expenses and revenues.

If you have never prepared a budget before or would consider this a weak area, request assistance from someone familiar with the budgeting process, such as someone in finance or another manager. Most organizations will utilize a standardized budgeting approach; therefore, while another manager may not be familiar with the laboratory, they should still be able to assist you with the budgeting process. By starting early, you will have a better chance of receiving help, especially from the finance department, as they tend to be overwhelmed during budgeting "season" by all the requests for assistance.

The laboratory manager should also obtain the assistance of each section supervisor. The section supervisor will be the best individual able to identify the nature and frequency of each expense. The section supervisor will also be capable of tracking and justifying variances to the current operating budget and if the variances are short-term or long-term and whether the variance correctly correlates with an increase or decrease in test volumes.

Seeking assistance from frontline staff is a good idea for many reasons: employees develop a better appreciation as they become aware of the expense involved with operating the laboratory, frontline staff have the best grasp of resources used during the course of laboratory operations, frontline staff are more apt to know if there is any waste in the process that may be able to be eliminated and many employees enjoy being a part of the decision-making processes involved in operating the laboratory.

Review Financial Reports

The organization's finance department should provide reports that can be used for financial analysis throughout the year, and especially during the budgeting process. Examples include expense reports including current period expenses (past month), fiscal year to date expenses, accruals (expenses incurred but not yet paid) and budget variance reports, which compare actual volumes and expenses to those that were projected.

As the invoice approval and submission process may be manual, transcription errors may occur resulting in some expenses assigned to the wrong account or sub-account. The following three examples demonstrate the need for thorough review on a regular basis:

1. Would it be acceptable for office supplies to be incorrectly charged to minor equipment repair?

2. Would hematology want to be charged for the transcription services budgeted for, and used by, histology?

3. Would the laboratory want to be charged for the new carpeting installed in the radiology offices?

The obvious answer to all three questions is "No." The expense reports should be reviewed periodically (whenever new reports are issued) to ensure all expenses have been codified and assigned to the appropriate account and/or subaccount.

This does two things: 1) it saves time, effort and energy not having to justify variances in accounts or sub-accounts that did not occur and 2) ensures accurate data for next year's budget preparation.

The laboratory manager should properly justify all variances, both negative and positive. Almost all managers realize that negative variances need to be justified and do so by documenting the reason(s) for the deviation from the projected values. Some managers, especially new managers, may figure a positive variance is favorable and does not need to be investigated or explained. This is simply not true. The laboratory manager should investigate and determine a reason for the deviation. Table 12-3 outlines some of the common reasons and categories for variances.

As most organizations' budget reports divide a budgeted expense equally across 12 months, the explanation may be a case of an expense not yet being incurred (see Table 12-4 Report 1 - Note). Note the positive YTD variances for account 6422 Instruments–QA. This is an example of some expense not yet being incurred, as a large QC order is due to be placed in May.

Please also note the negative monthly variance for 6408–Lab reagents and supplies. We will investigate and analyze this variance in depth later in this chapter.

Another example of an expected future expense not yet being incurred may be a positive variance in September's budget report for proficiency testing when the invoice will be submitted in November (not shown). When the invoice is submitted for payment in November, the charge will "hit" all at once as opposed to being spread out over the year. If the fiscal year ends in June, the manager will need to remember to explain the negative variance over the course of the remaining 7 months until the budgeted amount "catches up" to the amount of the expense incurred earlier in the year.

The manager should also ask himself/herself, "Has an expense been incurred, but not charged due to an invoice lost in inter-office mail, or sitting under a pile of papers on somebody's desk?" If the second scenario were to happen at the end of the fiscal year and the invoice was not submitted before the books closed

TABLE 12-3.   Common Reasons for Variances

1. The variance is a timing difference that will disappear in coming months. No action is needed.

2. The variance is correct and corresponds to a change in test volume.

3. The assumption in the budget was wrong, as proven by negative variance. The budget should be revised.

4. There was an error in the process that incorrectly assigned revenue or expense to the wrong account or subaccount.

5. Expenses are not being controlled. Corrective action is needed to eliminate the unfavorable trend.

for the year, the laboratory would be under budget in the first fiscal year and be over budget in the next, as the charges would hit the second year's budget. In any event, positive variances need investigation as well.

In Table 12-5 Report 2, by totaling the salary expenses and non-salary expenses, we can see how much cost is involved in staffing the department and the cost of supplies. We have also included the total number of tests performed as the Units of Measure and compare against the previous fiscal month's/year's statistics. We can now use these metrics in ratios that provide a good basis for productivity analysis including Salaries & Benefits Per Unit (cost of labor per test performed), Supplies Per Unit (cost of reagents, supplies, consumables, etc. per test performed) and Total Expenses Per Unit (total cost per test performed).

Please note that in many instances the financial reports provided by the organization contain only a summary of expenses by vendor and are not itemized (see Table 12-6 Report 3 & Table 12-7 Report 4). As such, we cannot tell what supplies are included on each invoice, unless we have cost per reportable contracts or standing orders that always contain the same amount of reagents and supplies.

It is also important to ensure the appropriate supplies are charged against the correct subaccounts. This will minimize the number of times that investigation, analysis and justification have to be performed for the current fiscal year's budget variance reports, as well as helping to ensure next fiscal year's budget is forecast and drafted with accurate data.

See Table 12-7 Report 4 for examples of incorrectly charged items. The finance department will need to be contacted to make the appropriate corrections and reclassify the expense to the correct subaccount.

Table 12-8 Report 5 is the monthly Inventory Expense Report generated and distributed by the storeroom. We can clearly see the supplies delivered for the month and year, the expense associated with each product and the subaccount to which each supply was charged.

It may be beneficial for each supervisor to use a spreadsheet to detail and track each item used in their section much like the Inventory Expense Report generated by the storeroom. Utilizing this approach, we can see in Table 12-9 Report 6 that this will provide the most accurate data to be used in evaluating resource utilization, efficiencies, etc. This will also be beneficial as we prepare our budgets for the next year, as we have also included a column for the subaccount into which we are expecting each expense to be charged. This also makes the budget variance investigation and analysis easier as misclassified charges will be clearly evident.

We can further simplify our task of tracking expenses by the addition of a column for each unit cost. A total column at the end will allow the laboratory manager to calculate how much is spent for each supply over the year by multiplying the unit cost by the total number of each supply used. Monthly totals for supplies can be tracked by the addition of a row on the bottom. Our formula would then multiply quantities for each supply by the unit cost and total all supply costs for each month. These totals can then be compared to the Budget Variance Reports for accuracy.

TABLE 12-4. Report 1–Sample of Hematology Budget Variance Report (BVR) Page 1

GROSS REVENUES EXPENSES	FY2011 April - Monthly Budget	Actual	Variance	Variance %	FY10 April Actual	FY10 April Actual	FY2011 Year-to-Date Budget	Actual	Variance	Variance %	FY10 Actual April-YTD
6000 Exist - Salaries and Wages	19,747	15,750	3,998	20.2%	22,099	22,099	200,106	207,052	(6,946)	(3.5%)	217,686
6021 Exist - Variable Salaries - Holiday	411	0	411	100.0%			4,164	3,470	694	16.7%	
6029 Exist - Fixed Salaries - Vacation	1,317	1,492	(175)	(13.30%)			13,343	9,273	4,070	30.5%	10,789
6030 Exist - Fixed Salaries - Sick	357	240	117	32.8%			3,621	1,475	2,146	59.3%	2,960
6032 Exist - Fixed Salaries - Holiday	281	0	281	100.0%			2,848	2,373	475	16.7%	3,329
6003 Exist - Salaries - Overtime	328	405	(77)	(23.50%)			3,322	3,810	(489)	(14.7%)	2,942
Total New & Existing Salaries	**22,441**	**17,887**	**4,554**	**20.3%**	**22,099**	**22,099**	**227,404**	**227,453**	**(48)**	**0.0%**	**237,706**
6304 - Total	5,049	2,140	2,909	57.6%	2,904	2,904	51,166	26,048	25,118	49.1%	39,449
6309 - Employers FICA		1,169	(1,169)		1,611	1,611		16,851	(16,851)		15,331
Employee Benefits Accts	**5,049**	**3,309**	**1,741**	**34.5%**	**4,515**	**4,515**	**51,166**	**42,900**	**8,266**	**16.2%**	**54,780**

(Continued)

313

TABLE 12-4. Report 1–Sample of Hematology Budget Variance Report (BVR) Page 1 (*Continued*)

FY2011 April - Monthly				FY10 April	GROSS REVENUES EXPENSES	FY2011 Year-to-Date				FY10 Actual
Budget	Actual	Variance	Variance %	Actual		Budget	Actual	Variance	Variance %	April-YTD
173		173	100.0%	209	6403 - Medical & Surgical Supplies	1,749	1,994	(245)	(14.0%)	2,105
17,027	21,443	(4,416)	(25.9%)	16,005	6408 - Lab Reagents & Supplies	172,539	136,333	36,206	21.0%	117,742
1,862	2,544	(690)	(37.2%)	3,215	6409 - Other Medical Supplies	18,790	15,740	3,050	16.2%	20,180
1,192	1,158	33	2.8%	1,456	6422 - Instruments-QA	12,077	9,990	2,087	17.3%	10,402
14	8	6	40.5%	10	6502 - Supplies - Other Non Med	142	116	26	18.3%	280
201	1,076	(875)	(434.3%)	70	6505 - Office Supplies	2,041	4,453	(2,412)	(118.2%)	1,614
41		41	100.0%		6603 - Forms	416		416	100.0%	4
52		52	100.0%		6902 - Minor Equipment	525	(7,558)	8,083	1540.0%	
					6509 - Others		36	(36)	–100.0%	
	(195)	195			6905 - Space & Building Rental		(195)	195	100.0%	
63	(881)	944	1509.6%	1,280	6909 - Minor Repairs/ Maint-Equipment	525	(585)	1,110	211.4%	1,367

Note: The positive YTD variances for account 6422 Instruments – QA. This is an example of some expense not yet being incurred, as a large QC order is due to be placed in May. Also note the negative monthly variance in the amount of $4,416 for subaccount 6408 – Lab Reagents & Supplies. Please note that due to rounding, some figures in charts may not total exactly as displayed.

314

TABLE 12-5. Report 2–April 2011 Hematology Budget Variance Report Page 2

	FY2011 April - Monthly				FY10 Actual	APRIL GROSS REVENUES EXPENSES	FY2011 Year-to-Date				FY10 Actual	April-YTD
	Budget	Actual	Variance	Variance %	Actual		Budget	Actual	Variance	Variance %		
	167		167	100.0%		7001 Educ/Confer/Seminars	1,667	258	1,408	84.5%	70	
	63	28	35	55.6%	49	7002 IS Direct Charges	625	341	284	45.4%	604	
	42		42	100.0%		7105 Travel, Meetings	417		417	100.0%		
	(1,475)		(1,475)	100.0%		7109 Other Direct Expenses	(11,800)		(11,800)	100.0%		
	125	46	79	63.2%		7110 Freight Expense	1,250	513	737	59.0%	1,167	
	19,547	25,226	(5,679)	−29.1%	22,294	Total Non-Salary Expense	200,963	161,436	39,526	19.7%	155,535	
	47,037	46,422	615	1.3%	44,539	Total Expenses	479,533	431,789	47,744	10.0%	448,021	
	13,600	12,100	(1,500)	(11.0%)	13,600	Units of Measure	135,000	123,900	(111)	(8.2%)	135,000	
	2.02	1.75	(0.27)	(13.4%)	1.96	Salaries & Benefits Per Unit	2.06	2.18	0.12	5.8%	2.17	
	1.44	2.08	0.64	44.4%	1.64	Supplies Per Unit	1.49	1.30	(0.19)	(12.8%)	1.15	
	3.46	3.84	0.38	11.0%	3.60	Total Expenses Per Unit	3.55	3.48	(0.07)	(2.0%)	3.32	

Note: The decrease in test volume and the corresponding decrease in salaries (variable cost) due to flexible scheduling. Implementation of new hematology analyzers (training) precluded the department from utilizing flexible scheduling for the full year. We also see a corresponding reduction (positive variance) in subaccount 6408 – Lab Reagents & Supplies (variable costs) because the test volumes have decreased. We see this relationship for the FY2011 YTD, but not for the April Monthly (Table 12-4). Investigation and analysis are indicated.

TABLE 12-6.   Report 3–2011 Year-to-Date Expense Report

Department: 04016 - Hematology

GL Subaccount: 6408 HEMA - Laboratory Reagents & Supplies

Voucher Number	Vendor Number	Vendor Name	Vendor Inv Number	Vendor Inv Date	GL Dist Date	Dist Period	P.O. Number	Amount
561791	57	Fisher Healthcare	1160021	02/01/2011	02/05/2011	8	294840	109.20
562001	17014	Sysmex America, Inc	90239318	01/20/2011	02/19/2011	8	288774	6.03
562493	17014	Sysmex America, Inc	90242751	02/02/2011	02/25/2011	8	288774	8,551.13
562598	15560	Diagnostica Stago Inc.	113044207	02/11/2011	02/25/2011	8	273984	4,417.96
563065	57	Fisher Healthcare	3993645	02/19/2011	03/03/2011	9	295240	122.79
563416	15560	Diagnostica Stago Inc.	113046746	02/24/2011	03/09/2011	9	273984	2,453.88
563792	57	Fisher Healthcare	7836606	03/01/2011	03/15/2011	9	295240	37.82
564687	57	Fisher Healthcare	1973344	03/25/2011	03/30/2011	9	296035	109.20
565343	17014	Sysmex America, Inc	90256721	03/09/2011	04/06/2011	10	288774	7,121.16
565344	17014	Sysmex America, Inc	90255152	03/05/2011	04/06/2011	10	288774	806.34
565849	15560	Diagnostica Stago Inc.	113048875	03/11/2011	04/13/2011	10	281167	4,417.96
565850	15560	Diagnostica Stago Inc.	113049523	04/11/2011	04/20/2011	10	285721	4,417.96
566200	17014	Sysmex America, Inc	90266693	04/07/2011	04/20/2011	10	288774	8,739.88
566783	13910	Precision Bio Logic	100001088	04/13/2011	04/23/2011	10	296549	435.00
566783	13910	Precision Bio Logic	100001088	04/13/2011	04/23/2011	10	296549	75.00
					Subaccount Subtotal			121,175.41

GL Subaccount: 6409 HEMA - Other Medical Supplies

547293	15560	Diagnostica Stago, Inc.	113004496	06/25/2010	07/22/2010	1	281167	618.55
547293	15560	Diagnostica Stago, Inc.	113004496	06/25/2010	07/22/2010	1	281167	43.00
549526	57	Fisher Healthcare	7251354	08/07/2010	08/20/2010	2	290837	59.49
550029	15560	Diagnostica Stago, Inc.	113004496	08/14/2010	08/31/2010	2	291000	63.86
550029	15560	Diagnostica Stago, Inc.	113004496	08/14/2010	08/31/2010	2	291000	36.00
552396	15560	Diagnostica Stago, Inc.	113004496	09/16/2010	10/05/2010	4	291736	22.20
552396	15560	Diagnostica Stago, Inc.	113004496	09/16/2010	10/05/2010	4	291736	37.00
552530	57	Fisher Healthcare	7251354	10/01/2010	10/06/2010	4	292038	170.52
554440	17014	Sysmex America, Inc.	90211921	10/26/2010	11/02/2010	5	292595	171.80
554440	17014	Sysmex America, Inc.	90211921	10/26/2010	11/02/2010	5	292595	5.01
557535	15560	Diagnostica Stago, Inc.	113004496	11/25/2010	12/22/2010	6	293400	37.00
557535	15560	Diagnostica Stago, Inc.	113004496	11/25/2010	12/22/2010	6	293400	507.00
557700	15560	Diagnostica Stago, Inc.	113004496	12/08/2010	12/17/2010	6	293660	283.00
557700	15560	Diagnostica Stago, Inc.	113004496	12/08/2010	12/17/2010	6	293660	366.00
557700	15560	Diagnostica Stago, Inc.	113004496	12/08/2010	12/17/2010	6	293660	38.00
558767	57	Fisher Healthcare	7251354	12/23/2010	01/04/2011	7	294032	170.52
560057	57	Fisher Healthcare	7251354	01/11/2011	01/22/2011	7	294287	50.04
563655	15560	Diagnostica Stago, Inc.	113004496	03/02/2011	03/11/2011	9	295474	148.00
563655	15560	Diagnostica Stago, Inc.	113004496	03/02/2011	03/11/2011	9	295474	35.00

(Continued)

TABLE 12-6. Report 3–2011 Year-to-Date Expense Report (*Continued*)

Department: 04016 - Hematology

Voucher Number	Vendor Number	Vendor Name	Vendor Inv Number	Vendor Inv Date	GL Dist Date	Dist Period	P.O. Number	Amount
564880	15560	Diagnostica Stago, Inc.	113004496	03/18/2011	03/31/2011	9	295941	60.10
565791	57	Fisher Healthcare	7251354	04/05/2011	04/13/2011	10	296373	296.37
566767	15560	Diagnostica Stago, Inc.	113004496	04/16/2011	04/23/2011	10	296726	129.00
566767	15560	Diagnostica Stago, Inc.	113004496	04/16/2011	04/23/2011	10	296726	35.00
					Subaccount Subtotal			3,382.46

Note: The GL Dist date (4/13/2011) of the Diagnostica Stago Invoice from March under subaccount 6408 for the amount of $4,417 for the current month. This invoice was received 03/11/2011 from the Vendor and should have been processed sooner.

TABLE 12-7. Report 4–2011 Year-to-Date Accounts Payable Distribution

Department: 04016 - Hematology

Voucher Number	Vendor Number	Vendor Name	Vendor Inv Number	Vendor Inv Date	GL Dist Date	Dist Period	P.O. Number	Amount
GL Subaccount: 6901 HEMA - Office Supplies								
552944	16764	Flo-Tech, LLC	MET0909	09/30/2010	10/13/2010	4		518.00
552944	16764	Flo-Tech, LLC	MET0909	09/30/2010	10/13/2010	4		304.00
553860	631	Staples	8013654004	10/03/2010	10/23/2010	4		676.83
556419	16764	Flo-Tech, LLC	MET0909	07/31/2010	11/30/2010	5	Reclass	881.00
566790	16764	Flo-Tech, LLC	MET1109	10/31/2010	12/30/2010	6	Reclass	195.00
566792	16764	Flo-Tech, LLC	MET0909	07/31/2010	04/26/2011	10	Reclass	881.00
					Subaccount Subtotal			3,455.83
GL Subaccount: 6902 HEMA - Minor Equipment								
546291	14308	Data Innovations	9537844	06/26/2010	07/07/2010	1	289347	4,326.38
551621	17014	Sysmex America, Inc.	90191737	08/24/2010	09/22/2010	3	288774	7.11
					Subaccount Subtotal			4,333.49
GL Subaccount: 6905 HEMA - Space & Building Rental								
555254	16764	Flo-Tech, LLC	MET1009	10/31/2010	11/11/2010	5		144.00
555254	16764	Flo-Tech, LLC	MET1009	10/31/2010	11/11/2010	5		51.00
566790	16764	Flo-Tech, LLC	MET1109	10/31/2010	12/30/2010	6	Reclass	(195.00)
					Subaccount Subtotal			0.00

(Continued)

TABLE 12-7. Report 4–2011 Year-to-Date Accounts Payable Distribution (*Continued*)

Department: 04016 - Hematology

Voucher Number	Vendor Number	Vendor Name	Vendor Inv Number	Vendor Inv Date	GL Dist Date	Dist Period	P.O. Number	Amount
GL Subaccount: 6909 HEMA - Minor Repairs/ Maintenance								
546405	39	Beckman Coulter, Inc.	3275412	06/24/2010	07/07/2010	1	274693	160.00
549013	16764	Flo-Tech, LLC	MET0709	07/31/2010	08/14/2010	2		881.00
556419	16764	Flo-Tech, LLC	MET0709	07/31/2010	11/30/2010	1	Reclass	(881.00)
563131	4280	Clearview Microscope Service	5031	01/29/2011	03/10/2010	4	294926	135.00
566792	16764	Flo-Tech, LLC	MET0709	07/31/2010	04/26/2011	1	Reclass	(881.00)
					Subaccount Subtotal			(586.00)
GL Subaccount: 7110 HEMA - Freight Expense								
547828	1601	Abbott Diagnostics	928441505	07/22/2010	07/27/2010	1	290401	41.03
549381	1601	Abbott Diagnostics	927100121	03/09/2010	08/19/2010	2	287206	51.56
551342	57	Fisher Healthcare	8424363	09/14/2010	09/18/2010	3	291636	12.00
553654	57	Fisher Healthcare	9389033	10/14/2010	10/21/2010	4	292404	12.00
555867	57	Fisher Healthcare	7906665	11/16/2010	11/20/2010	5	293153	21.50
556616	57	Fisher Healthcare	1090533	11/23/2010	12/01/2010	6	293330	12.00

Note: The incorrectly classified office supplies (Flo-Tech, LLC provides toner for copiers) under subaccounts 6905 & 6909. A simple email to finance and they are correctly classified to sub-account 6901 Office Supplies. Correct classification of charges will help ensure an accurate budget.

TABLE 12-8.   Report 5–April 2011 Inventory Expense Report

Department: 04016 - Hematology

For Period 10/2011

Item Number	Description	Loc Code	PTD Net Issued	Net Expense PTD Amount	YTD Net Issued	Net Expense YTD Amount	Item Type
Expense Subaccount: 6502							
15390	Tissue Facial	SR	0	0.00	10	5.00	S
25560	Kimwipe 13×21	SR	0	0.00	1	71.00	S
60175	Bleach Gallon	SR	4	8.00	19	38.00	S
		Subaccount Totals:		8.00		114.00	
Expense Subaccount: 6502							
43605	Paper Xerox 8 1/2×11″	SR	0	0.00	186	566.00	S
		Subaccount Totals:		0.00		566.00	
		Department Totals:		2,741.00		27,228.00	

Note: The itemized list for items obtained from the stockroom (SR). This report clearly details each supply used, the quantities and the cost. The reports generated by the hospital's financial system only listed a summarized invoice expense by vendor.

Predict or Obtain Predictions of Future Test Volumes

In many cases, predictions of future volumes will be provided by senior management to department managers at the start of the budgeting process. This is oftentimes advantageous as senior management is aware of all changes in programs or services in the organization and has discussed what the changes will mean to overall volumes. In addition, outside factors, such as the state of the economy, will factor into projecting future volumes. For example, the high unemployment rate caused by the current recession, which began in 2008, has caused many Americans to lose their insurance coverage. Consequently, many of these uninsured patients have chosen to delay their elective surgeries and other medical procedures, including laboratory testing. This has resulted in flat or contracted future volume predictions. Occasionally the laboratory manager will be responsible for estimating future volumes.

Predict or Obtain Expense Increases

Unless under contract for a fixed price, most vendors adjust pricing for inflation on an annual basis. Price increases are generally in the 2–4% range.

TABLE 12-9. Report 6–FY 2011 Hematology Supplies & Consumables

Hematology FY 2011 Supplies & Consumables														
2010-2011	Subacct	Jul	Aug	Sep	Oct	Nov	Dec	Jan	Feb	Mar	Apr	May	Jun	Total
Sedi-plast West Polymed	6408	1		1		1			1		1		1	6
WBC-diluting fluid Fisher	6408							2				2		4
Retic pack Coulter	6408	1												1
Isoton Coulter	6408	8												8
Scatter pack Coulter	6408	1												1
Wright-Giemsa stain Fisher	6408	3	1	3	2	3		3	3		2	1	3	24
Coulter clenz Coulter	6408	3												3
Frosted slides Fisher	6409		1			3					2	2		8
Immersion oil Fisher	6409		2											2
Platen tubing-stainer Fisher	6409					1								1
Pump tubing-stainer Fisher	6409					1								1
Stainer cannulas Fisher	6409										2			2

Item	Code						Total
Filter concentrators **Fisher**	6409		2		2	3	7
Spinalscopic controls **Quan**	6422				1		1
ESR 1&2 control **Polymed**	6422	3	3		6		21
Manual sed-chek 2	6422		1	1		1	5
Cytofuge filter clips **Fisher**	6409	1			1		1
Rubber plate **Sysmex**	6409	2	2				2
Piercer-set **Sysmex**	6409				1		1
Toner-stago 1 **Okidata**	6505				1	2	3
Toner-stago 2 **Okidata**	6505				1		1
Hyaluronidase **Fisher**	6400		1	3		4	8
Methanol **Fisher**	6409			1			1

Note: Accurate Data will help ensure a successful budgeting process. Use of a spreadsheet will allow each section supervisor to track expenditures and know exactly how much and where money is spent. This data can then be compared to each month's Budget Variance Report for accuracy. Please also note that this chart will require revision as the laboratory's change in Hematology Instrument vendors is evident.

Notification is usually given via a letter sent 30–90 days in advance (within the terms of the vendor contract) indicating the adjustment in pricing. These increases should be factored into the cost of reagents, consumables, blood and blood products.

The human resources or personnel in the laboratory usually receive an adjustment to pay as well, be it in the form of a cost of living increase, merit raise or combination of both. These increases raise the employees' pay for the year the adjustment is received, as well as all subsequent years. Employees may also receive bonuses based on performance, project completion or some other goal attainment. These adjustments usually pertain only to the current period in which the bonus is given and do not recur. However, some hospitals have implemented bonus programs in which bonuses may recur based on goals attained from a balanced scorecard or some other metric. In these cases, guidance from senior administration or the chief financial officer would be appropriate.

Provide Documentation

Documentation should accompany all significant adjustments to the budget. Documentation should be clear and concise, yet sufficient to properly explain the adjustment. In many instances, the budget review and approval process will require the budget to be scrutinized by senior administration and possibly the hospital's board. Some managers, especially new managers, may be nervous in situations such as these. Adequate documentation may be explanation enough for the parties reviewing the budget, or at the very least, will assist the nervous laboratory manager in explaining the adjustments. For example, an increase of $250,000 in the Blood Bank budget would be warranted for a projected increase in blood to support the new Oncology and Infusion Program in our case scenario.

Historically, organizations have tracked and trended data such as volumes, revenues and expenses on an internal basis. Many organizations are now incorporating external benchmarking into their productivity comparisons. External benchmarking is designed to compare productivity between laboratories similar in size, scope, personnel, equipment, etc. The external benchmarking data can be very useful in justifying additional FTE's or capital equipment.

Compare the Proposed Budget with the Existing

Compare the proposed budget to the existing budget and ask yourself the following questions: Does the new budget make sense? Is it consistent with previous budgets? Have you accounted for any significant adjustments? Did you remember everything? Will you be satisfied being held accountable to the figures submitted?

Senior administration realizes emergencies and unexpected occurrences can happen in operating a business, just as in running a household. However, proper planning, including accurate record-keeping and realistic projections, can help minimize the impact these events have in causing variances to a budget.

TABLE 12-10.   Report 7–Non-Salary Expense Worksheet for Proposed Budget

Subacct	Description	thru 12/1/2010	2012 Budget	Notes
6403	Medical & Surgical Suppl (Owens & Minor Conglomeration)	1331	2700	
6408	Polymedco (Sed Rates)	2200	5000	
6408	Diagnostica Stago (Coag - PT/ PTT/Fib/D-Dimer)	35000	70000	Includes Latest Controls
6408	AJP Scientific (WBC Diluting Fluid)	250	500	
6408	Sysmex	50000	110000	(Includes Service & Ctrls & OP Infusion)
6408	Fisher (Hematology Stain, Urine Multistix, IctoTest)	3500	8000	
6408	Laboratory Supplies	90950	193500	
6409	MarketLab	100	1000	
6409	Stockroom (Saniclothes, Gloves, Alcohol, Paper)	2178	4400	
6409	Polymedco (Thermal Paper)	80	160	
6409	Diagnostica Stago (Needles, O Rings, Stir Bars, Suction Tips)	1450	3000	
6409	Fisher (Hematology Stain, Stainer Tubing, CSF Clips, Filter Conc, Clinitek Printer Paper)	6700	15000	
6409	Other Medical Supplies	10508	23560	
6422	Orasure Rapid HIV QC	1000	2000	
6422	Quantimetrix (CSF Cell Count Controls)	100	200	
6422	Polymedco (Sed Rate Controls)	2200	4500	
6422	Fisher (Kovatrol)	1773	3600	
6422	Instruments-QA	5073	10300	
	Stockroom (Bleach, Kimwipes, Tissues)	85	170	
6502	Supplies-Other Non Med	85	170	

(Continued)

TABLE 12-10.   Report 7–Non-Salary Expense Worksheet for Proposed Budget (*Continued*)

Subacct	Description	thru 12/1/2010	2012 Budget	Notes
6505	FloTech (Toner)	1000	2000	
6505	Staples (Binders, Folders, Markers, etc.)	700	1250	
6505	Office Supplies	1700	3250	
6603	Forms	0	500	New OP Infusion Center Forms
6902	Minor Equipment (Pipettes, Heating Blocks, Vortex)	0	750	
6909	Minor Repairs/Maint-Equi (Peter Potter)	500	750	
7001	Educ/Conference/Seminar (ASH or AACC)	2000	2000	
7002	IS Direct Charges	220	500	
	Diagnostica Stago Service Contract (included in CPR)		0	
	Sysmex Service Contract included in CPR)		0	
7008	Outside Services		0	
7105	Travel, Meetings-Domestic	500	500	
7109	Other Direct Expenses	0	250	
7110	Freight Expense	200	750	
	TOTAL	113067	239480	

Note: The concise, streamlined view of each subaccount with just enough detail that should suffice for most applications. It includes notes for any significant changes that may draw attention as the budget is submitted for approval.

COMMON BUDGET PROBLEMS AND POSSIBLE SOLUTIONS

Losing sight of real objectives occurs when too much emphasis is placed on completing a complex procedure in a short time, involving endless revisions and paperwork. People are so pleased that this process is over, they often forget that it is only actually beginning. Once the budget is approved, it will serve as the standard for the time it is in place.

To avoid losing sight of the reason for budgeting, it is important to remember the following:

- Focus decisions toward clear objectives.
- Think of the budget as a standard and focus performance against it.
- Involve the staff by communicating the goals set forth in the budget and seeking input from the staff for any cost reductions that may be able to be implemented
- Analyze monthly variances by comparing actual expenses to budget expenses and examining causes (both negative and positive variances need to be explained).
- Periodically analyze the services provided by the laboratory for specific keys to higher profits and identify ways to either reduce expenses or improve income.

Budgeting above 100% of the previous year is known as **historical-based budgeting** and is the easiest way to budget without major effort. To budget in this way, the total spent in the previous year is divided by 12. The number obtained plus a percentage for inflation is used to budget for the upcoming year. Accepting this approach builds lack of control into the process and encourages further spending. As today's economic climate has become more challenging, historical-based budgeting has been replaced by other methods that are based less on assumptions, and more on periodic thorough analysis.

Other factors, when used as the only criterion, may result in a poorly developed budget and include:

- Using historical information as the only assumption source.
- Only examining the accounts that show unfavorable variances.
- Looking for solutions not to increase the budget but to enforce realistic spending limits.
- Making budget increases automatically.

Another important aspect of the budgetary process to consider is that individuals who prepare budgets and develop assumptions rarely have the final word (approve their own budgets). No matter how carefully the budget is analyzed and prepared, it is not possible to prevent a superior from changing the budget. However, proper and sufficient documentation of justification will reduce capricious budget reductions.

TABLE 12-11.   Report 8–Summarized Salary Expense Worksheet for Proposed Budget

Clinical Laboratory

Salary	Description	FTE Expense Proposed	FTE Expense Target	FTEs
1	S-Level Management Reg.	228,384	218,384	3.00
2	M-Level Management Reg.	232,791	222,791	3.00
3	Lab/Tech Staff Union Reg.	1,910,629	1,900,629	34.00
4	Lab/Tech Staff Union OT	98,000	88,000	1.51
5	Lab/Tech Staff Non Union	55,159	45,159	1.10
6	Lab/Tech Staff Non Union OT	18,480	8,480	0.22
7	Clerical Employees Reg.	113,355	103,355	3.00
8	Clerical Employees OT	1,620	1,620	0.03
9	Service Employees 1199 Reg.	118,439	108,439	4.00
10	Service Employees 1199 OT	1,650	1,650	0.04
11	Casual A-Level Management	1,620	1,620	0.03
12	Casual Office/Clerical Emp.	1,620	1,620	0.03
	Salary-Total:	**2,781,747**	**2,701,747**	**49.96**

Note: Please note that this is a summarized overview of salaries. Each section supervisor should have a detailed list outlining their direct report's salaries and the department manager should have a detailed list outlining every employee's salary.

To help ensure approval of a budget, the following points may be helpful to consider:

- Present a strong case based on sound assumptions.
- Do not defend a budget that has been changed randomly.
- Use discretion in discussing any issue with a superior. Know when to accept their answer and above all remain composed.

Realistic expectations help explain the inevitable variances that may arise. A variance is a sign that control over expenses is needed. A problem can be solved only if it is identified. Budgets should be a tool not for blame but for improvement.

Follow the steps below when explaining variances:

- Always go back to the assumption when writing a variance explanation, and base it on a comparison.
- Realize that some variances are expected, especially given a variance in workload, and should show correlation to an increase or decrease in test volumes.

- Identify real problems and recommend solutions.
- Recognize the budgeting process as one that monitors process.
- Acknowledge that budget is only a guideline and no one can do better than estimate.

Furthermore, the explanations that do not identify causes but rather attempt to indicate a trend, do not drill down and identify the cause of the variance. If the laboratory manager is not able to identify a cause, solutions that address the root cannot be developed and implemented.

Avoid the following:

- Don't try to excuse the previous year's excessive variances by referring to a previous period. Confront the problems that exist each year.
- Don't ask for a budget increase this year based on not being able to meet last year's budget.
- Try not to use weak assumptions. It leads to an inability to identify or explain problems.

Table 12-12 lists the major areas of concern for planning the additional workload the Outpatient Infusion Center will bring to the laboratory. One problem with budgeting is that problems are often left unresolved and allowed to continue. Changes must be suggested immediately to respond to major budget errors. Management must understand that problems will not go away and must be solved. If the manager does not have a voice in the decision-making process, it is important to point out the problem to those in a position to make changes. Try to meet a challenge by asking for authority. Keep all lines of communication open with internal and external customers to ascertain the necessary information. Always attempt to develop joint solutions rather than being an adversary.

TABLE 12-12. **Major Aspects to Consider in Planning a Significant Increase in Test Volume**

Increased Test Volume	Capacity – Analyzers
Computer system	Compatibility with other systems
Space	Adequacy
Specimens	Transport
Specimen processing	Location/convenience
Staffing	Number of employees – additions?
Cost justification	Expense/Savings/Growth
Implementation	Schedule/Training

SURVIVING BUDGET JUSTIFICATION EXPLANATION

In most organizations, proposed budgets are presented to the finance department and/or senior management for approval. Depending on the size of your organization, you may either present the proposed budget to a single individual who will then, in turn, present to a panel of finance personnel and senior administration, or you may present the proposed budget directly to the panel of finance personnel and senior administration. This justification process can be unnerving to say the least. Many people are nervous in everyday conversations with senior management, especially when they are relatively new to an organization or have just recently been promoted to a managerial role. In a formalized presentation such as presentation of a proposed budget, nervousness can cause "amnesia."

In order to ensure a smooth, pain-free presentation, the laboratory manager should, prior to the formal presentation:

1. Follow the organizational format
2. Ensure the data used to develop the budget is accurate
3. Make sure you have evidence to support your data
4. Practice, Practice, Practice

Follow the Organizational Format

In many organizations, there will be a formalized process for preparing, submitting, presenting and approving a proposed budget for approval. As stated earlier, seek advice from another manager or finance personnel who have been through the process in the organization before. Carefully read the instructions provided by the finance team. Utilize any tools that may be provided, such as spreadsheets or forms. While you may only be responsible for a single budget, the Chief Financial Officer, senior administration or the Board will be responsible for reviewing and approving every budget in the hospital. In large organizations, this may number over 100 budgets! It will be much easier and take less time to receive approval if your presentation is in the format they will be expecting to review.

Ensure the Data Used to Develop the Budget Is Accurate

Consult with purchasing and accounts payable to ensure all invoices have been accounted for, especially the most recent invoices. The most recent invoices will need to be accounted for as an expense or an accrual (expense incurred, not yet paid). Review the appropriate portion of the proposed budget with each section supervisor to ensure you have a thorough understanding of all projected revenues and expenses. Soliciting a "second set of eyes" will not only aid in the review, the discussion generated will help in gaining a better familiarity of each department's expenses and operations.

Make Sure You Have Evidence to Support Your Data

Budget presentation is similar to a regulatory agency inspection in many ways: proper preparation, organization and the ability to provide supporting documentation when requested is paramount to either's success. Be prepared to discuss any significant variances from last year's figures. You should be able to provide enough documentation to support your calculations or conclusions. Prepare neat and organized notes for each budget you must present. When questioned and unsure, refer to your notes to provide accurate answers. It is far better to pause, gather and communicate accurate information, than to rapidly spew forth information that may not be accurate.

Practice, Practice, Practice

Practicing the presentation serves many purposes. Practicing is an essential element of delivering a professional, polished presentation. Practicing also serves to more thoroughly familiarize yourself with each section's budget, thereby having to refer to your notes less. Work with each section supervisor and try to anticipate any questions that may be asked and prepare answers. Final practices could include all supervisors and/or other department managers to simulate presenting before the finance personnel and senior administration.

Justification does not end after your proposed budget has been approved. As stated earlier, most organizations prepare a monthly report that lists both actual and budgeted costs, highlighting the variances. In many instances, in an effort to meet the goals of the existing budget, investigation and explanation of variances is required of each department manager and is reviewed by senior administration. A good **budget justification** report analysis not only identifies the reasons for variances; it also proposes concrete solutions or alternatives to prevent the variance from recurring. One of the proposed corrective action plans should be implemented with proper follow-up in the next monthly or quarterly budget review period.

TABLE 12-13.   Common Causes of Variance

Causes of Variances	Example	Action Needed
Periodic large expenditures	Equipment maintenance	No action needed
Increased usage due to special circumstances	Increase in volume of tests	Document
Incorrect budgeting	Forgetting to account for expenses or revenues	Document
Changes in method of testing not known at the time of budgeting process	Modification of existing assay testing due to changes in the analyzer	Rebudget appropriately & inform administration

MONTHLY BUDGET VARIANCE JUSTIFICATION EXERCISE

Problem

As noted earlier in this chapter, review of the April 2011 Hematology Budget Variance Report shows a $4,416 budget variance for Account 6408 – Lab Reagents & Supplies. Refer to Table 12-4 Report 1 – Sample of Hematology Budget Variance Report (BVR) Page 1 earlier in the chapter.

Investigation

After reviewing Table 12-4 Report 1 and finding $4,416 variance, investigation of Table 12-6 Report 3–2011 Year-to-Date Expense Report, shows that the Diagnostica Stago invoice for March ($4,417) was incorrectly expensed in April. The April Invoice ($4,417) was correctly expensed, and is also found on the April Expense Report. Further investigation yielded a positive budget variance in the 6408 subaccount for the month of March in the amount of $4,417. This invoice was received 03/11/2011 from the Vendor and should have been processed in March.

Analysis

From this, we can discern that two months of Diagnostica Stago invoices were processed for the current month, one properly expensed (as displayed on the April Expense Report) and one incorrectly expensed (the March Invoice is expensed on the April Expense Report). Further investigation and analysis determined the March invoice was found amongst other paperwork (policy and procedure revisions) on the Hematology Supervisor's desk. In addition, the Hematology supervisor had been on vacation when the previous month's budgets were reviewed, so that section's review was tabled to the following month. Consequently, the Diagnostica Stago invoice was not expensed in March and was incorrectly expensed in April.

It is important to be mindful of various causes of variances. Some common causes of variance are listed in Table 12-13. In our analysis above, we found we were guilty of overlooking or forgetting to account for an expense, one of the examples in our list of common causes. The ability to effectively identify and investigate budget variances provides the necessary information for the laboratory manager to analyze and come to the appropriate conclusions on why the variance(s) occurred.

Recommendations

Quality Assurance and Performance Improvement should not just be reserved for quality control, but should be applied to all processes within the laboratory including paperwork. Regularly scheduled dates and times (15th of every month, 2nd Thursday of every month, etc.) will encourage monthly review of the laboratory's performance. In the supervisor's absence, lead techs will serve as "backups" to ensure the process continues normally and costs are expensed in the months incurred. This also serves to involve and educate key people in each department as to expenses incurred; the work involved projecting and tracking expenses; and justifying variances.

SUMMARY

Budgeting is a process in which every manager must become proficient. It is a way to take control of the laboratory environment, master the financial aspects of a department, and solve problems before they become critical. The budget is a tool to reassure, to clarify, to lower risk, to keep on track, and to assist in attaining goals. The budget defines the steps taken in the annual cycle to keep the plan on target. It is a management resource that defines the fiscal plan for the department and informs management of progress in achieving targets.

If properly prepared, a budget can increase revenues, decrease spending, and identify ways to make improvements. For the significant amount of effort that is invested into the budgetary process, it should generate recognizable results. Variances (negative and positive) need to be identified, investigated, and documented. Corrective action may or may not need to be developed and implemented, based upon the justification for the variance (Corrective action would not be needed for an increase in reagent expense due to an increase in test volumes).

The goal of the budget is to set standards. Those standards must then be communicated to the staff with a plan of how revenues will be maximized and expenses minimized. The success of meeting goals relies on everyone that is assigned to the section that the budget covers including the manager, supervisors and frontline staff. A budget variance report reflects the accuracy of assumptions. It also demands that problems must be identified and explained, and solutions recommended. By knowing the common budgetary problems, one can develop a sense of what to avoid and how to make the budget succeed. Reports 1 & 2 are examples of this.

The real test of a budget's merit is how it compares to actual expenses monthly and overall at the end of the fiscal year. Thorough budget variance analysis on a regular basis (at a minimum monthly), will assist in maximizing the accuracy of the forecast and whether problems can be identified and solved during the year.

SUMMARY CHART:
Important Points to Remember

➤ As reimbursement rates shrink, hospitals will need to become even more business-oriented, placing an increased emphasis on quality, the cost of non-quality, and the bottom line.

➤ A budget is an outline of projected revenue and expenses.

➤ There are many different types of operating budgets including fixed, flexible, program, appropriation, rolling, incremental, and zero-based.

➤ There are three important segments for the complete budget: income forecasting, expense budget, and cash flow projections.

➤ The budget may change due to changes within the laboratory, changes outside the laboratory, and changes outside the organization.

➤ Total Cost (expense) includes fixed and variable costs.

➤ Generally speaking, variable costs should change in relation to test volumes, i.e. as test volumes increase, cost should increase (the laboratory will need more reagents to perform the additional tests).

➤ Expenses and revenues must be periodically compared to the budget.

➤ Variances, both positive and negative, should be investigated, analyzed, and plausibly explained.

➤ As problems or causes of budget variances are identified, processes should be improved to prevent recurrence of the problem or cause.

➤ Process Guidelines for Preparing a Budget

• Start early
  ◦ The proposed budget may require multiple reviewers
  ◦ Allow enough time to analyze thoroughly

• Utilize your resources—Seek assistance
  ◦ Consult experienced directors from other departments
  ◦ Consult finance—budget analyst
  ◦ Engage section supervisors and staff to ensure every expense is accounted for

• Preparation is key—Year round activity
  ◦ Review Budget Variance Reports on a monthly basis
  ◦ Investigate, analyze, and be able to explain negative and positive variances
  ◦ Track expenses and revenues to sufficient detail

- Ensure accuracy of data
  - Ensure volumes and pricing are accurate
  - Analyze contracts for adjustments
    - Increase/decrease due to change in volume
    - Inflationary increases
- Documentation—Not too little or too much
  - Should be concise yet must be able to explain clearly
  - Should be able to answer questions and justify budget
- Compare proposed budget to existing revenues/expenses
  - Scrutinize—ensure the proposed budget makes sense
  - Focus on large adjustments and be able to explain/justify
- Practice your presentation
  - Reduces nervousness
  - Provides familiarity with budget
  - Ensures a smooth presentation—potentially less questions

SUGGESTED PROBLEM-BASED LEARNING ACTIVITIES

Chapter 12: Effective Budgeting in the Laboratory: Practical Tips

Instructions: Use Internet resources, books, articles, colleagues, etc., to present solutions to the problems listed below. There is no one correct solution to any problem.

Note to Instructor: Students in class may be divided into groups and given the problem-based learning activity to discuss and solve. Once the group has reached consensus as to a solution the group may present it to the other students in the class. This activity will provide all students with information regarding solutions to the problem.

Problem #1

Suppose your laboratory budget is cut. Indicate how you as the laboratory manager would maintain your current level of quality laboratory testing.

Problem #2

Prepare a laboratory budget forecasting an 8.5% increase in patient admissions.

Problem #3

Suppose that administration informed you that you must reduce your operating/personnel budget by 10%. As laboratory manager, you have been asked to design a plan indicating how you will handle and survive this cut.

REFERENCES

1. Ledue C: Number of Uninsured Americans Could Grow by 10M in Five Years. *Healthcare Finance News*. Princeton, NJ, 2010. Retrieved June 26, 2010, from: http://www.healthcare financenews.com/news/number-uninsured-americans-could-grow-10m-Five-Years

2. American Hospital Association, Uncompensated Hospital Care Cost Fact Sheet: *National Uncompensated Care Based on Cost: 1980–2008 (in Billions), Registered Community Hospitals*. Nov 2009. Retrieved June 26, 2010, from: http://www.aha.org/aha/content/2009/pdf/09uncompensatedcare.pdf

3. OECD Health Data 2010: How Does the United States Compare. OECD, 29 June 2010. Retrieved June 29, 2010, from: http://www.oecd.org/dataoecd/46/2/38980580.pdf

4. The World Bank, 2009 United States GDP. Retrieved June 26, 2010, from: http://search. worldbank.org/data?qterm=2009+united+s tates+gdp&language=EN&format=html

5. Bartlett B: Health Care: Costs and Reform. *Forbes, 3* July 2009. Retrieved June 26, 2010, from: http://www.forbes.com/2009/07/02/ health-care-costs-opinions-columnists-reform.html

6. Health Care, Health Reform in Action. The White house, 25 June 2010. Retrieved June 26, 2010, from: http://www.white house.gov/issues/health-care

7. Fenter T, Lewis S: Pay-for-Performance Initiatives. Supplement to *Journal of Managed Care Pharmacy* 2008: 14(6) (suppl S-c); S12–S15. Retrieved June 26, 2010, from: http://www.amcp.org/data/jmcp/Aug%20 suppl%20C_S12-S15.pdf

BIBLIOGRAPHY

Andersen RM, Rice TH, Kominski GF: *Changing the U.S. Health Care System: Key Issues in Health Services Policy and Management*. Jossey-Bass, A Wiley Company, San Francisco, CA, 2001.

Drucker P: *Management Challenges for the 21st Century*. HarperCollins Publishers, New York, NY, 1999.

Fenter T, Lewis S: Pay-for-Performance Initiatives. Supplement to *Journal of Managed Care Pharmacy*. 2008:14(6)(suppl S-c): S12–S15. Retrieved June 26, 2010, from: http://www. amcp.org/data/jmcp/Aug%20suppl%20C_ S12-S15.pdf

Groppelli A, Nikbakht E: *Finance (Barron's Business Review Series)*. Barron's Educational Series, Inc., Haupaugge, NY, 2006.

Kimmel PD, Weygandt JJ, Kieso DE: *Accounting and Finance: Managerial Use and Analysis*. John Wiley & Sons, Inc., New York, NY, 2000.

Label W: *Accounting for Non-Accountants*. Sourcebooks, Inc., Naperville, IL, 2010.

Powanga L, Marshall DH, McManus WW, Viele DF, Peter JP, Donnelly JH: *Effective Business Decisions*. McGraw-Hill Primis Custom Publishing, New York, NY, 2001.

Sobel M: *MBA in a Nutshell*. McGraw-Hill Professional, New York, NY, 2010.

Zelman WN, Mccue MJ, Millikan AR, Glick ND: *Financial Management of Health Care Organizations: An Introduction to Fundamental Tools, Concepts, and Applications*. Blackwell Publishing, Malden, MA, 2004.

INTERNET RESOURCES

American Hospital Association (AHA)
http://www.aha.org/aha_app/index.jsp

Global Health Observatory (GHO), World Health Organization
http://www.who.int/gho/en/

Google, Public Data, Gross Domestic Product (GDP)
http://www.google.com/publicdata?ds=wb-wdi&met=ny_gdp_mktp_cd&idim=countr y:USA&dl=en&hl=en&q=american+gross +domestic+product

Health Care Reform, The White House
http://www.whitehouse.gov/issues/health-care

Healthcare Finance News
http://www.healthcarefinancenews.com/

Overview. Clinical Laboratory Improvement Amendments (CLIA), Centers for Medicare and Medicaid Services (CMS)
http://www.cms.gov/CLIA/

Overview. Hospital-Acquired Conditions (Present on Admission Indicator), Centers for Medicare and Medicaid Services (CMS)
https://www.cms.gov/HospitalAcqCond/

Payback Period, Investopedia ULC
http://www.investopedia.com/terms/p/paybackperiod.asp

Static (Fixed) Budget. Business Glossary, Allbusiness.com
http://www.allbusiness.com/glossaries/static-fixed-budget/4947372-1.html

Tampa Bay Associates, Healthcare Consulting
http://www.e-tba.com/flexible-budgeting.htm

U.S. Department of Health and Human Services, Hospital Compare
http://www.hospitalcompare.hhs.gov

CHAPTER 13

The Cost of Quality

Lucia M. Berte, MA, MT(ASCP)SBB, DLM;
CQA(ASQ)CMQ/OE

CHAPTER OUTLINE

Objectives
Key Terms
Case Study
Introduction
The Concept of Quality Costs
Prevention Costs
Appraisal Costs
Failure Costs

Managing Quality Costs
Summary
Summary Chart: Important Points
 to Remember
Suggested Problem-Based Learning
 Activities
References
Internet Resources

OBJECTIVES

Following successful completion of this chapter, the learner will be able to:

1. Discuss the relationship between quality, cost, and variation.
2. Name four types of quality costs.
3. Identify at least 3 examples of each type of laboratory quality cost.
4. Describe the division point between the two types of failure costs.
5. Explain what happens to the total cost of quality and why, as the issue or problem progresses through the laboratory's path of work flow.
6. Diagram the financial relationship between prevention, appraisal, and failure costs.
7. Summarize the concept of using an iceberg to describe quality costs.
8. Explain how management can use prevention and appraisal to improve quality and reduce cost.

9. Locate prevention, appraisal, and failure costs on the laboratory's budget.
10. Illustrate the three components of a charge for a laboratory test.
11. Name at least 5 quality indicators for which failure costs could be tracked.
12. Given direct labor and supplies costs and the margin, calculate the failure cost for a given indicator.
13. Paraphrase at least 5 actions management can take to reduce failure cost.

KEY TERMS

Appraisal Cost
External Failure Costs
Failure Costs
Internal Failure Costs

Prevention Costs
Quality Indicators
Total Quality Cost
Variation

Case Study — Cost of Quality in Laboratory Management

You are the administrative director of a medium sized community hospital laboratory. The vice-president of ancillary services tells you that your laboratory continues to be overbudget and wants an explanation as to why. In a budget-cutting measure the previous year, the laboratory's inpatient phlebotomy team was disbanded and replaced with nurse's assistants at each inpatient location who were trained in blood sample collection, and who are under the nursing staff's control and budget. You begin to formulate your defense of the laboratory's overbudget condition.

Issues and Questions to Consider:
1. *Why might the budget-cutting decision described above cause cost overruns in the laboratory?*
2. *What are the four types of quality costs experienced by any organization?*
3. *Where on the budget would you find "good" quality costs?*
4. *Where on the budget would you find "bad" quality costs?*
5. *How can the cost of quality be calculated for any given laboratory activity?*

INTRODUCTION

"Quality is doing the right thing right—the first time and every time."
"It's cheaper to do the job right the first time than to recover from an error."

—Phillip Crosby, Industry Quality Expert

These two quotes were made by an important quality management expert who was instrumental in helping American businesses understand the financial impact of scrap, waste, and rework on their respective costs and revenues.[1] All of the principles of quality costs and cost management applied to business and industry today can also be applied to the economics of laboratory medicine. Laboratory managers often have a limited understanding of the costs associated with quality improvement processes. This knowledge is vital to making operational and financial decisions to ensure high quality laboratory services.[2]

A simple example that illustrates the value of these two quotes in laboratory medicine is that of an unacceptable sample that needs recollection. A "quality" collection consists of obtaining the correct sample from the correct patient at the proper time in the correct container that is properly labeled. A "quality" collection uses the correct amount of resources—one time only. According to Dr. Westgard, "the measure of quality is termed *unquality*; which is the lack of conformance to requirements, and universally described by defectives, defects, or defect rates."[3] Any recollection of an "unquality" sample for any reason adds to the laboratory's operating expenses without providing any value to the patient, ordering practitioner, or the laboratory. "Unquality" expenses are multiplied every time a sample recollection is needed. Likewise for any laboratory activity; it always costs less when the correct amount of resources is only expended once.

Healthcare economics is such that laboratories often have only the minimum necessary resources to provide basic services. Wasting resources significantly erodes the operating budget because the amount and negative impact of "unquality" expenses is considerable. Therefore, a basic understanding of the four different types of quality costs is vital to comprehending the value of their impact on the quality of laboratory services and the laboratory's operating budget.

THE CONCEPT OF QUALITY COSTS

Quality costs are the costs connected with both attaining and missing the desired level of quality in a service or product.[4] They are a measure of the costs specifically associated with the achievement or nonachievement of laboratory service quality—including all requirements established by the laboratory as well as regulatory requirements, laboratory accreditation requirements, and professional standards.

Quality costs may be seen as the cost of preventing quality problems, the cost of measuring, controlling and/or inspecting quality levels, and the cost of failing to accomplish the desired quality levels.[4] Quality costs can also be defined as—and represent—"the difference between the actual cost of a product or service and what the reduced cost would be if there was no possibility of substandard service, failure of products, or defects in their manufacture."[5] **Total quality cost** is a measure of both "good" and "bad" quality costs.

Another industry quality management expert, Dr. Genichi Taguchi, published a philosophy on cost and quality, reproduced here with applicable laboratory examples:[6]

- *We cannot reduce cost without affecting quality.* (What would happen to patients if a phlebotomist decided to wash and reuse blood collection needles to save money?)
- *We can improve quality without increasing cost.* (What would happen to turnaround time of STAT testing if the testing process was streamlined?)
- *We can reduce cost by improving quality.* (What would happen to the quality of blood samples if they were collected by trained, certified phlebotomists rather than by minimally trained nurses aides?)
- *We can reduce cost by reducing variation. When we do so, performance and quality will automatically improve.* (What would happen if, for each process in every laboratory job, there was a documented work flow [flow chart], concise procedures [instructions], and a documented training plan that competent trainers would follow?)

One of the many definitions of quality is "lack of variation." Therefore, if unwanted variation is reduced, quality is improved. When quality is improved, cost is reduced because the laboratory is not paying for variation and the resulting nonconformances.

The four types of quality costs are summarized in Figure 13-1 which represents an overview of quality costs. Each type and its respective laboratory examples are discussed in the sections that follow.

PREVENTION COSTS

Prevention costs represent the costs of laboratory activities specifically designed to prevent poor quality in laboratory services. Prevention costs are considered "good" quality costs because the related activities prevent errors or problems altogether. If errors or problems occur downstream, they are much more expensive to detect and correct. Therefore, these problems could compromise the quality of laboratory services or patient safety.

Examples of Laboratory Prevention Costs

Quality Planning
The time spent by the laboratory's management team in periodically reviewing the status of laboratory quality and setting forth and following up on documented laboratory quality objectives develops a focus on quality and a vision for what to strive for in the coming year.

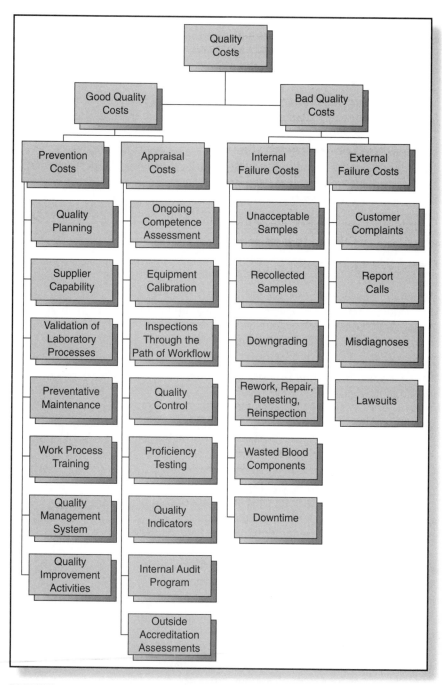

FIGURE 13-1. **Overview of Quality Costs with Laboratory Examples**

Supplier Capability

Carefully establishing the responsibilities of the laboratory (as a customer) and those of a supplier (such as a referral laboratory or device manufacturer) in a documented agreement for supplies or services before purchasing anything prevents costly assumptions and misunderstandings. The same is true for establishing responsibilities in agreements, where the laboratory will provide laboratory services (supplier) to physicians' office laboratories or other laboratories (customer).

Validation of Laboratory Processes

The time and cost expended in installing and challenging the performance of a new instrument before commencing patient testing (known as "process validation") help ensure that the instrument and tests performed on it will work as expected when "going live." Likewise for validating laboratory computer system functions.

Preventive Maintenance

By its very name, preventive maintenance programs ensure that instruments and equipment will perform as expected when needed, likely preventing costly breakdowns that compromise the laboratory's ability to provide timely service to users and patients.

Work Process Training

The time spent in training new employees in their respective work processes and procedures, whether they have previous experience or not, and ensuring initial competence to perform independently provides for uniformity in work performed. Training reduces personal variation that could lead to poor quality and time expended in counseling and retraining of an employee who has performance problems.

Quality Management System (QMS)

Maintaining an effective quality management system costs far less than having to repeatedly respond to customer problems and inspection deficiencies. (See Chapter 1.)

Quality Improvement Activities

Time spent in acquiring quality skills (such as auditing), teaching staff about quality concepts, attending quality improvement meetings, and participating in improvement projects all contribute to preventing problems that negatively affect the quality of services provided to users and patients.

A small amount of money spent in the prevention activities described above greatly reduces the chance of process problems later. Every budget should contain funds for prevention activities. Prevention activities are readily identified in a laboratory budget and can be quantitated.

APPRAISAL COSTS

Appraisal costs represent the costs of laboratory activities associated with measuring, evaluating, or auditing products or services to assure conformance to regulatory, accreditation, and customer requirements. Appraisal costs are considered "good" quality costs because the related activities help the laboratory catch and correct nonconformances before they adversely affect the quality of laboratory service or patient safety.

Examples of Laboratory Appraisal Costs

Ongoing Competence Assessment

Verifying ongoing competence of staff to perform their assigned tasks correctly ensures that personal variations that can cause nonconformances does not creep back into staff performance.

Equipment Calibration

Money spent in time, calibration materials, and calibration instruments (e.g., a NIST-traceable thermometer) ensures that equipment and instruments are measuring accurately, thus providing accurate test results.

Inspections Throughout the Path of Workflow

Preanalytic: Time taken at sample receiving to perform a thorough evaluation of samples and requests and resolve any problems shortens throughput time because only samples acceptable for testing are passed on for analysis.

Analytic: Sample inspection by testing staff at the time of sample analysis ensures proper conditions exist on sample entry into the test system.

Postanalytic: Review and evaluation of test results before verification identifies results needing further investigation (e.g., instrument warnings or flags, absurd values, delta checks, critical values, etc.) so that only accurate results are released.

Quality Control (QC)

Use of quality control (QC) reagents and materials is required on a scheduled basis for all analytic methods. This quality cost needs to be inherent in every laboratory budget.

Proficiency Testing (PT)

Laboratories are required to pay for participation in interlaboratory proficiency testing (PT) programs to verify performance comparable to that of their peers for the same instruments and methods. This quality cost needs to be inherent in every laboratory budget.

Quality Indicators

The laboratory is required to measure how well its preanalytic, analytic, and post-analytic processes are working and take action to reduce or eliminate any identified problems.[7] Laboratories often measure the number and types of unacceptable samples; the turnaround time for selected tests to key customers, such as cardiac markers to the emergency department or blood component delivery in trauma cases; and the number of reporting errors and their impact on patient care.

Internal Audit Program

A program of internal audit of management and technical processes verifies that requirements are being met. The time and cost of performing internal audits that trace laboratory samples or records through preanalytic, analytic, and postanalytic workflow processes reduces the embarrassment and cost of responding to customer issues and inspection deficiencies—especially those frequently repeated.

Outside Accreditation Assessments

Regulation requires that the laboratory obtain and maintain successful accreditation from specified accreditation organizations. Such assessments are conducted by persons outside the laboratory trained to review objective evidence that the laboratory meets applicable regulatory and accreditation requirements.

The laboratory's budget usually always contains funds for calibration, inspection, QC, PT, and accreditation activities because these are mandated by regulatory and accreditation agencies. However, laboratories should also add to their budgets the "good" quality costs of indicator development, data collection and analysis, and the training for and maintenance of an internal audit program. Appraisal helps ensure that problems are caught and corrected in an effort to eliminate or minimize any negative impact on customers and patients.

FAILURE COSTS

Failure costs are those resulting from products or services not conforming to requirements or customer/user needs; they are the costs resulting from poor quality. Failure costs are divided into internal and external failure cost categories. The distinction occurs when the product (ie, the laboratory test results and/or report) or the provision of a laboratory service to a customer (e.g., a pathology consultation) leaves the laboratory's control.

Internal Failure Costs

Internal failure costs are considered "bad" quality costs and represent costs incurred *before* delivery of the product or provision of a service.

Examples of Laboratory Internal Failure Costs

Unacceptable Samples. Any time a blood, body fluid, tissue or other type of sample is received in the laboratory and is not acceptable for testing, the organization has incurred the procurement costs and cannot perform testing or charge for its services to that point. All procurement costs must be expended a second time to get an acceptable sample.

Downgrading. These are the costs incurred when laboratorians need to consult with practitioners, record special comments, or perform other workarounds regarding testing samples that are less than acceptable (e.g., inadequate cell material on an outpatient Pap smear), difficult to replace (e.g., spinal or amniotic fluid) or irreplaceable (e.g., biopsy tissue).

Rework, Repair, Retesting, Reinspection. The dictionary defines the prefix "re" as "again, renew, over again."[8] A common occurrence is the retesting of QC and patient samples when the controls do not give the proper results. Another common occurrence is instrument failure, which incurs both repair time and retesting costs.

Wasted Blood Components. The hospital must still pay the blood center (or expend the collection and testing costs if it maintains its own donor center) whenever labile blood components such as thawed plasma or cryoprecipitate or pooled or apheresis platelets are prepared for transfusion but are not transfused and exceed their expiration time. Red cell units into which administration sets have been spiked are also wasted if not transfused within their 4 hour expiration time.

Downtime. Downtime occurs any time the laboratory cannot provide its regular services, such as when the computer is unavailable, an instrument is not functioning, or when an accident or other disaster causes laboratory service restrictions or closures. Costs include having other laboratories provide services in the interim, such as sending samples to referral laboratories, lost revenue, loss of customers, and verifying correct system functioning after service is reinstated.

Internal failures are those caught and corrected before they adversely affect customers or patients. Operating funds have been expended and wasted because the activity was not performed correctly the first time.

External Failure Costs

External failure costs are considered "bad" quality costs and occur *after* release of laboratory test results or reports and during or after the furnishing of a laboratory service to a customer (e.g., blood collection, pathology consultation, etc.).

Examples of Laboratory External Failure Costs

Customer Complaints. Labor and materials are expended to rectify the customer's concern when complaints are resolved. Until the root cause of the problem is identified and removed, the rectification costs are likely to recur with the same or a different customer. Often, workarounds are enacted; that is, management issues policies or memos that change what staff do under certain circumstances or for certain customers—or staff devise their own means around the problem. Workarounds usually add more complexity to already complex processes, thus increasing the likelihood of more variation that can lead to more nonconformances and more complaints. Workarounds directly add to labor costs.

Report Recalls. The discovery of a wrong result on a laboratory report after its release obligates the laboratory to investigate and rectify the error and issue a corrected report. In addition, action may have been taken on the patient as a result of the erroneous information; therefore, appropriate practitioners must be notified of the error and its correction. The cost to correct a reporting error erodes the laboratory's operating budget and significantly erodes customer and user confidence in the laboratory's quality and credibility.

Misdiagnoses. Misdiagnoses can result in patients receiving unnecessary treatment or patients not receiving a necessary treatment. In the first case, resources are consumed with no benefit to the patient. In the second case, the cost for treating the patient after delay in obtaining a correct diagnosis is usually always greater than for a timely intervention, not to mention the extensive adverse cost on the patient's well-being, outcome, and personal finances.

Lawsuits. This is the most expensive failure cost, far exceeding all "good" quality costs. Lawsuits can usually be completely avoided if the laboratory realizes the value of prevention and appraisal costs.

"Bad" quality costs are the most expensive and hard to measure because they include both actual and intangible costs incurred to correct a nonconformance that has reached the customer.

MANAGING QUALITY COSTS

A health care study reported that as much as 30% of all direct health care outlays are the result of poor quality health care including, but not limited to, overuse, misuse, and waste.[9] The Makerere University and John Hopkins University reported the first study which quantified the cost of quality (COQ) for a clinical laboratory in a resource-limited environment (Uganda).[2] Their report indicated that 32% of total laboratory expenses and 94% of total COQ was spent on creating and following procedures that ensure good laboratory practices (GLP), thereby contributing high-quality outcomes. Therefore, 94% represented the cost of good quality and 6% of the costs were for "bad" quality.[2] The COQ in this clinical laboratory in Uganda is much different than the COQ reported at a hospital clinical laboratory in the United States. In this study, the overall COQ was about 35% of the operating expenses, with the cost of good quality approximately 10% and the cost of poor quality, 25%.[10]

There are two significant aspects in looking at laboratory quality costs. First, the cost of quality for a given issue grows larger as the issue progresses through the laboratory's path of workflow toward the user or customer. From prevention through measurement, detection, follow-up, and possibly to litigation, each level results in a significant increase in quality costs (failure costs)—said to be as much as a ten-fold increase at each level. Not all issues make it to the litigation stage; however, all issues increase in cost every time they move forward. A graphic representation of this concept is presented in Figure 13-2.

The second significant aspect in looking at laboratory quality costs is that many are not obvious. These are called hidden quality costs and often represent the amount of easily measured laboratory costs. An iceberg analogy is often used to illustrate the concept of "10% visible and 90% hidden." The tip of the iceberg represents easily identified and measured good and bad quality costs, while the remainder of the iceberg under the surface represents many of the really bad quality costs in laboratory operations and service delivery. Figure 13-3 shows the iceberg of visible and hidden laboratory quality costs. The costs shown are not meant to be all-inclusive.

It's easy for management to blame workers for making mistakes that lead to failure costs. What's harder is for management to accept that all quality management literature supports the conclusion that decisions management make—and do not make—lead to unnecessarily complex or bad processes that set workers up for problems to occur. Workers are not the issue—processes are. The best way for management to remove the cost of poor quality is to design good processes that meet requirements (prevention), train staff to follow the processes (prevention), ensure ongoing staff competence (appraisal), measure process performance (appraisal), and improve processes that have problems.

A Quality Cost Approach for the Laboratory

The total cost of quality is the sum of prevention, appraisal, internal failure, and external failure costs. Prevention and appraisal costs are the price the laboratory pays for conforming to regulatory, accreditation, user and customer requirements and should be considered as investments in providing quality products and services. The laboratory is required to perform calibrations, maintenance, quality control, proficiency testing, and participate in accreditation assessments. The laboratory should further invest in planning for quality, delivering effective training, ensuring staff competence, monitoring quality indicators, auditing laboratory processes, and participating in quality improvement projects. These costs are measurable and, as previously mentioned, can be found as line items in a laboratory budget.

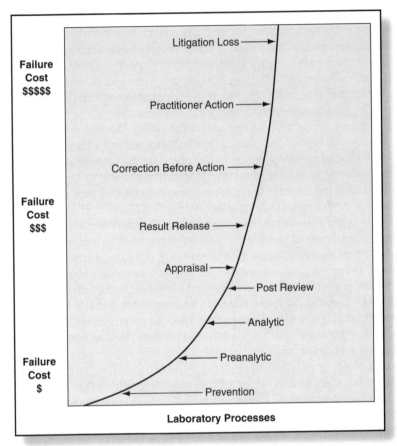

FIGURE 13-2.   **Failure Cost as a Function of Detection Point in Laboratory Processes**

Adapted from: Campanella J, ed: *Principles of Quality Costs*, ed 3. ASQ Press, 1999.[5]

A relatively modest increase in prevention costs realizes a significant reduction in the cost of failure. When the cost of failure is reduced, the cost of appraisals to catch constant failures is also reduced, thus further reducing the total cost of quality.

Failure costs are the price the laboratory pays for nonconformance and are considered losses. Unfortunately, budgets don't contain line items for failure costs. Instead, the cost to rectify failures is spread over the applicable line items; for example, overtime in the labor budget and additional reagents and QC materials when repeating testing due to a failure. Failure costs are hidden across many line items disguised as routine expenditures and therefore are not readily apparent and not easily separated from valid costs. Managers are often at a loss to explain budget overruns because they cannot see the buried failure costs.

A laboratory example best illustrates the effect of failure cost on the laboratory's budget. When an outpatient blood sample is received in the laboratory and

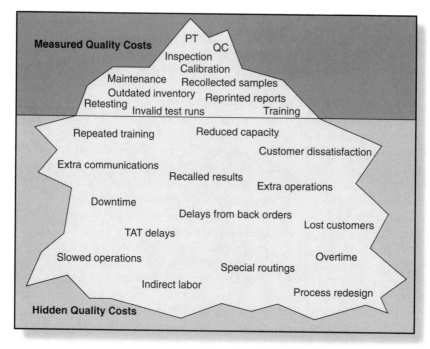

Measured Quality Costs

PT QC
Inspection
Calibration
Maintenance   Recollected samples
Outdated inventory   Reprinted reports
Retesting
Invalid test runs   Training

Repeated training   Reduced capacity

Customer dissatisfaction

Extra communications
Recalled results
Extra operations

Downtime
Delays from back orders
Lost customers
TAT delays

Slowed operations   Overtime
Special routings
Indirect labor
Process redesign

Hidden Quality Costs

FIGURE 13-3.   The Iceberg of Measured and Hidden Quality Costs

Adapted from: Wood DC: *The Executive Guide to Understanding and Implementing Quality Cost Programs.* ASQ Press, 2007.[4]

found unacceptable for testing, the laboratory has already expended: 1) outpatient receptionist labor to greet and register the patient; 2) phlebotomist labor to collect the sample; and 3) sample receiving clerk labor to evaluate and accession the sample. The laboratory has also expended the cost of both the collection supplies and printed sample requests and labels. Whatever the total amount expended thus far, the fact remains that the sample cannot be used for testing, therefore the laboratory cannot enter a charge for the sample collected and generate the small margin usually added. To get a viable sample for testing, the laboratory must incur the labor and supply costs a second time—now having two collection expenses for only one sample. Also consider that the funds to collect a second sample the first time come from the existing budget. Every time a sample needs recollection, funds that could be used for a different patient sample the first time are used out of the existing budget. There are also the hidden costs of patient dissatisfaction in having to return for recollection and prerequisites of test results, to which no dollar amount can be accurately attributed.

The sample recollection problem is an example of a common significant internal failure cost. Anytime a laboratory activity—from test ordering through report delivery—needs to be repeated, the cost of poor quality increases. However, laboratories often control their budgets by reducing spending in all line items—including the good quality costs of prevention and appraisal, such as cutting back on maintenance, shortening training, and postponing a laboratory audit program. When that happens, it's likely that poor quality costs are high. Said in another way: When the amount spent on prevention and appraisal is low, the amount spent on failure is high.

Figure 13-4 looks at the sum of quality costs from the perspective of a single laboratory activity. First, there are the acceptable real direct costs of labor and supplies. Then there are the unseen failure costs buried in the budget that add to the real cost of production to generate the actual cost of production, shown as "waste." Also added is a margin; in the laboratory environment, the margin helps offset direct operating costs and provides revenue to the laboratory's owner (e.g., hospital, physician's office or physician, commercial company, etc.). In the laboratory environment, margins are often added to charges for phlebotomy collections, laboratory tests, and anatomic pathology services. The sum of the actual cost of production and the margin becomes the charge to the customer for the product or service. The cost of failure is built into the charge! Failure costs erode the margin—the more internal and external failure costs, the smaller the realized margin. Reducing or removing cost of failure represents the opportunity to increase the margin/profit if the charge stays the same or allows for the charge to be reduced to compete in the market while still preserving the margin. However, government and private health care reimbursement organizations are only willing to reimburse the real cost with perhaps a small margin, which is why reimbursement fees are often below a laboratory's "actual" cost.

Using Indicators to Determine Failure Cost

The quality indicator for the number of unacceptable samples received in the laboratory can be converted to a failure cost indicator in the following manner. First, the direct variable costs of labor and supplies to collect the different types of samples are calculated (e.g., blood, blood culture, urine, stool, Pap smear, etc.).

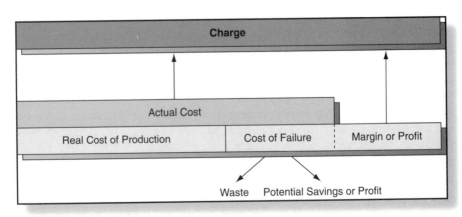

FIGURE 13-4.   The Components of Charge and Cost

Then, the number of unacceptable samples of each type is tallied on a regular basis, such as monthly. A spreadsheet function can calculate the failure cost for one instance of an unacceptable sample and multiply it times the number of unacceptable samples of that type tallied for the month. This application can be used to calculate the failure costs for other laboratory indicators such as repeating a test run or replacing a lost report. (For a discussion of laboratory indicators, see Chapter 1.) A worksheet for calculating the tangible failure cost of almost any laboratory indicator is presented in Table 13-1.

It is one thing for management to have failure cost information and another thing to do something about it. In the words of another industry quality management expert, Taiichi Ohno, "Costs do not exist to be calculated. Costs exists to be reduced."[4]

Reducing the Cost of Failure

The best way to reduce the cost of failure is for laboratory management to devote efforts to prevention and appraisal—that is, put money and time into the good quality costs.

Plan for Quality

The laboratory should document new or changed processes (e.g., a new analyzer, bar-coded patient samples, etc.). This is usually done with a quality tool called a flowchart.[11] Staff should review the flowchart and at every action ask the question, "What could go wrong here and how could we prevent that?" This is a systematic method of identifying and preventing process problems before they occur and allows for designing failure prevention or controls into the process.

Streamline Processes

The act of documenting the laboratory's processes with a flowchart provides a common understanding of the correct sequence of necessary activities and responsibilities. The further application of "Lean" thinking removes wasted time, effort, and resources from work processes, therefore reducing the cost of work. (See Chapter 16.)

Validate Processes

Before "going live," the laboratory should verify that any new process works as intended, so that any problems can be identified and resolved. This prevents the customers from experiencing any problems in the "live" environment; thereby, avoiding dissatisfaction and failure recovery costs.

Write Effective Documents

Properly validated and written process flowcharts, procedures, and job aids that are used by the staff in laboratory work provide powerful tools to prevent errors. Documents are the means that laboratory management uses to communicate with staff; therefore, the time and attention paid to providing good documents prevents staff and process problems later.

TABLE 13-1.   Worksheet for Calculating the Failure Cost of a Laboratory Quality Indicator

Name of Item Being Measured:			
Cost Type	Unit Cost	Number of Units	Extension
Direct Labor	$ ____ per hour	_____ hours	$ _____
Direct Supplies A:	A:	A:	A:
B:	B:	B:	B:
C:	C:	C:	C:
etc.	etc.	etc.	etc.
Cost for original (direct labor and supplies)			$
Margin/profit foregone			$
Cost to replace (direct labor and supplies)			$
Borrowed from the budget (direct labor and supplies)			$
TOTAL COST FOR THE FAILURE OF ONE INSTANCE Insert this number above in the spreadsheet or calculation program to get the product of the frequency of instances and the failure cost for the designated time period.			
Date worksheet prepared: Prepared by:			

Improve Training

Poorly trained employees make errors, revert to techniques used in previous employment, or invent their own creative means to accomplish tasks—all of which lead to highly variable work and high failure cost. Effective training is based on the laboratory's work processes and procedures.[12] Initial assessment of competence before employees work unsupervised in the live environment ensures that staff has the knowledge and uses the skills needed to perform tasks correctly.

Measurement, Monitoring, and Improvement

The effort and costs of measurement and monitoring should not be regarded with dread but rather be strongly supported as a means to identify and reduce or eliminate more costly errors. The laboratory should invest in measuring work processes (i.e., quality indicator tracking), comparing the laboratory's performance to others of like kind, and auditing internal processes—and then take appropriate follow-up actions to minimize or eradicate failure. As failures are revealed, they should be examined for root causes. Corrective action taken to eliminate root causes means permanent removal of the problem. Whereas the laboratory only pays for corrective action one time, it pays for failure to take corrective action over and over again.

SUMMARY

The good quality costs of prevention and appraisal efforts lead to reduction in the bad quality costs of laboratory errors and dissatisfied customers. The strategy for using quality costs is simple to understand.

1. Directly attack internal and external failure costs and attempt to drive them to zero.
2. Invest in the appropriate prevention activities to bring about improvement.
3. Reduce appraisal costs according to results achieved.
4. Continuously evaluate and redirect prevention efforts to gain further improvement.[5]

The following cost management philosophy supports the strategy described above and bears remembering:

- For each failure there is a *root cause.*
- Causes are *preventable.*
- Prevention is always *cheaper.*[5]

SUMMARY CHART:
Important Points to Remember

➤ Quality costs are the costs of preventing quality problems, measuring quality levels, controlling and/or inspecting quality levels, and failing to accomplish the desired quality levels.

➤ There are four types of quality costs: prevention, appraisal, internal failure, and external failure.

➤ Prevention costs are "good" quality costs. Laboratories should invest money and time in prevention activities because prevention of errors or problems is far less expensive than rectification downstream.

➤ Appraisal costs are "good" quality costs. Appropriately applied internal monitoring and assessment helps the laboratory identify problems or errors and rectify them before they reach users and customers.

➤ Internal failure cost is higher than the cost of prevention and appraisal combined, and erodes the laboratory's budget with rework that does not add value to laboratory services or patient safety.

➤ External failure costs are the most expensive and public, and can be avoided through diligent application of prevention and appraisal.

➤ A significant portion of a health care organization's operating budget is spent in failure cost and recovering from failures.

➤ The cost of quality grows larger as the issue progresses through the laboratory's path of workflow.

➤ Hidden quality costs can be many times larger than easily measurable prevention, appraisal, and failure costs.

➤ Laboratory quality indicators can be used to determine measurable failure costs.

➤ A small amount of money invested into prevention and appraisal greatly reduces the cost of failure.

Suggested Problem-Based Learning Activities

Chapter 13: The Cost of Quality

Instructions: Use Internet resources, books, articles, colleagues, etc. to present solutions to the problems listed below. There is no one correct solution to any problem.

Note to Instructor: Students may be divided into groups and given the problem-based learning activity to discuss and solve. Once the group has reached consensus on a solution, the group may present it to other students in the class, thus providing all students with information about potential solutions.

Problem #1

Use the information in this chapter to identify all the cost elements that would go into calculating the cost of testing a batch of 20 samples on a selected analyzer.

Problem #2

Formulate the defense of your laboratory's over-budget condition using the concepts of prevention, appraisal, and internal and external failure costs. Construct your argument as to why an inpatient phlebotomy team should be restored to laboratory control.

Problem #3

You want to describe to the vice president the hidden quality costs not shown on nursing's budget for their nursing assistants' phlebotomy activities. Identify these hidden quality costs, explain where the cost amounts might be found, and describe the impact of these costs to the hospital's external and internal customers. (See Chapter 1 for a discussion about external and internal customers.)

REFERENCES

1. Crosby PB: *Quality Is Free*. McGraw-Hill, New York, NY, 1979.

2. Elbireer A, Gable AR, Brooks, JJ: *Cost of Quality at a Clinical Laboratory in a Resource-Limited Country*. ASCP LabMed 2010: 41(7); 429-433.

3. Westgard JO: *Testing Equivalent Quality: A Better Way—Westgard QC*. Westgard Web - Westgard QC. Feb. 2004. Accessed 1 Mar 2011 from: http://www.westgard.com/es say61.htm#2

4. Wood DC: *The Executive Guide to Understanding and Implementing Quality Cost Programs*. American Society for Quality Press, Milwaukee, WI, 2007.

5. Campanella J, ed.: *Principles of Quality Costs*, ed 3. American Society for Quality Press, Milwaukee, WI, 1999.

6. Byrne DM, Ryan NE, eds.: *Taguchi Methods and QFD*. ASI Press, Dearborn, MI, 1988.

7. Centers for Medicare and Medicaid Services: Code of Federal Regulations, Title 42, Parts 430 to end. U.S. Government Printing Office, Washington, D.C., revised annually.

8. Neufeldt V, Guralnik DB, eds.: *Webster's New World Dictionary*, ed 3. College Edition. Simon & Schuster, New York, NY, 1988.

9. Midwest Business Group on Health: *Reducing the Cost of Poor Quality in Health Care Through Responsible Purchasing Leadership*. Midwest Business Group on Health, Chicago, IL, 2002.

10. Menichino T: A Cost-of-Quality Model for Hospital Laboratory. *MLO Med Lab Obs* 1992: 24; 47-50. Accessed 1 Mar. 2011 from: http://www.findarticles.com/p/articles/mi_ m3230/is_n1_v24/ai_11815914/

11. Cardelino C, Harkins M, Johnson C, Brassard M, Ritter D: *The Memory Jogger II™ for Laboratory Operations*. GOAL/QPC and COLA, Methuen, MA, 2007.

12. Clinical and Laboratory Standards Institute: *Training and Competence Assessment; Approved Guideline*, GP21-A3. Wayne, PA, 2009.

INTERNET RESOURCES

Agency for Healthcare Research and Quality (AHRQ)
http://www.ahrq.gov/

American Society for Quality (ASQ)
http://www.asq.org

American Society for Quality (ASQ): Knowledge Center
http://www.asq.org/knowledge-center/

Centers for Medicare and Medicaid Services (CMS)
http://www.cms.gov/

Clinical and Laboratory Standards Institute (CLSI)
http://www.clsi.org

Juran Institute
http://www.juran.com/

Juran Institute—Solutions for Reducing Costs
http://www.juran.com/solutions_reduce_ costs_index.html

Juran Institute—Solutions, Reduce Costs, Quality Control
http://www.juran.com/solutions_reduce_ costs_quality_control.html

Midwest Business Group on Health (MBGH)
http://www.mbgh.org/

CHAPTER 14

Healthcare
Reimbursement

Jeanne M. Donnelly, MBA, RHIA
Matthew M. Anderson, MS

OBJECTIVES

Following successful completion of this chapter, the learner will be able to:

1. Identify and discuss the following reimbursement methodologies used by the Center for Medicare and Medicaid Services (CMS):
    a. Diagnostic Related Groups (DRGs)
    b. Resource Based Relative Value Scale (RBRVS)
    c. Ambulatory Payment Categories (APCs)
2. Calculate the payment rate for each methodology based on CMS formulas.
3. Discuss other payment methodologies such as:
    a. Fee-for-service
    b. Capitation

c. Per diem
d. Per case
e. Carve out
4. Calculate payment based on a capitated rate.
5. Identify reasons why healthcare costs have escalated and discuss how the healthcare industry has responded.
6. Critically analyze healthcare reform and how it may impact reimbursement in the future.

KEY TERMS

Ambulatory Payment Categories (APCs)
Capitation
Carve Out (Carved Out)
Co-payments
Deductibles
Diagnostic Related Groups (DRGs)
Fee-for-Service
Governmental Payers
Managed Care

Payer
Per Case
Per Diem
Premiums
Prospective Payment System (PPS)
Private Payers
Provider
Resource Based Relative Value Scale (RBRVS)
Self Payers

Case Study Healthcare Reimbursement

As the manager of a clinical laboratory, you have been asked to calculate the reimbursement rates for certain laboratory tests with Ambulatory Payment Categories (APCs) under the new Outpatient Prospective Payment System. You must estimate what your laboratory will receive for Medicare patients under this system to assist you in the budget process.

Issues and Questions to Consider:

1. *What coding system is used to assign APCs?*
2. *What allied health professional is preferred for assigning code numbers?*
3. *What is the formula for calculating the payment rate?*
4. *Where can you find the most current information regarding the APC rates and the conversion factor used in determining the payment rate?*
5. *How can this information be used in planning for the budget?*
6. *What is another way that laboratory tests are billed for non-Medicare patients?*

INTRODUCTION

This chapter provides the reader with a basic understanding of healthcare reimbursement. A brief history of healthcare costs shows why costs have escalated and how payers have responded. The different types of reimbursement mechanisms are discussed. These are broken down into governmental and private sectors. It is important to note that more than one of these mechanisms may be used by the payers.

Certain terms related to reimbursement are used throughout the chapter. A **provider** refers to the hospital, the outpatient department, the physician or other healthcare professional who furnishes care to the patient. A **payer** refers to the **governmental payers** (such as Medicare, Medicaid, and other public sources of funds), **private payers** (such as Blue Cross and other commercial insurers) or **self payers** who do not have any other type of insurance.

HISTORICAL PERSPECTIVE

In 2008, healthcare represented 16.2% of the Gross Domestic Product (GDP) or the equivalent of $2.3 trillion. Clinical laboratory costs account for approximately $30 to $40 billion of that amount. It is estimated that total healthcare costs will increase to 19.6% of the GDP or $4.5 trillion by the year 2019.[1] Yet, in 1965, healthcare accounted for only 5.5% of the GDP. How did healthcare come to consume such a large portion of our national expenditure? Several elements have contributed to the increase in healthcare costs.

1. *Increase in technology:* Technology advances in testing, surgical procedures, and diagnostic procedures required new, cost intensive equipment. Not only did equipment need to be purchased, but in some cases, new facilities needed to be built to house the equipment.

2. *Increase in skilled personnel:* These new technologies required staff with different skill sets to operate the equipment. This resulted in new categories of allied health personnel that needed to be educated, trained, and hired.

3. *Aging population:* As we age, we access healthcare services more frequently. In addition, the improved technology resulted in a longer life span and increased the need for skilled nursing care to accommodate an elderly population.

4. *Consumer awareness and expectations:* The consumer expected and demanded the high-priced technology. Where an x-ray study would have sufficed in the past, now a magnetic resonance imaging (MRI) or positron emission tomography (PET) scan is the expectation.

5. *The uninsured/underinsured:* Individuals who do not have readily available access to insurance use more expensive services, such as emergency room

services or physician specialists to receive routine care. Even worse, these individuals may wait until they are very ill before accessing the healthcare system.

As the cost of healthcare continued to rise, the cost of health insurance increased as well. Government and private insurance plans had to increase their premiums to keep pace with the rising costs. Employers sponsoring the health insurance benefits for employees initially covered the cost increase; however, as time went on, the employee had to share in the increased cost of insurance through higher premiums, deductibles, and co-payments, or face a decrease in benefits. **Premiums** are the amount charged by the insurer to insure against specific risks. **Deductibles** represents the amount the insured must first pay (usually annually) before benefits are payable. **Co-payments** are the proportion of total medical costs, or a pre-determined dollar amount that the insured must pay out of pocket each time health services are received after the deductible has been paid. As the employer and consumer become responsible for more of the cost of healthcare, they tend to focus more on cost efficiency regarding the use of healthcare dollars. The healthcare industry has responded in several ways to try to manage such a large segment of spending. There is an increased emphasis on preventive medicine and alternative care options. Employers have initiated programs to decrease occupational health hazards and increase employee wellness. Spending limitations and benefit exclusions have been added to insurance plans to try to slow the growth of spending. The main sources of healthcare funding are federal government programs and private insurance. Both have sought new ways to curb costs. The private sector has incorporated parts of the federal programs and the federal programs have seen value in the private arena. But the goal is the same in both cases: obtain the best quality care at the correct level of service for the least cost.

FEDERAL AND STATE REIMBURSEMENT SYSTEMS

As seen in Figure 14-1, state and federal governments pay for approximately 48% of healthcare expenditures through Medicare, Medicaid, and other public programs. Medicare came into being as an amendment to the Social Security Act (SSA) in 1965. It is funded by the federal government through a payroll tax and is administrated by the Center for Medicare and Medicaid Services (CMS). Medicare pays for healthcare for persons 65 and over, disabled individuals entitled to Social Security benefits, and patients with end stage renal disease. The Medicare Program benefits were originally separated into two parts. "Part A" covers certain hospital and outpatient costs; "Part B" covers certain individual physician costs. In recent years, "Part C" managed care plans were added as options for many beneficiaries, which were modeled after private sector managed care plans.

Medicaid, also created by the SSA of 1965, is a state-run healthcare plan for the poor. It is funded jointly by state and federal funds based on income levels for each state. Each state has a different methodology for reimbursement, but all must meet

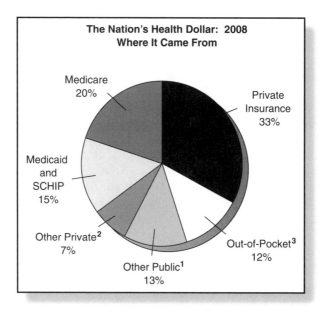

FIGURE 14-1. **The Nation's Healthcare Dollar: 2008**
Note: Numbers shown may not add to 100 because of rounding.
[1]Other Public includes programs such as workers' compensation, public health activity, Department of Defense, Department of Veterans Affairs, Indian Health Service, State and local hospital subsidies and school health.
[2]Other Private includes industrial in-plant, privately funded construction, and non-patient revenues, including philanthropy.
[3]Out of pocket includes co-pays, deductibles, and treatments not covered by Private Health Insurance.
SCHIP – State Children's Health Insurance Program
Source: Centers for Medicare and Medicaid, Office of Actuary, National Health Statistics Group.[3]

the funding limitations set by the federal government. Each state must also provide certain basic health services as mandated by the federal government. Most states reimburse under a fee-for-service basis; however, one third of the states use a managed care program. Under the Balanced Budget Act (BBA) of 1997, states were given the authority to mandate managed care enrollment for Medicaid beneficiaries.

Another component of the BBA of 1997 was the implementation of the State Children's Health Insurance Program (SCHIP), which was later shortened to the Children's Health Insurance Program (CHIP). The CHIP is a program jointly funded by state and federal governments to provide healthcare to children in families who are not qualified for Medicaid, but with incomes too low to afford insurance. Initially the program provided coverage to over 5 million uninsured children, but the number of uninsured children continued to rise. In February of 2009, President Barack Obama signed into law the Children's Health Insurance Program Reauthorization Act of 2009, expanding insurance coverage to an estimated additional 4 million children.[2]

Other types of public health aid funded by federal and state governments include: programs for veteran's health care, Indian health care, school health programs, and maternal and child health services. Because the government subsidized such a large portion of healthcare expenditures, it became evident that the rapid growth of healthcare costs needed to be controlled. The first area to be addressed, hospital costs, accounted for one third of total healthcare dollars.

"My costs are higher because I have sicker patients," was the rallying cry for hospitals in the 1970s to explain their higher costs, but there was no mechanism to justify this claim. Data was collected on patients' diagnoses and procedures, but there was not a way to relate the diagnosis and treatment to costs.

Prior to the early 1980s, hospitals were reimbursed on a *fee-for-service* basis. This meant that the provider was paid by the government, the commercial insurance company, or patients themselves for all services the physicians ordered. Each test, shot, examination, and procedure generated a separate charge. During this time, there were no controls or incentives to order only the tests that were deemed necessary for the patient, because the physician and hospital would get paid for any test ordered. Tests were also ordered to prevent litigation and to provide teaching opportunities. Medicare spending was increasing at a rate that outpaced inflation. Between 1980 and 1990, healthcare spending increased from approximately $247 billion to $699 billion—a 183% increase. The government needed a mechanism to control the increase in spending. The CMS researched a patient classification system for the tests being ordered to assist in controlling expenditures, known as the diagnostic related groups.

Diagnostic Related Groups (DRGs)

Diagnostic Related Groups (DRGs) are a patient classification system initially developed to evaluate quality and resource consumption in a hospital setting. In 1982, the Tax Equity and Fiscal Responsibility Act (TEFRA) stated that Medicare reimbursement would be based on DRGs, and in 1983, the Social Security Act was amended to include a DRG-based reimbursement system for all Medicare patients. This system is referred to as the **Prospective Payment System (PPS)**. Under the PPS, hospitals would receive a set amount of reimbursement per patient discharge.

DRGs are used to reimburse hospital costs for Medicare inpatients only (Part A services). They are not used for physician services. As patients are discharged, the hospital provider assigns code numbers for the diagnoses and procedures relevant to that hospital admission. The codes utilized for this process are referred to as the International Classification of Diseases, 9th Revision, Clinical Modification (ICD-9-CM) classification system. These code numbers, along with certain patient demographic information are "grouped" via decision trees into a DRG specific to the patient's episode of care. There are currently more than 500 DRGs. The CMS assigns a weight to each DRG based on the severity of the diagnoses, type of procedure, number of laboratory and diagnostic tests, number and type of drugs prescribed, and presence of complications or co-morbid conditions.

Each hospital is assigned a specific rate by the CMS that has been calculated based on several factors: type of hospital (community versus teaching), setting (urban versus rural), and location (Western United States versus Northeast). These factors determine the case mix of the facility. The DRG weight multiplied by the hospital rate determines how much the hospital will be reimbursed for the care of patients who have been grouped to the DRG. See Table 14-1 for example.

The hospital's rate does not vary greatly from year to year unless there has been a dramatic change in the case mix. The DRG weights are evaluated annually and modified based on changes in treatment. Additional DRGs have been added over the years to account for new diseases and updated treatment methodologies.

Once a hospital's base rate has been established, the CMS accounts for several variables to adjust payment to the hospital. First, a wage index is applied to a hospital to reflect the vast differences in salaries throughout the country. Hospitals in locations with higher average salaries receive more reimbursement. The CMS also reimburses hospitals for the costs associated with training future healthcare professionals through an Indirect Medical Education (IME) payment. Hospitals that treat low-income patients also receive an additional level of reimbursement through a disproportionate share payment, since treating these patients is more costly to the hospital. Finally, hospitals may be compensated for patients whose costs far exceed the average for a given case. In these instances, the hospital must make a request to the CMS and justify the elevated reimbursement.

Using PPS, hospitals are now able to determine how much reimbursement they will receive for Medicare patients. If a hospital can treat a patient for less than the reimbursed amount, it will make a profit. If it costs more to treat the patient than the amount it receives, the hospital must absorb the cost. The patient cannot be billed for the excess cost.

Assume that we are evaluating two patients who have been categorized to DRG 126 from the preceding example (see Table 14-1). The reimbursement rate for a patient in this DRG at Community Hospital is $3,908. To determine if the hospital will make a profit or loss we compare the cost with the reimbursement rate.

It is now possible for hospitals to estimate the amount of reimbursement they would receive from Medicare. Historically, if they discharged 150 patients annually in DRG 126, they could estimate $586,200 worth of reimbursement. With this kind of information, hospitals can begin to evaluate all aspects of care

TABLE 14-1. Example of Using DRGs to Calculate a Hospital's Reimbursement (FY 2005)

Community Hospital has a rate of $1500			
DRG	Definition	DRG Weight	Hospital's Reimbursement
126	Acute endocarditis	2.6051	$3,908
235	Fracture of femur	.7512	$1,127

Source: DRG Relative Weights Final Version 22. Centers for Medicare and Medicaid Services, 2006.[4]

to ensure all tests and drugs ordered are necessary; thereby increasing efficiency in providing those services. Any nonessential services, or extended length of stay due to inefficiency, will cost the hospital more money.

Resource Based Relative Value Scale (RBRVS)

While hospitals were dealing with DRGs and their impact, physician's finances were not directly affected because they were still reimbursed by payers on a fee-for-service basis. Physicians were responsible for ordering the laboratory tests and diagnostic procedures reimbursed to hospitals under PPS, but their services were reimbursed under a separate payment system. Once the DRG system was in place and operational, CMS turned its attention to physician services.

In 1985, the Consolidated Omnibus Budget Reconciliation Act (COBRA) mandated that Congress explore a new payment system for physician reimbursement and in 1992, CMS began implementation of a physician payment schedule using the **Resource Based Relative Value Scale (RBRVS)**. The program was fully operational by January 1996.

The RBRVS is used to reimburse physicians for their services under Part B of Medicare. Each patient visit receives a code number using the Current Procedural Terminology (CPT-4) or CMS Common Procedure Coding System (CCPCS). The code numbers are usually assigned by either a Health Information Management professional or a staff member trained in coding. Each code has three relative value units (RVUs) associated with it: work, practice expense or overhead, and malpractice expense. In addition, a geographic index is applied to each of these RVUs to account for cost differences based on locality (Tables 14-2 and 14-3).

Each RVU is multiplied by the geographical practice cost index (GPCI) for each RVU to calculate an unconverted number. This unconverted total is then multiplied by a national conversion factor, determined annually by CMS, to establish the amount of reimbursement for the physician. The conversion factor, RVUs and geographical index are published in the *Federal Register* that can be located at *http://www.cms.gov*. The conversion factor for the year 2010 is $36.0846.

TABLE 14-2.   Relative Value Units (RVUs) for Three Selected CPT Codes (2010)

Relative Value Units				
CPT Code	Description	Work RVU	Practice RVU	Malpractice RVU
88104	Cytopathology, fluids	0.56	1.11	0.02
88305	Tissue examination by pathologist	0.75	2.05	0.02
88319	Enzyme histochemistry	0.53	3.20	0.03

TABLE 14-3. **Geographic Index by Relative Value Units (RVUs) for Three Selected Localities**

Geographic Index by RVU			
Locality	Work GI	Practice GI	Malpractice GI
St. Louis	0.993	0.931	1.075
Los Angeles	1.041	1.225	0.804
Manhattan	1.064	1.298	1.010

Note: GI, Geographical Index.

TABLE 14-4. **Calculation of RBRVS Payment for Cytopathology, Fluid in Two Localities**

Locality	CPT Code	RBRVS Calculation	Payment
St. Louis	88104	$[(0.56 \times 0.993) + (1.11 \times 0.931) + (0.02 \times 1.075)] \times \$36.0846$	$58.13
Manhattan	88104	$[(0.56 \times 1.064) + (1.11 \times 1.298) + (0.02 \times 1.010)] \times \$36.0846$	$74.22

The formula for calculating payment for a given CPT code is:

Payment = [(RVU work × GPCI work)
+ (RVU practice expense × GPCI practice expense)
+ (RVU malpractice × GPCI malpractice)] × CF

Table 14-4 illustrates what the different payment rates would be for different localities.

As with the DRG system, physicians could look at historical data and determine what impact the RBRVS would have on their practice.

Ambulatory Payment Categories (APCs)

As hospitals absorbed the impact of DRG-based reimbursement, certain procedures that had been performed on an *inpatient* basis were moved to the *outpatient* setting. Improved technology and changes in practice protocols allowed this to occur without compromising the quality of care. Hospital-based outpatient care (including the emergency room) was still being reimbursed on a fee-for-service basis, and resulted in higher revenue for the facility. This was the next area that CMS was to target to control expenditures. The Omnibus Budget Reconciliation Act (OBRA) of 1986 mandated that Congress investigate an outpatient prospective payment system. However, it was not until the Balanced Budget

Act of 1997 that CMS was mandated to implement an Outpatient Prospective Payment System (OPPS) using **Ambulatory Payment Categories (APCs)**.

APCs are based on a combination of the CCPCS and the ICD-9-CM coding systems. Services performed during an outpatient or emergency room visit are coded using the CCPCS/CPT-4 coding system. In addition, diagnoses are coded using the ICD-9-CM classification system to justify medical necessity for the treatments and laboratory tests ordered. Services that are similar clinically and in terms of resource consumption are then grouped into APCs. Laboratory tests have been grouped into certain levels based on time and supplies needed to run the tests. Unlike the inpatient DRG system, it is possible for one patient encounter to generate more than one APC. As with DRGs, CMS has assigned weights to each APC. This weight is then multiplied by a national conversion factor determined annually by CMS to calculate reimbursement for the hospital. The conversion factor for the calendar year 2010 is $67.406. (See Table 14-5.)

Summary of Medicare Payment Systems

The federal government has adopted three payment methodologies (DRGs, RBRVS, APCs) to help control the rate of growth in healthcare expenditures. *DRGs* are used to pay hospitals for inpatient services. *RBRVS* is used to calculate payments to physicians for inpatient and outpatient visits or services. *APCs* are used to pay hospitals for outpatient services and emergency room care. CMS evaluates and adjusts the programs on a continual basis to ensure that they remain viable mechanisms for healthcare payment. Some private insurers have adapted these or similar payment systems for their beneficiaries.

Moving forward, the CMS plans to update its current coding systems. By the year 2013, Medicare plans to update its diagnosis system from ICD-9-CM to ICD-10-CM, which reflects new diagnoses and advances in medical knowledge.

PRIVATE INSURERS/MANAGED CARE REIMBURSEMENT

Increases in healthcare costs were also affecting the private sector of health insurance. As seen in Figure 14-1, private insurance accounted for one third of the total healthcare dollar. The increase in healthcare costs and consumer demand for

TABLE 14-5. Calculation of APC Payment for Two Procedures

CPT/ CCPCS	Description	APC	Weight	Payment Rate
88305	Tissue examination by pathologist	0343	0.5301	$35.73
88319	Enzyme histochemistry	0342	0.1546	$10.42

APC, Ambulatory Payment Category; CPT, Current Procedural Terminology; CCPCS, CMS Common Procedure Coding System higher technology in treatment forced the private sector to evaluate its reimbursement methodologies. Increased premiums affected employers who were providing health insurance for employees. Employees, therefore, were now expected to pay for an increased portion of the premium, a deductible, and a co-payment for healthcare. Individuals without employer-sponsored insurance found it very difficult and expensive to obtain health insurance. Private insurers began to take a greater interest in the type, amount, and cost of healthcare services being provided to their beneficiaries.

Managed care is a "means of providing health care services within a network of health care providers. The responsibility to manage and provide high quality and cost effective health care is delegated to this defined network of providers."[5] Although there are different types of managed care plans, the common denominator is that the insured individual must see a physician who participates in the managed care plan, or else they must pay a higher co-payment to obtain services outside the network. A health maintenance organization (HMO) is the most common type of managed care organization.

Types of Reimbursement

Managed care plans are reimbursed in several ways. The more common methods are described here. A managed care plan will typically use a combination of these methodologies.

Capitation is a prospective payment agreement between an insurance plan and a provider. Under capitation, a physician is paid x dollars per member per month (PMPM). From this amount, the physician agrees to provide services to all of their patients covered by the plan. For example, assume Dr. Williams has 200 active patients who belong to Community HMO. She has agreed to a reimbursement rate of $20.00 PMPM. That means she will receive $4,000 per month or $48,000 per year to treat those 200 patients. Dr. Williams' contract may state that this amount includes outpatient care and any necessary diagnostic or therapeutic tests. Any office visit, laboratory test, or radiology study ordered for any of the 200 patients during the year will come from the $48,000. If Dr. Williams can see her patients and treat them for less than $48,000, then she makes a profit; but if she orders too many tests, or sees the patients too frequently, she may experience a loss of income by the end of the year.

Capitation can also be established for individual treatment areas. Insurance plans may contract separately with a laboratory to provide outpatient testing for plan members served by the laboratory. The laboratory supervisor may be asked to determine the PMPM payment rate the laboratory is willing to accept. Assume that a laboratory provides only three levels of tests. Based on the data in Table 14-6, the annual cost to the laboratory for these tests would be $105,900 as depicted in Table 14-7.

If there were 2,000 patients in the Community HMO, the laboratory would need to receive from the HMO a fee of at least $4.41 per member per month to cover their costs. If the laboratory performs less than the estimated number of tests, or

TABLE 14-6.   Sample Average Cost and Volume Data for Three Different Levels of Laboratory Testing

Level of Testing	Average Cost	Average Number of Tests Performed
Level I	$11 per test	3,000
Level II	$19 per test	2,100
Level III	$33 per test	1,000

TABLE 14-7.   Example Calculation of Annual Cost and Per Member Per Month Cost

Level of Testing	Average Cost	Average Number of Tests Performed
Level I	$11.00 per test	3,000
Level II	$19.00 per test	2,100
Level III	$33.00 per test	1,000

Annual Cost per Patient: $105,900 ÷ 2,000 = $52.95
Per Member per Month: $52.95 ÷ 12 = $4.41

can lower their unit cost, they can realize a profit on testing. If testing orders exceed estimation, the lab would be responsible for absorbing the additional costs.

Capitation agreements may include provisions for adjustments or minimum payments. For example, a health care provider may have a stratified group of patients varying significantly in age. Since age is largely indicative of health care utilization, the capitation arrangement might include different PMPM payments for the different patient groups. An agreement might also include the possibility of adjusting the PMPM rate if the characteristics of the patient population significantly change.

Per Diem

Inpatient care may be reimbursed on a **per diem**, or "per day" basis. The hospital may negotiate, with the managed care program or other insurers, a set amount of reimbursement per day while the patient is in the hospital. Assume a hospital had 39,652 patient days during the year. The cost for treating these patients, including meals, laboratory tests, and ancillary services, was $5.7 million. The average cost per patient day is $144. The hospital will use the cost per day to negotiate the per diem rate. If the hospital can decrease the services provided without compromising the quality of care, or lower the unit cost of providing the care, it will have an increased profit.

Per Case

Reimbursement on a **per case** basis is similar to the federal prospective payment systems. The cost for certain diagnoses or procedures that have a relatively similar treatment protocol can be determined. The provider and the managed care plan or private insurer can then agree on a per case reimbursement rate for those specific diagnoses or procedures. This method may be used for physician reimbursement as well as hospital reimbursement.

Carve Out ("Carved Out")

There may be some instances where certain types of care will be **"carved out"** of the set reimbursement amount. In the discussion under per diem, the contract may state $1438 per diem *except* special care unit days (ICU, CCU, NICU, etc.). Those "carved out" days may have a separate per diem rate, or they may be reimbursed on a **fee-for-service** basis.

For laboratories, it may be critical to "carve out" certain tests from a prospective payment arrangement. Cytogenetic testing, molecular diagnostic assays, and esoteric testing sent to a reference laboratory all have significantly higher unit costs that cannot be covered by the usual PMPM negotiated rate.

THE FUTURE OF REIMBURSEMENT

As time passes and health care costs continue to rise, significant changes are likely to occur in the landscape of reimbursement. On March 23, 2010, President Barack Obama signed into law the Patient Protection and Affordable Care Act (PPACA), widely considered the largest expansion of health care benefits since the enactment of Medicare in 1965. With an estimated cost of $115 billion, there are likely to be many ramifications on reimbursement in an attempt to curb expenses.[6]

Reductions in Payment

Providers can expect to see financial penalties for excess readmissions for certain conditions, such as heart failure and pneumonia. Whereas hospitals used to be reimbursed for these return visits by Medicare or Medicaid, they will now face increased financial burdens for patients readmitted with these afflictions. Additionally, the PPACA contains a provision for a reduction in federal payments for certain hospital acquired conditions (HACs). When a hospital now falls in the highest quartile for certain HACs, they will experience a one percent reduction in payment from CMS.

Paying for Quality

Perhaps the most important impact for reimbursement moving forward is the shift in philosophy from simply paying a provider per service, to mixing a physician or hospital's compensation for the quality of care provided within the reimbursement. Payers, both public and private, are expected to move toward pay for performance and bundled payment models, potentially reducing the mutual exclusivity of quality and cost.

One example of these new reimbursement strategies is the CMS Acute Care Episode Demonstration Project. The CMS will reimburse a single bundled payment to the hospital (Part A) and physicians (Part B) for select inpatient orthopedic and cardiovascular procedures. If the patient can be treated for less than the bundled payment, the hospital and physicians will both share the cost savings. The theory behind this model is that health care providers will have incentives to treat patients more efficiently.

While efficiency is important, quality care will play a role in how much reimbursement a provider can expect to receive. The PROMETHEUS Payment® model is one of the best examples of pay for performance reimbursement.[7] A single evidence-based case reimbursement rate (ECR) is assigned to a condition, similar to the prospective payment models currently employed by Medicare and Medicaid. A single ECR covers all inpatient and outpatient care the patient receives related to that condition. Once the base rate is determined, an additional amount may be paid based on the results of a quality scorecard, which analyzes outcomes, complications, and patient satisfaction. Once each of these components is calculated, a final bundled payment amount is determined for all providers delivering care to a particular patient.

Implications

Given the recent developments in health care reform and changing attitudes towards reimbursement, health care providers will be expected to "do more for less." In other words, hospitals and physicians will need to find ways to improve the quality of care delivered to patients, while also realizing lower levels of reimbursement. Organizations will be forced to find new and innovative ways to improve financial efficiency, while also improving the quality of patient care.

SUMMARY

The federal government, managed care plans, and private insurers may use all of the reimbursement methods described in this chapter to provide healthcare coverage for their plan members. Hospitals, physicians, laboratories, and other ancillary departments must understand what their services actually cost to perform in order to negotiate appropriately with the insurers. These areas must also know the level of activity at which they are operating. Hospitals must know the number of patients, patient days, diagnoses, and procedures. Physicians must know the number of visits. Laboratories must know how many and what types of tests they perform, as well as how many and why duplicate tests are done. The reimbursement area of healthcare is complex and data driven. If the manager of a department cannot supply the information needed to adequately estimate costs, then that department is at risk of negotiating an arrangement that will not provide adequate reimbursement for their services.

Moving forward, laboratory managers will need to also understand the changing environment of reimbursement. They will need to understand how tests might fit into bundled payments, and as a result may need to determine more efficient methods of delivering the same services.

SUMMARY CHART:
Important Points to Remember

➤ Healthcare costs have steadily increased due to improvements in technology, increases in skilled personnel, an aging population, expanded consumer awareness, and a growing group of uninsured/underinsured individuals.

➤ Individuals pay for their health insurance through premiums, deductibles, and co-payments.

➤ Employers have initiated programs to improve employee wellness and decrease medical costs.

➤ Approximately 48% of total healthcare expenses are paid for by state and federal governments through programs such as Medicaid and Medicare.

➤ Medicare pays for healthcare for persons 65 and over, disabled individuals entitled to Social Security benefits, and patients with end stage renal disease.

➤ Medicaid, also created by the SSA of 1965, is a state-run healthcare plan for the poor that is funded jointly by state and federal dollars.

➤ The Children's Health Insurance Program (CHIP) expanded coverage to 4 million additional children in 2009 under legislation signed into law by President Barack Obama.

➤ The Centers for Medicare and Medicaid Services (CMS) developed a patient classification system to control rapidly increasing healthcare expenditures.

➤ Diagnostic Related Groups (DRGs) were developed as a Prospective Payment System (PPS), where hospitals received a set amount of reimbursement per Medicare inpatient discharge.

➤ CMS pays hospitals varying DRG rates based on factors such as hospital type, setting, and location.

➤ PPS allows hospitals to more easily predict Medicare revenues based on projected patient volumes in defined service lines.

➤ The federal government implemented a Resource Based Relative Value Scale (RBRVS) in 1985 to reimburse for physician services to Medicare patients. Reimbursement rates vary based on geographic location.

➤ Advances in technology created an increase in outpatient treatment.

➤ To curb outpatient expense, CMS implemented an Outpatient Prospective Payment System (OPPS) using Ambulatory Payment Categories (APCs).

➤ APCs differ from DRGs because certain tests and procedures are grouped into categories based on material costs and testing times, as opposed to groupings based on a single diagnosis.

➤ Private insurers have moved away from the fee-for-service model of reimbursement, implementing new reimbursement types to control costs.

SUGGESTED PROBLEM-BASED LEARNING ACTIVITIES

Chapter 14: Healthcare Reimbursement

Instructions: Use Internet resources, books, articles, colleagues, etc., to present solutions to the problems listed below. There is no one correct solution to any problem.

Note to Instructor: Students in class may be divided into groups and given the problem-based learning activity to discuss and solve. Once the group has reached a consensus as to a solution, the group may present it to the other students in the class. This activity will provide all students with information regarding solutions to the problem.

Problem #1

Research the history of laboratory reimbursement from Medicare and Medicaid services. Itemize and discuss relevant issues.

Problem #2

What problems are generated with DRG reimbursement?

Problem #3

Suppose your institution is providing glucose and occult blood point-of-care testing. Explain how you will charge for this service and why.

REFERENCES

1. *National Health Expenditure Projections 2009-2019 (September 2010) Forecast Summary.* Centers for Medicare and Medicaid Services, Baltimore, MD, 2010. Retrieved Sept. 13, 2010, from: http://www.cms.gov/ National HealthExpendData/Downloads/ NHEProjections2009to2019.pdf

2. *National CHIP Policy, 2010.* Centers for Medicare and Medicaid Services, Baltimore, MD, 2010. Retrieved May 14, 2010, from: http://www.cms.gov/NationalCHIPPolicy/

3. Office of Actuary, National Health Statistics Group: *Nation's Health Dollar – Where It Came From, Where It Went.* Centers for Medicare and Medicaid Services, Baltimore, MD, 2008. Retrieved Sept. 2010, from: http://www.cms.gov/National-HealthExpendData/downloads/PieChart-SourcesExpenditures2008.pdf

4. DRG Relative Weights Final Version 22. Centers for Medicare and Medicaid Services, Baltimore, MD, 2006. Retrieved Sept. 10, 2010, from: https://www.cms.gov/AcuteInpatientPPS/FFD/itemdetail.asp?filterType= none&filterByDID=99&sortByDID=2&sor tOrder=ascending&itemID=CMS022597&i ntNumPerPage=10

5. Samuels DI: *New Opportunities in Healthcare Delivery.* McGraw Hill Companies, Boston, MA, 1996: 20-21.

6. CMS Health Reform Center. Centers for Medicare and Medicaid Services, Baltimore, MD, 2010. Retrieved Sept. 8, 2010, from: https://www.cms.gov/Center/healthreform. asp

7. Satin D, Miles J: *Benefits and Burdens of This Pay-for-Performance Strategy.* Special Report, 2009. Retrieved Sept. 10, 2010, from: http:// www.minnesotamedicine.com/CurrentIssue/ SpecialReportOct2009/tabid/3209/Default. aspx

BIBLIOGRAPHY

Behal R: *Quality, Healthcare Reform and Outcomes Research: Start Your Engines!* Presentation delivered to the College of Health Sciences at Rush University Medical Center on May 27, 2010.

Burns L: *The Business of Healthcare Innovation.* Cambridge University Press, New York, NY, 2005.

Casto A, Layman E: *Principles of Healthcare Reimbursement.* AI-DMA, Chicago, IL, 2006.

Cleverly W, Cameron A: *Essentials of Health Care Finance,* ed 6. Jones and Bartlett, Sudbury, MA, 2007: 134-137.

DRG Diagnosis Related Groups-Definitions Manual. 3-M Health Information Systems, 1999: 1.

Elevitch F: Impact of Managed Care on Laboratory Economics. *Lab Medicine* 1998: 29; 747-752.

Fuller R, Clinton S, Goldfield N, Kelly W: Building the Affordable Medical Home. *Journal of Ambulatory Care Management* 2010: 33(1); 71-80.

Gallagher P, ed.: *Medicare RBRVS: The Physician's Guide.* American Medical Association, Chicago, IL, 2000: 4-10.

Gapenski L: *Cases in Healthcare Finance,* ed 3. Health Administration Press, 2005.

Levit KR, et al: National Health Expenditures, 1994. *Health Care Financing Review* 1996: 19; 220.

Nowinski M: *The Financial Management of Hospitals and Healthcare Organizations.* American College of Healthcare Executives, Chicago, IL, 2004.

Rowell J, Green M: *Understanding Health Insurance: A Guide to Professional Billing.* Delmar Learning, Clifton Park, NY, 2004.

Shi L, Singh D: *Delivering Health Care in America: A Systems Approach,* ed 3. Jones and Barlett Publishers, Sudbury, MA, 2003.

Shi L, Singh DA: *Delivering Health Care in America.* Aspen Publication, Gaithersburg, MD, 1998: 178-179, 185-187.

Sultz HA, Young KM: *Health Care USA— Understanding Its Organization and Delivery,* ed 2. Aspen Publication, Gaithersburg, MD, 1999: 209-211.

INTERNET RESOURCES

American Medical Association (AMA)
http://www.ama-assn.org/

ASC Addenda Updates, 2010
http://www.cms.gov/ASCPayment/11_Ad
denda_Updates.asp

ASC Regulations and Notices, 2010
http://www.cms.gov/ASCPayment/ASCRN/
itemdetail.asp?filterType=none&filterBy
DID=-99&sortByDID=3&sortOrder=des
cending&itemID=CMS1230100&intNum
PerPage=10

Data Compendium 2009 Edition. Centers for Medicare and Medicaid Services, Baltimore, MD, 2009
http://www.cms.gov/DataCompendium/
15_2009_Data_Compendium.asp#Top
OfPage

Hospital Outpatient Prospective Payment System, *Changes.* Centers for Medicare and Medicaid Services, Baltimore, MD, 2010
http://www.cms.gov/HospitalOutpatient
PPS/HORD/itemdetail.asp?filterType=non
e&filterByDID=99&sortByDID=3&sortOr
der=descending&itemID=CMS1237082&i
ntNumPerPage=10

Medical Group Management Association (MGMA)
http://www.mgma.com/

Medicare Reimbursement under RBRVUs
http://www.mgma.com/policy/default.
aspx?id=5658

National Health Expenditures 2008 Highlights. Centers for Medicare and Medicaid Services, Baltimore, MD, 2008
http://www.cms.gov/NationalHealthExpend
Data/downloads/highlights.pdf

Organization for Economic Co-Operation and Development (OECD)
http://www.oecd.org/

Overview. *Medicare Physician Fee Schedule (MPFS).* Centers for Medicare and Medicaid Services, Baltimore, MD, 2010. Updated Aug. 2010
http://www.cms.gov/PhysicianFeeSched/
01_Overview.asp

Overview. *Medicare Physician Fee Schedule (MPFS) Search Tool.* Centers for Medicare and Medicaid Services, Baltimore, MD, 2010
http://www.cms.gov/apps/physician-fee-
schedule/overview.aspx

Operations

Today's healthcare environment demands attention to operation details by laboratory managers. The reasons for this are many and include the following:

- There are more compliance and regulatory issues.
- Creative workflow and staffing have resulted from an administrative mindset that laboratories must work more and better with less (the staffing shortage affects these issues even more).
- Information technology is the wave of today as well as of the future.
- Private laboratories must now market themselves to customers, such as hospitals, private physician practices and clinics.

Section IV of this text covers four important aspects of laboratory operations: compliance issues, process designs, laboratory information systems, and marketing. An introduction to the concepts, as well as tips on ways to address the various issues, are included. These chapters are designed to equip learners with the knowledge, tools, and advice necessary to tackle managerial operations and situations.

Section IV Contents:

Compliance Issues—The Regulations

Sharon S. Ehrmeyer, PhD, MT(ASCP)

OBJECTIVES

Following successful completion of this chapter, the learner will be able to:

1. In the framework of CLIA, discuss the concepts of:
   a. Site neutrality
   b. Certification
   c. Test complexity categories
   d. Proficiency testing
   e. Quality systems for nonwaived testing
2. Compare and contrast CLIA, COLA, TJC, and CAP testing requirements for waived and nonwaived testing.

3. Formulate strategies for meeting the regulations that are applicable to his or her healthcare organization.
4. Describe the OSHA requirements in terms of laboratory testing.
5. Discuss the laboratory requirements for meeting the HIPAA legislation.

ABBREVIATIONS

CAP	College of American Pathologists
CDC	Centers for Disease Control and Prevention
CLIA	(or CLIA'88) Clinical Laboratory Improvement Amendments of 1988
CMS	Center for Medicare and Medicaid Services
COLA	Formerly the Commission on Laboratory Accreditation
FDA	Food and Drug Administration
HHS	Health and Human Services
HIPAA	The Health Insurance Portability and Accountability Act of 1996
TJC	The Joint Commission
LAP-CAP	The Laboratory Accreditation Program of the College of American Pathologists
OSHA	Occupational Safety and Health Administration
POCT	Point-of-Care Testing
PT	Proficiency Testing
QC	Quality Control
USDHHS	United States Department of Health and Human Services
WT	Waived Tests

KEY TERMS

Accreditation
Centers for Medicare and Medicaid Services (CMS)
Clinical Laboratory Improvement Amendments of 1988 (CLIA)
Compliance
High Complexity Testing
Moderate Complexity Testing
Nonwaived Testing

OSHA's Standard Precautions
Proficiency Testing (PT)
Provider-Performed Microscopy Procedures (PPMP)
Quality Control (QC)
The Joint Commission (TJC)
Waiver
Waived Testing

Case Study

Compliance Issues—The Regulations

You are a supervisory level, clinical laboratory scientist (10 years of experience) in a 300+ Bed, The Joint Commission (TJC) accredited hospital. The laboratory director informs you that the organization's administrator has asked the laboratory to assess the institution's overall approach to meeting its regulatory responsibilities including point-of-care testing (POCT). In addition to the main laboratory testing, POCT is performed on inpatients, outpatients, at off-site clinics, and through outreach (e.g., visiting nurses). The laboratory director asks you to assume the overall responsibility for this reevaluation.

Issues and Questions to Consider:

1. *What regulations govern point-of-care testing?*

2. *What type of quality control for point-of-care testing must be implemented?*

3. *What kind of complexity testing does point-of-care fall under?*

4. *What kind of tests does point-of-care testing offer?*

5. *What is the benefit of point-of-care testing?*

6. *Who is allowed to perform point-of-care testing? What type of training is required?*

INTRODUCTION

This chapter explores the regulations by which laboratory testing, including point-of-care testing (POCT), is performed. Central to this discussion are the Clinical Laboratory Improvement Amendments of 1988, referred to as CLIA'88 or just CLIA. CLIA is a federal mandate that identifies laboratory testing standards and supersedes the requirements outlined in the Clinical Laboratory Improvement Act of 1967. This chapter describes this CLIA mandate, discusses the CLIA certificates, and provides an overview of the actual regulations to provide the learner with information that is essential for clinical laboratory and POCT compliance. Voluntary accreditation, through professional organizations, is a means by which many laboratories prove that *the entire* CLIA laboratory standards are being met, is also described. Three well-known and respected accrediting organizations are profiled. The regulations related to safety, that is, the Occupational Safety and Health Administration (OSHA) requirements, are also discussed along with the protection of patient medical information by the Health Insurance Portability and Accountability Act (HIPAA).

Due to the nature of this chapter, numerous terms that have abbreviations are used. To assist the learner in familiarizing him or herself with these terms, in addition to serving as an easy reference, an alphabetized listing of these abbreviations and their meanings is located at the beginning of this chapter.

THE CLINICAL LABORATORY IMPROVEMENT AMENDMENTS OF 1988 (CLIA)

Definition

All laboratory testing is regulated by the **Clinical Laboratory Improvement Amendments of 1988 (CLIA)**. (Public Law, 1988) Because of real and perceived problems in test quality, primarily with Pap smear evaluation, Congress passed CLIA to establish quality standards for all laboratory testing to ensure accuracy, reliability, and timeliness of patient test results. CLIA is "test site neutral," meaning that the same regulations apply regardless of the location of testing. Every site examining "materials derived from the human body for the purpose of providing information for the diagnosis, prevention, or treatment of any disease. . ." is subject to CLIA. (USDHHS, 1992)

CLIA was signed into law in 1988 by President Reagan and supersedes all former laboratory regulations. (Public Law, 1988) The initial testing requirements to meet the intent of the law were published on February 28, 1992 in the *Federal Register*. (USDHHS, 1992) [The testing requirements are based on the complexity or difficulty to perform a test method. The three categories of tests methods are: waived; moderate complexity (which includes the subcategory of provider performed microscopy procedures (PPMP) for clinicians and midlevel practitioners only); and high complexity.] The most stringent requirements are for methods in the high complexity category. These 1992 CLIA requirements have been modified and clarified in a series of *Federal Registers*. The most up-to-date (2003) version of the CLIA requirements that include all of the changes, can be downloaded from the **Centers for Medicare and Medicaid Services (CMS)** website (see Internet reference list). CMS with the Centers for Disease Control and Prevention (CDC) were charged originally with developing and promulgating the CLIA regulations. CMS continues to be responsible for the following activities: registering laboratories for CLIA certificates, collecting fees, on-site and self-inspection surveys, surveyor guidelines and training (for enforcement actions when needed), approving proficiency testing providers, accrediting professional organizations, and exempting states. The Food and Drug Administration (FDA) categorizes test methods for complexity.

CLIA Certificates

All laboratory testing must be done under an appropriate CLIA certificate. Each certificate has a fee schedule, which is dependent on the number of test specialties and test volume. As mentioned previously, CLIA regulations divide test methods into three categories: waived, moderate complexity, and high complexity. However, if a site develops its own test procedure, or chooses to modify an existing FDA-approved procedure (which includes not following the manufacturer's directions), the test automatically falls into the high complexity category and is subject to CLIA's most stringent requirements. Depending on the test complexity, laboratories will receive one of the following CLIA certificates: 1) **waiver,** which permits a site to perform only those tests methods identified as waived; 2) **provider-performed microscopy procedures (PPMP),** a certificate issued to a laboratory for physicians, midlevel practitioners, or dentists to perform PPMP procedures, or those tests on specimens collected during a physical examination along with waived tests; or 3) *registration,* a certificate issued to enable laboratories to conduct waived, moderate, and/or high complexity laboratory testing. Once the laboratory is judged to be in compliance with the requirements through inspection, a permanent certificate of **compliance** is issued to those laboratories inspected by an agent of CMS or a certificate of **accreditation** is issued to laboratories seeking accreditation by a CMS-deemed professional organization. As of June 2010, approximately 220,000 CLIA certificates have been issued. Information on applying for a CLIA Certificate (the CMS 116 form), along with associated certificate fees, is available on CMS's website: *http://www.cms.gov/CLIA.*

OVERVIEW OF CLIA REGULATIONS

CLIA and Waived Testing

The CLIA Law (Public Law, 1988) specifies that laboratory requirements are to be based on complexity of the test method performed and established provisions for categorizing a test as waived, which are test methods waived from regulatory oversight, provided they meet certain requirements established by the statute. CLIA defines waived as "tests cleared by the FDA for home use" (patients can purchase the product over the counter) and "tests using such simple and accurate methodologies that the likelihood of erroneous results is negligible." In 1992, when the requirements for meeting CLIA were first published in the *Federal Register,* only simple and foolproof methods for eight analytes were waived: dipstick/tablet reagent urinalysis (visually read), fecal occult blood, visual urine pregnancy and ovulation tests, nonautomated erythrocyte sedimentation rate, blood glucose by monitoring devices cleared by FDA for home use, hemoglobin by copper sulfate (automated), and spun hematocrit. (USDHHS, 1992) Beginning in 1997, Congress instituted revisions to the CLIA waiver provisions (see FDA website) and under the current process, waiver may be granted to 1) any test listed in the regulation, 2) any test system in which the manufacturer provides scientifically valid data to meet the waiver criteria, and 3) test systems cleared by the FDA for home use. Currently, the number of analytes on the waived list has expanded to over 100, and includes hundreds of methodologies to test these analytes. The categories for all test methods are available on CMS's web site: *http://www.cms.gov/CLIA/downloads/waivetbl.pdf.* Reagent and instrument manufacturers also have current information on the classification of their products. For sites using test methods classified as waived, CLIA has no specific personnel, **quality control** or quality assurance requirements other than to follow the manufacturer's directions. CMS inspectors responsible for determining adherence to CLIA regulations will not inspect waived testing facilities unless a specific complaint has been lodged, or fraudulent activities are suspected.

CLIA and Moderate and High Complexity Testing

Each specific laboratory test system or methodology is graded for level of complexity by assigning scores of 1, 2, or 3 to each of seven criteria: 1) knowledge; 2) training and experience; 3) reagents and materials preparation; 4) characteristics of operational steps; 5) calibration, quality control, and proficiency testing materials; 6) test system troubleshooting and equipment; and 7) interpretation and judgment. These criteria are considered key elements to perform a test correctly (see FDA website). A score of 1 indicates the lowest level of complexity (**waived testing**), and a score of 3 is the highest level (**high complexity testing**) when applying scores to the seven criteria. For the seven criteria, test systems receiving a total score of 12 or less are categorized as **moderate complexity testing**. Methods receiving scores above 12 are categorized as high complexity. Of the test systems currently being marketed, more than one-half are classified as moderate complexity and the remaining, excluding those in the waived category, are high complexity. CLIA requirements, as well as those of accrediting agencies, vary with test complexity.

Personnel

For sites performing moderate complexity testing, individuals with the proper qualifications must be identified for the positions of director, technical consultant, clinical consultant, and testing personnel. The director, as listed on the CLIA certificate, can range from a physician to an individual with a bachelor's degree in medical technology/clinical laboratory science or a degree in chemical, physical or biological science and having two years of laboratory training/experience and two years of laboratory supervisory experience. The director is responsible for all aspects of laboratory operation and administration. Although the director may delegate the duties to qualified individuals, the director is ultimately responsible for ensuring that all duties are properly performed. When the director is a physician, she or he typically also serves as the clinical consultant or as the liaison between the patient and clinician. The laboratory must employ one or more individuals who are qualified by education and training (or experience) to provide technical consultation for each of the specialties and subspecialities of service in which the laboratory performs moderate complexity test procedures. The technical consultant establishes the quality standards of the laboratory through selecting and monitoring the laboratory's methods/instrumentation, and evaluating and documenting the competency of the personnel. Qualifications for the technical consultant range from a clinician to an individual possessing a bachelor's degree in chemical, physical, biological, or medical technology/clinical laboratory science and one year of laboratory training (or experience) in the designated specialty of responsibility. The clinical consultant must be a clinician or have a doctorate in chemical, physical, biological, or medical technology/clinical laboratory science and serve as the liaison between the laboratory and its customers. This individual must be qualified to consult with clinicians and patients, and give opinions concerning the diagnosis, treatment, and management of patient care. Testing personnel are responsible for specimen processing, test performance, and reporting test results. Minimum requirements for testing personnel include a high school education (or equivalent), plus appropriate director-approved training, and continued (at least yearly) competency assessment.

For sites performing high complexity testing, individuals with the proper qualifications must be identified for five positions: director, technical supervisor, clinical consultant, general supervisor, and testing personnel. As with moderate complexity testing, the director is responsible for the overall operation and administration of the laboratory. In addition to laboratory training or experience, to qualify as a director, an individual must be a licensed doctor of medicine, osteopathy, or podiatry; have a doctorate in chemical, physical, biological, or medical technology/clinical laboratory science. For those hired after February 24, 2003, the individual must also be certified by a board approved by the Health and Human Services (HHS); or have qualified as a director on or before February 28, 1992. The technical supervisor establishes the quality standards of the laboratory by selecting and monitoring methods and instrumentation, and evaluating and documenting the competency of its personnel at least once per year after the first year of employment. The qualifications for this position range from a clinician to an individual possessing a bachelor's degree in medical technology/clinical laboratory science or chemical, physical, or biological science plus specified training (and/or experience). The role and qualifications of the clinical consultant are the same as those for moderate complexity testing. The general supervisor provides day-to-day supervision of testing personnel and reporting of results. Requirements range from individuals who qualify as a clinician, to persons possessing an associate degree in a laboratory science or medical laboratory technology, and two years of laboratory training and experience. Furthermore, personnel who have served, or would be qualified to serve as a general supervisor on or before February 28, 1992, can fill this position. Testing personnel performing high complexity testing must possess: an associate degree in laboratory science or medical laboratory technology, or education and training equivalent to an associate degree. (USDHHS, 2003)

Proficiency Testing

Under CLIA, regulatory **proficiency testing (PT)** plays a key role in assessing the internal quality for CLIA-regulated analytes in test sites performing moderate and/or high complexity testing. Successful participation in PT is a requirement for maintaining the CLIA certificate of compliance. All laboratories must be enrolled in a CMS-approved PT program for at least the CLIA-specified regulated analytes tested (see CMS website). CLIA requirements identify the minimum performance limits for passing each analyte in the three PT events that occur yearly and mandates that PT samples be treated, as much as possible, like patient specimens. Testing sites failing the same analyte in two of three consecutive PT events can be subject to sanctions ranging from being required to submit a plan of correction to mandatory suspension of testing for the failed analyte. However, CMS views PT as more educational and has indicated that its intent is to help laboratories improve performance rather than to revoke CLIA certificates, except in cases of clear danger to patients.

Quality Systems for Nonwaived Testing

On January 24, 2003, CMS published the latest "final" rule to CLIA (USDHHS, 2003), which includes a revised Subpart K, Quality Systems for Nonwaived testing. The specified requirements are for all **nonwaived testing**, applicable to both the moderate and high complexity test categories. *(http://www.cdc.gov/clia/regs/toc.aspx)* This revised section, which consolidates quality requirements found in multiple sections and revisions of the February 28, 1992 version of the CLIA regulations, is organized to follow the path of patient specimens through the testing process—preanalytical, analytical, and postanalytical. The preanalytical requirements specify the information needed on each test request and the policies and procedures that must be in place for specimen submission, handling and referral. CLIA is concerned with maintaining sample integrity and positive patient identification throughout the testing process. The analytical requirements address the procedure manual, all components associated with a particular test system/instrument, verification of methods' performance specifications before routine implementation, maintenance and function checks, calibration and calibration verification, and quality control procedures. This section also includes additional requirements for specialty testing such as bacteriology and immunohematology. Postanalytical requirements include the systems that need to be in place to ensure accurate, reliable and timely-reported patient data along with the needed information on the test report.

The requirements for each of the three phases of testing have identical quality assessments and continuous quality improvement mandates. Section '493.1200 states: *establish and maintain written policies and procedures that implement and monitor quality systems for all phases of the total testing process meaning the preanalytical, analytical, and postanalytical phases of the testing process* [and, as part of this ('493.1200(b)] *each of the laboratory's quality systems must include an assessment component that ensures continuous improvement of the laboratory's performance and services through ongoing monitoring that identifies, evaluates and resolves problems.* (USDHHS, 2003)

Procedure Manual

Failure to follow manufacturers' directions (procedures) is one of the top deficiencies identified by inspectors for CLIA compliance. As a consequence, high quality "standard operating procedures" or SOPs are essential. Procedures, in written or in electronic form, must be available to all testing personnel for all tests performed. The necessary elements of the manual that need to be included are detailed in section §493.1251 of the January 24, 2003 *Federal Register.* (USDHHS, 2003) All procedures for nonwaived testing must at least include written policies and procedures for patient preparation, specimen collection, labeling, preservation, transportation, referral, specimen acceptability and rejection; step-by-step performance of the procedure; instrument calibration and calibration verification; reportable range; quality control and corrective actions; limitations to the methodology; reference intervals; panic values; literature references; reporting of patient results; and course of action when a test system becomes inoperable. Manufacturers' product inserts or operator manuals may be used to partially meet this requirement, however, additional information specific to the laboratory must be included. Initially, the procedures must be approved, signed, and dated by the laboratory director. Any changes to the procedures or changes in directorship require re-approval by the current director.

Method Verification of Performance Specifications

Method verification for unmodified, FDA-approved, nonwaived test methods means collecting data that document the method's performance in the test site by the site's analysts. This enables the site to make decisions on how to manage the method. The performance characteristics that need to be evaluated include accuracy, precision, reportable range, and identification of appropriate reference intervals. Sites can use the manufacturer's reference ranges or those from other literature sources, as long as the director determines that they are suitable for the testing site's clientele. Test sites developing their own methods or modifying FDA-approved test systems must also determine, in addition to the above, analytical sensitivity and specificity, appropriate reference ranges, and any other performance characteristics required for test performance.

Quality Control

Section §493.1256 specifically describes a series of quality control procedures for nonwaived testing. (USDHHS, 2003) The section begins with the following statement: "*For each test system, the laboratory is responsible for having control procedures that monitor the accuracy and precision of the complete analytical process.*" This section describes what the control procedures must do: 1) detect immediate errors that occur due to test system failure, adverse environmental conditions, and operator performance; and 2) monitor over time the accuracy and precision of test performance that may be influenced by changes in test system performance and environmental conditions, and variance in operator performance. Section §493.1256(d) goes on to break new ground by allowing test sites to use routinely manufacturers' approaches to quality control—process, electronic, on-board liquid, etc. Test sites must first qualify these and have data to prove that the manufacturer's approach provides information on method performance equivalent to that provided by traditional, liquid, external quality control.

Inspection

CLIA requires those sites performing nonwaived testing (moderate and high complexity tests) to be inspected every two years for compliance to the regulations. CMS assesses a fee for this process. (USDHHS, 2003) These inspections are unannounced, but must be conducted while the laboratory's CLIA certificate is still valid.

VOLUNTARY ACCREDITATION

Many testing sites decide to meet the CLIA requirements through professional accreditation. This is possible because CLIA regulations allow CMS to approve or deem nonprofit, professional organizations having laboratory testing and inspection standards that are essentially equivalent to, or more stringent than, those of CLIA (USDHHS, 1992). Testing sites voluntarily choose to be accredited by a CLIA-deemed organization and pay the required fees, which are in addition to the ongoing CLIA fees. In 2010, approximately 220,000 testing sites received CLIA certificates (CMS website); 8% of these are accredited and inspected by deemed organizations. The three principal organizations are the TJC, the Laboratory Accreditation Program of the College of American Pathologists (LAP-CAP), and COLA (formerly the Commission on Office Laboratory Accreditation). When these sites meet the accrediting agency's requirements, as assessed through inspection every two years, the test site is, in essence, meeting CLIA requirements. CMS, however, has the right as a quality check to re-inspect up to 5% of testing sites accredited by deemed organizations. The choice of accrediting organization is the decision of the laboratory.

The Joint Commission

The Joint Commission (TJC) is a voluntary organization that accredits more than 80% of U.S. healthcare organizations (see TJC website). Test sites in a TJC accredited institution need to adhere, at minimum, to the standards identified in the latest TJC *2010 Comprehensive Accreditation Manual for Laboratories and Point-of-Care Testing* (CAMLAB). These testing standards focus on quality improvement and are designed to promote quality outcomes. Inspection for *compliance* is conducted every two years by inspectors hired and trained by TJC. TJC recognizes the test categories including waived test (WT) methods as defined by CLIA, but unlike CLIA, TJC has specific requirements, including personnel training and quality control criteria, and inspects waived testing. These (2010) include the following:

Standard WT.01.01.01: Policies and procedures for waived tests are established, current, approved, and readily available.

Standard WT.02.01.01: The person named on the CLIA certificate identifies the staff responsible for performing and supervising waived testing.

Standard WT.03.01.01: Staff and licensed independent practitioners performing waived tests are competent.

Standard WT.04.01.01: The [organization] performs quality control checks for waived testing on each procedure. Note: Internal QC may include electronic, liquid, or control zone. External QC may include electronic or liquid.

Standard WT.05.01.01: The [organization] maintains records for waived testing. TJC quality testing requirements for nonwaived testing are identified in Table 15-1.

The Laboratory Accreditation Program of the College of American Pathologists (LAP-CAP)

The Laboratory Accreditation Program of the College of American Pathologists (LAP-CAP) accredits only laboratory testing sites and not the entire healthcare organization (see CAP website). LAP-CAP spells out its requirements in a series of specialty related checklists. All test sites must follow the Laboratory General Checklist (GEN) and then the specific checklists appropriate to the specialty of testing. (Checklists, 2010) For high complexity testing, CAP accredited test sites must identify a director, clinical consultant, technical supervisor, general supervisor, and testing personnel. The qualifications are identified in CLIA, Section §493.1441–1495, for high complexity testing. The director, as listed on the CLIA certificate, needs to be a physician (preferably a pathologist) or a doctoral scientist with appropriate experience. When test sites cannot find qualified testing personnel, LAP-CAP will allow less qualified personnel to perform tests as long as they meet the CLIA personnel requirements identified for the specific complexity classification of testing and have appropriate "general" supervision. (Checklists, 2010) For example, there are no specific educational requirements for personnel performing waived tests under CLIA. Proficiency testing has long been an important component of LAP-CAP inspection philosophy. CAP-accredited sites, including POCT sites and those performing only waived testing, must participate in PT (when available) through CAP surveys or other CAP-approved PT surveys for each analyte tested. LAP-CAP, like TJC, emphasizes an overall total quality management approach and continuous quality improvement for the entire analytical process, including management of pre-analytical, analytical and postanalytical errors. CAP inspections are intended to be educational and are unique in that they are conducted primarily by a team of "peer" laboratory professionals. More quality testing requirements are identified in Table 15-1.

COLA

COLA, formerly the Commission of Office Laboratory Accreditation, initially focused on accrediting physician office laboratories (COLA website; Laboratory Accreditation Manual, 2007). Today COLA accredits many other types of test sites including those in small hospitals. COLA's philosophy is one of education and problem solving. Inspectors usually are medical technologists/clinical laboratory scientists who are prepared to assist test sites in meeting the regulations and generating quality test results. To prepare for the accreditation process COLA provides sites with an initial, preinspection (self-inspection) checklist. The COLA inspector then uses this same checklist during the on-site inspection. COLA's requirements essentially follow the CLIA regulations. COLA does not inspect sites performing only waived testing. More quality testing requirements are identified in Table 15-1.

TABLE 15-1.   Comparison of Testing Requirements (CLIA, COLA, TJC, LAP-CAP)

Requirement	CLIA	COLA Accreditation (2007)	TJC Accreditation (2010)	LAP-CAP Accreditation (2010)
General requirements for (WAIVED test methods)	Follow manufacturer's directions	Same as for CLIA	Follow WT standards in current Laboratory Accreditation Standards	Follow applicable standards in current GEN and POC Checklists
General requirements for (NONWAIVED test methods)	Follow manufacturer's directions; have policies and procedures in place for the pre-analytical, analytical and post-analytical phases of testing	Same as for CLIA	Same as for CLIA	Same as for CLIA
Procedure manual (standard operating procedures [SOP]) (NONWAIVED test methods)	Written policies and procedures, as appropriate from patient preparation to reporting (§493.1251) Approved by director initially and with any changes	Same as for CLIA	Same as for CLIA; approved by director initially and with any changes; reapproved annually	Same as for CLIA; approved by director initially and with any changes; reapproved annually
Quality Control (NONWAIVED test methods)	Follow section §493.1256 for general requirements and §493.1261, .1267, .1269 and .1254 for analyte specific requirements. General requirement— 2 QC levels/test/day	Follow, as applicable, general QC section and test specialty requirements in current COLA Laboratory Accreditation Criteria manual	Follow, as applicable, general QC and test specialty standards in current Laboratory Accreditation Standards	Follow, as applicable, QC and test specialty standards in current POC Checklist

Accepts manufacturer's internal/procedural/on-board alternative QC approach to fulfill daily QC requirements (NONWAIVED test methods)	Yes, once qualified by one of 3 Evaluation Options (identified in the CMS 2004 SOM)	Yes, qualify approach by either a 10- or 30-day evaluation	Yes, qualify approach for routine chemistry or hematology with a 10- or 30-day evaluation	Yes, qualify approach with a 25-day evaluation study
Proficiency testing in a CMS-approved PT program/accuracy assessment (NONWAIVED test methods)	Yes, follow, as appropriate §493.801–865 for regulated analytes; when PT is not performed, than an accuracy assessment (§493.1236(c)) must be made at least every 6 months	Essentially the same as for CLIA, but follow COLA standards	Essentially the same as for CLIA, but follow TJC standards	For all analytes tested, when PT is available; when not available, assess accuracy at least every 6 months
Personnel qualifications (NONWAIVED test methods)	Follow §493.1403–.1425	Same as for CLIA	Same as for CLIA	Same as for CLIA; pathologist preferred for high complexity testing
Testing personnel training and on-going competency assessment (NONWAIVED test methods)	Yes, technical consultant (or director) is responsible for identifying (initial) training needs and ongoing competency assessments (§493.1403(7)(8))	Same as for CLIA	Same as for CLIA	Same as for CLIA

(Continued)

TABLE 15-1. Comparison of Testing Requirements (CLIA, COLA, TJC, LAP-CAP) (*Continued*)

Requirement	CLIA	COLA Accreditation (2007)	TJC Accreditation (2010)	LAP-CAP Accreditation (2010)
Initial method verification at start-up (unmodified FDA-approved NONWAIVED test methods)	Follow §493.1253 (accuracy, precision, reportable range, and approve acceptability of reference range)	Same as for CLIA	Same as for CLIA	Same as for CLIA
Ongoing assessment of reportable range (every 6 months) (NONWAIVED test methods)	Yes, §493.1255(b)(3) (accomplished through calibration verification)	Same as for CLIA	Same as for CLIA	Same as for CLIA (termed analytical measurement range—AMR)
Method correlations (at least every 6 months) (NONWAIVED test methods)	Between all methods under same CLIA certificate (§493.1281)	Same as for CLIA	Comparison across all test sites and CLIA certificates in entire organization	Same as for CLIA

OCCUPATIONAL SAFETY AND HEALTH ADMINISTRATION (OSHA) REQUIREMENTS

In addition to the CLIA regulations and requirements from the various professional organizations (TJC, LAP-CAP, and COLA), the U.S. Department of Labor, under the **Occupational Safety and Health Administration (OSHA)**, is responsible for regulations relating to general workplace safety and protecting the health of U.S. workers. These regulations are most commonly known as the "OSHA Bloodborne Pathogens Standard 1910.1030." In general the handling of biological specimens, fall under the part of the OSHA regulations addressing "Universal Precautions." They require that all blood, body fluids, tissue and other potentially infectious materials be treated as equally hazardous. OSHA regulations require facilities to devise an exposure control plan for blood-borne pathogens that is updated annually. Facilities must have a classification system in place for each job based on the level of exposure to blood-borne pathogens. In addition, the facility must develop and implement procedures that are in compliance with OSHA regulations, to protect workers and minimize the risk of exposure. Employees must be informed of the occupational hazards, provided with personal protective equipment (such as goggles, masks, gloves, gowns, and laboratory coats), and monitored to ensure compliance with safety procedures. Employees at risk for exposure must receive employer-financed hepatitis B vaccinations, unless they sign an affidavit stating that they refused the vaccine. Upon employment, employees must participate in an on-the-job training program that minimally covers the facility's exposure control plan, use of personal protective equipment, procedures to be followed in the event of exposure to a blood-borne pathogen, and the labeling system for biohazardous materials. The training program is repeated on an annual basis for all employees or more frequently whenever changes occur. OSHA inspectors may choose to make an unannounced inspection; they cannot (legally) be refused admittance to the workplace. An extended discussion of workplace safety requirements is beyond the scope of this chapter. The reader, unfamiliar with OSHA requirements, is referred to the agency's website: *http://www.osha.gov/*.

HEALTH INSURANCE PORTABILITY AND ACCOUNTABILITY ACT (HIPAA)

The Health Insurance Portability and Accountability Act of 1996 (HIPAA), was the result of efforts by President Clinton's Administration and healthcare reform proponents. The primary goal of this "health insurance focused" legislation was to make it easier to detect and prosecute fraud and abuse and enable workers of all professions, even those with pre-existing medical conditions, to change jobs without loss or interruption of health insurance protection. Safeguarding patient privacy, with respect to health related information was a paramount concern. As part of this legislation, HIPAA established new privacy rules for "covered entities" including laboratories, which took effect April 14, 2003. While not all information needs to be protected under HIPAA, most patient information is considered protected and is subject to HIPAA requirements. For example, laboratories must ensure confidentiality when transmitting health information electronically. This rule requires healthcare organizations (laboratory test sites are part of this), insurers and payers using any electronic means of storing patient data and performing claims submission to comply with the Final Rule for National Standards for Electronic Transactions.

The full scope of HIPAA related requirements is beyond this text. However, larger institutions are required to have a "HIPAA Privacy Officer" to provide information. The following are some general principles. Access to patient information must be limited to a "need to know basis" making records that are accessible through open folders, laboratory notes, unsecured computer terminals, etc., not acceptable. Written patient data needs to be shredded before disposal. The extensive *Standards for Privacy of Individually Identifiable Health Information* are designed to help guarantee privacy and confidentiality of patient medical records. Healthcare providers must be in HIPAA compliance, which means that staff needs to be educated and trained and documentation for these activities available to demonstrate compliance with the HIPAA requirements. Staff also is subject to ongoing compliance monitoring and application of appropriate sanctions when necessary.

For more details on HIPAA, the government has prepared a website: *http://www.hhs.gov/ocr/privacy/hipaa/understanding/index.html*

SUMMARY

Today's laboratories must meet multiple regulations—CLIA, HIPAA, OSHA and others. With CLIA, all laboratories are required to implement minimum standards to ensure quality laboratory test results that are available in a reasonable time frame. Meeting these standards, which may be achieved through CLIA-deemed professional organizations, is critical in providing high quality laboratory services to the healthcare community. Laboratory managers must be familiar with *all* applicable regulations and constantly work toward ensuring that they are met at minimum and preferably at an exceeded level.

SUMMARY CHART:
Important Points to Remember

➤ All clinical laboratory testing regardless of where it is performed is regulated by the Clinical Laboratory Improvement Amendments of 1988 (CLIA), and must be performed under an appropriate CLIA certificate.

➤ The testing requirements delineated in CLIA are based on test complexity or difficulty to perform the test. The test complexity categories are waived, moderate and high. In the 2003 revision of CLIA, the moderate and high complexity categories are grouped together and called nonwaived; personnel requirements for each remain separate with high complexity having the more stringent requirements.

➤ CLIA defines waived testing as tests cleared by the FDA for home use, or tests using such simple and accurate methodologies that the likelihood of erroneous results is negligible; and CLIA has no specific personnel, quality control or quality assurance requirements for waived testing other than to follow manufacturer's requirements.

➤ Any method that is modified by the user, automatically is considered to be highly complex and must meet the more stringent personnel and method validation requirements.

➤ Under CLIA, proficiency testing plays a key role in assessing the internal quality of CLIA-regulated analytes for test sites performing moderate and high complexity testing. CLIA quality systems approach to testing focuses on maintaining sample integrity and positive patient identification throughout the testing process.

➤ Policies and procedures must be in place for the three phases of testing—pre-analytical, analytical, and post-analytical—and each phase of testing must be subjected to quality assessment for continuous quality improvement.

➤ The competence of staff in performing their assigned job tasks needs to be assessed twice; the first year of testing and at least once annually thereafter.

➤ CLIA requires those sites performing nonwaived testing to be inspected every two years for compliance to the regulations.

➤ The Occupational Safety and Health Administration (OSHA) is responsible for regulations relating to general workplace safety and protecting the health of U.S. workers. The handling of biological specimens under OSHA's "Universal Precautions," require that all blood, body fluids, tissue and other potentially infectious materials be treated as equally hazardous.

➤ Under the Health Insurance Portability and Accountability Act (HIPAA) of 1996, most patient information is considered protected and laboratories must ensure confidentiality.

Suggested Problem-Based Learning Activities

Chapter 15: Compliance Issues—The Regulations

Instructions: Use Internet resources, books, articles, colleagues, etc., to present solutions to the problems listed below. There is no one correct solution to any problem.

Note to Instructor: Students in class may be divided into groups and given the problem-based learning activity to discuss and solve. Once the group has reached consensus as to a solution, the group may present it to the other students in the class. This activity will provide all students with information regarding solutions to the problem.

Problem #1

Suppose you are told that your central laboratory will soon have a CAP/ AABB inspection and a TJC inspection for POCT. As the laboratory supervisor, you must develop a plan to prepare for and initiate this process.
Note: AABB stands for the American Association of Blood Banks, an organization that issues standards for blood bank practices, conducts inspections, and accredits blood bank laboratories.

Problem #2

Correlate your laboratory practices to the CLIA regulations for your type of operations.

Problem #3

Identify and explain the OSHA regulations that apply to your laboratory operations.

BIBLIOGRAPHY

Checklists: Laboratory Accreditation Program— College of American Pathologists (LAP-CAP), Northfield, IL, 2010.

The Joint Commission (TJC): *Comprehensive Accreditation Manual for Laboratory and Point-of-Care Testing.* The Joint Commission (TJC), Oakbrook Terrace, IL, 2010.

Laboratory Accreditation Manual. COLA, Columbia, MD, 2007.

Public Law 100-578, Section 353 Public Health Service Act (42 U.S.C. 263a). October 31, 1988.

U.S. Department of Health & Human Services: Centers for Medicare & Medicaid Services. *Appendix C, Survey Procedures and Interpretive Guidelines for Laboratories and Laboratory Services.* Available at: http://www.cms.hhs.gov/CLIA/03_Interpretive_Guidelines_for_Laboratories.asp#TopOfPage

U.S. Department of Health and Human Services: Centers for Disease Control and Prevention. *Current CLIA Regulations (including all changes through 01/24/2004).* Accessed Sept 2010 at: http://wwwn.cdc.gov/clia/regs/toc.aspx

U.S. Department of Health and Human Services: Medicare, Medicaid and CLIA Programs: Regulations implementing the Clinical Laboratory Improvement Amendments of 1988 (CLIA); Final rule. *Fed Reg* 1992: 57; 7002-7186.

U.S. Department of Health and Human Services: Medicare, Medicaid and CLIA Programs: Laboratory Requirements Relating to Quality Systems and Certain Personnel Qualifications; Final rule. *Fed Reg* 2003: 68; 3640–3714. Accessed Mar 2011 at: http://www.cdc.gov/clia/docs/CMS-2226-F.htm

U.S. Department of Health and Human Services: Medicare, Medicaid and CLIA Programs: Regulations implementing the Clinical Laboratory Improvement Amendments of 1988 (CLIA); Final rule. (Codified 10-1-03 edition including all changes from 1992). Accessed Mar 2011 at: http://www.cdc.gov/clia/pdf/42cfr493_2003.pdf

INTERNET RESOURCES

Centers for Medicare & Medicaid Services (CMS)
http://www.cms.gov

Centers for Medicare & Medicaid Services. *Clinical Laboratory Improvement Amendments (CLIA)*
http://www.cms.gov/CLIA/

COLA
http://www.cola.org/

College of American Pathologists (CAP)
http://www.cap.org

The Joint Commission (TJC)
http://www.jointcommission.org/

The Joint Commission Resources
http://www.jcrinc.com/

United States Department of Health and Human Services (USDHHS). *Understanding Health Information Privacy,* HIPAA, Office for Civil Rights.
http://www.hhs.gov/ocr/privacy/hipaa/understanding/index.html

United States Department of Labor. Occupational Safety and Health Administration (OSHA)
http://www.osha.gov/

United States Food and Drug Administration (FDA)
http://www.fda.gov/

chapter 16

Process Designs— Workflow and Staffing

Sandra S. Brown, MBA, MT(ASCP)
Kelly L. McLeay, RN, MSN
Dale C. Scutro, BS, MT(AMT)

CHAPTER OUTLINE

OBJECTIVES

Following successful completion of this chapter, the learner will be able to:

1. Explain the relationship between process design, workflow, and staffing.
2. Identify the factors that must be considered when developing a process design.
3. Construct a table that contains the three phases of workflow and discuss the components of each.
4. Define Process Management and identify various process improvement methodologies.
5. Compare and contrast the written application with the oral interview.

6. Develop a generic schedule using:
   a. 8/80 work rule
   b. 40-hour workweek rule
   c. Self-scheduling guidelines
7. Discuss the importance of retention in the workplace.

KEY TERMS

40-Hour Workweek Rule
8/80 Work Rule
Analytical Phase
Flowchart
FOCUS-PDSA
Postanalytical Phase
Preanalytical Phase

Process Designs
Process Management
Process Management Tools
Self-Scheduling
Six Sigma
Staffing
Workflow

Case Study — Process Designs—Workflow and Staffing

You are the manager of a small to medium-sized city hospital laboratory. A small rural hospital within an hour's drive has decided to close its microbiology department and has asked if your facility can do the work for them. This would mean a 50% increase in the workload of your department. To determine if this is feasible a process design must be developed, and the workflow analyzed. Staffing must be reviewed and if needed additional employees hired, trained, and scheduled to work.

Issues and Questions to Consider:

1. What factors should be considered when developing a process design?

2. How does process design differ from and relate to workflow?

3. What are the three phases of workflow?

4. What is the purpose of the application and the interview in the hiring process?

5. What is the 8/80 work rule? The 40-hour workweek rule?

6. How do the two work rules differ?

7. How is a generic schedule developed and what purpose does it serve?

INTRODUCTION

Process Designs are broad overall plans used to develop and design a process or way of completing work or doing a task. Once the process design is developed, workflow can be analyzed. **Workflow** is the pathway the work follows from the beginning to the end of the task. **Staffing** is the hiring, training, scheduling, and retaining of the employee who will be doing the work or task.

Each of these is interrelated and must be developed and studied if the work or task is to be successfully completed. Process designs can be complex or simple depending on the size of the task, or the amount of work that needs to be done. In this case study, the addition of a 50% workload is large so it will be fairly elaborate; but it will cover all the thoughts, designs, and processes necessary for this to be a successful endeavor.

Process Management is a systematic data based approach to improving the performance of business. It is a method of continuously seeking improvement opportunities without sacrificing quality and it is necessary to be successful in the dynamic environment of health care.

This chapter explores in detail how to develop a process design. Then using the process design it explores in-depth workflow, staffing, and the interrelationships of each. Process management is introduced along with a variety of tools that can be used to improve processes.

To best illustrate the concepts in this chapter, the chapter case study is referred to and discussed throughout. Learners are thus encouraged to revisit the case along with the issues and questions to consider during the study of this chapter.

PROCESS DESIGNS

Process designs are the broad plans or overall designs that are developed to provide a blueprint for completing work or a task. They are not unlike an outline in a textbook. To design a process you must know what work or task needs to be completed.

Many factors, which are discussed in the following paragraphs, influence every process design. Each must be identified, understood, and applied if the process design is to be successful. Moreover, each factor is related to the other in such a manner that one by itself is not complete. In the laboratory the reliability (i.e., the accuracy and timeliness of test results), is only as good as the process design that produces that result. A process design may be large or small depending on the task, but all must: 1) be cost effective; 2) be within organizational needs and budgets; 3) be customer friendly; and 4) produce quality results.

Sometimes to make the process easier to understand, it is helpful to draw a **flowchart** (Figure 16-1), which is a picture or diagram of a process. Flowcharts can be simple or complicated and of various designs, depending on the work or task that needs to be completed. In this case a fishbone flowchart is used for illustration. This flowchart has been developed to present all possible factors that can influence a process design in the laboratory and is therefore somewhat complicated. It is global in nature, and not all factors on the chart are relevant to our case study, but they may be applicable in other situations. Managers should choose those that work best in their setting.

Referring to Figure 16-1, Flowchart of Process Design, you will note that there are eight "global" factors numbered 1 through 8, which can influence the workflow process design. There are also arrowed lines that represent the interrelationships between each of the global factors. From the global factor lines are additional lines. These are subdivisions, which further define or influence the global factors.

Process designs are influenced by the following eight global factors:

1. *Size and setting of the laboratory or department:* Is it large or small? Is it in a hospital or is it off site? Is it a commercial or specialty laboratory? In our case study, it is a small to medium-sized hospital department.

2. *Design of the laboratory:* Is it centralized (all of it is located in one area of a building) or decentralized (parts are located throughout the building or even in different buildings)? Is it a core laboratory design (the routine or most commonly performed tests in the areas of hematology, chemistry, coagulation and urinalysis are grouped together in one area of the laboratory), or is it departmentalized (all tests in one discipline such as hematology are grouped into one area or department)? If it is a core laboratory design, nonsimilar tests, tasks, or instruments are grouped in such a way that one person can do many things. If it is departmentalized, people will need to be assigned to each department. In the case study, microbiology is the department that will be affected. Microbiology is a specialized area of a laboratory and is usually separate because regulatory issues require that some of the work processes must be isolated from other work areas.

3. *Equipment:* What type of equipment is used? Is it fully automated (it does most of the work with very little interaction from the employee), or is it semiautomated (it does some of the work and the employee does the rest manually)? Is it a batch analyzer (it does only one type of test at a time), or is it a discrete analyzer (it can process many different tests at the same time or in any order)? In this case study, the microbiology department has a semiautomated piece of equipment that assists with culture processing.

4. *Test methodology:* Is the test performed manually or is it automated? Is it Clinical Laboratory Improvement Act (CLIA) waived or moderate/highly complex testing? (see Chapter 15) Most of the work in microbiology is considered highly complex under CLIA.

5. *Regulations:* Regulatory issues are complex and a laboratory must answer to many: CLIA, the Joint Commission (TJC), College of American Pathologists (CAP), Food and Drug Administration (FDA), state and local authorities

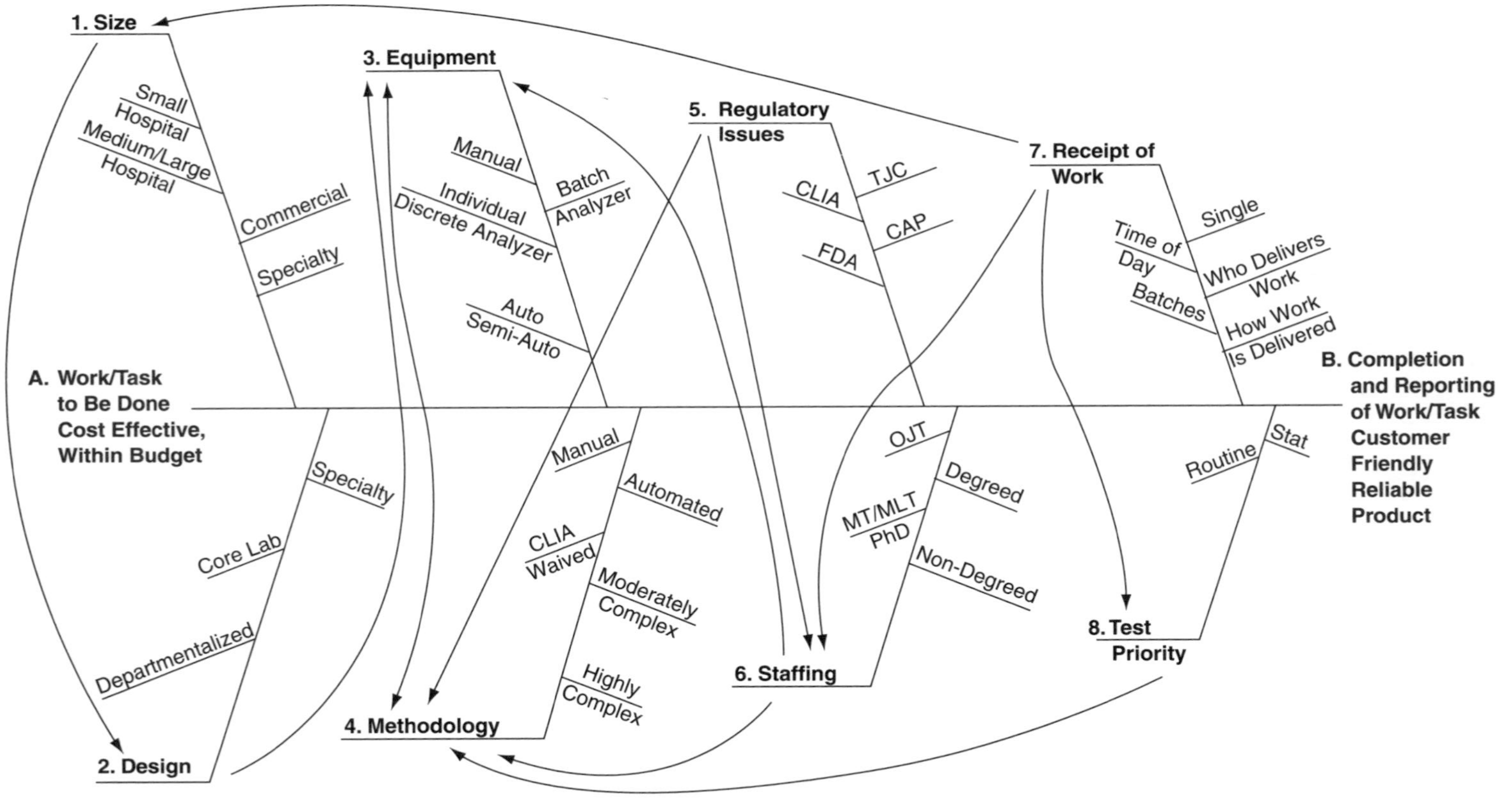

FIGURE 16-1. Flowchart of Process Design

KEY: OJT, On job-trained; CLIA, Clinical Laboratory Improvement Act; FDA, Food and Drug Administration; TJC, Joint Commission on Accreditation of Hospital Organizations; CAP, College of American Pathologists; Auto, Automated; Semi-auto, Semi-automated.

402

may all apply depending on the process or testing method used. In this case study, the microbiology department has interactions with each of the organizations listed.

6. *Staffing:* How many and what type of employees are needed to do the work? Do they need to have a degree (PhD, MT, MLT), or no degree (technical assistant, phlebotomist or on-the-job trained)? What is the availability of each type? In this case study, most of the work in microbiology must be done by someone with a degree in laboratory sciences.

7. *When/how will the work be received?* Will the work come one or two times during the day? Will it be received in off hours? Will it come in batches or one test at a time? Who delivers the specimens (i.e., laboratory or non-laboratory personnel)? In this case study, we will look at this issue under workflow and staffing.

8. *Test priority:* Is the test to be performed routinely or is it STAT? If it is STAT, can it be performed/reported immediately, or within a short period of time, as that term implies? Most microbiology work can be collected STAT but not performed immediately.

Developing a process design can be complex as seen by the flowchart. It may look confusing, but all the factors must be considered and they are interdependent. Work experience, and in some cases, additional education may be necessary to complete all the parts of a process design; therefore this chapter is limited to introducing the learner to basic concepts.

To return to the case study, you as the manager need to develop a process design for the 50% increase in work. To do this, you must ask many questions, and then try to answer them.

- What needs to be done?
- What costs are associated with increasing the workload, and is there a benefit to the organization if this work is completed?
- How will the work be completed, and will it affect the current workload?
- Will new equipment be needed?
- Will more staff be needed and at what level?
- Will the department need remodeling?
- When and how will the work get to the laboratory, and then to the microbiology department?

After further examining Figure 16-1, Flowchart of Process Design, it can be seen that each of these questions falls under one or more of the global factors (numbers 1 through 8 in the flowchart). These are the subdivisions of the global factors.

1. *What needs to be done?*

The answer may seem obvious—it must be the work. On the flowchart, this question is represented by the "A – B" line. The question must consider not only the work but also the kind of work. In the microbiology department, cultures such as wounds are much more complex to process than a voided urine culture. In our case study, the work that will need to be done is similar to that already being done in the department. There will just be more of it.

2. *What costs are associated with increasing the workload, and is there a benefit to the organization if this work is completed?*

Remember that the work needs to be cost effective (best product for the lowest cost), within the budget (historical data usually provides this information such as cost/test and projected costs—see Chapter 11), timely (increased workload does not mean it takes longer to complete the work), customer friendly, and reliable (easily available and understood).

3. *How will the work be completed, and will it affect the current workload?*

Adding a fifty percent increase to the current workload sounds like a lot of work, and it may be a burden to the existing processes. A burden on the department would exist if the staff is unable to perform the tests within acceptable time frames or incurs overtime in completing the work. On the flowchart, this question is represented by the numbers 3, 4, 5, and 6. In our case study, the department has a semiautomated instrument that assists with culture processing. Everything else is done manually. All processes except culture setups are considered highly complex by CLIA. It must be determined if there is room for expansion i.e., will the department be able to do more work as it now stands. Also when referring to a fifty percent increase, do not forget to express this as a number. Fifty percent may be only two cultures, or it may be 150 cultures per week. In the case study, the increase represents 75 cultures per week. The department with a current workload of 150 cultures per week is close to capacity with the existing processes. To handle the increased work, the processes will need to be changed. This may mean adding staff, getting new equipment, or remodeling the department to be more efficient. A combination of all three considerations will probably be needed, but until everything is studied the answer is uncertain.

4. *Will new equipment be needed?*

On the flowchart, this question is represented by the number 3. The department has a semi-automated piece of equipment that assists with processing cultures. It will be able to do the type of work projected in the increase because it is doing similar work now. It can also handle the extra capacity. It is not interfaced with the laboratory computer and cannot be interfaced. Every result produced must be manually entered on a departmental log and in the computer. With the workload nearly at capacity, an automated piece of equipment should be considered. When considering new equipment, determine the age and value of the current instrument, the cost of purchasing the new instrument, the cost of operating both, and how much more work can the new piece do than the old. Also when choosing an instrument, do not get the biggest and most expensive one on the market. Instead choose a reliable instrument with a throughput (number of tests completed in one hour) matched to the needs of the work. Another consideration is the ability of the new instrument to interface with the computer. This ability reduces the need for manual entry, which is often time consuming and fraught with clerical errors. This could also influence a staffing decision.

5. *Will more staff be needed and at what level?*

On the flowchart, this question is represented by numbers 5 and 6. In the case study, it has been determined that with the current workload and present staff, the department is working at nearly full capacity. The type of work in microbiology requires it to be done or supervised by a person with a laboratory science degree. Some of the work could be done by an assistant such as setups, Gram staining, and ordering supplies. Would an employee at this level allow the technical staff more time to perform the rest of the work? An assistant's salary expense is less than that for technical staff, but there is less flexibility because the employee cannot do all tasks within the department. A technical employee's salary expense is higher but this person can perform all tasks. The equipment decision will influence the type of employee needed. If a new instrument is obtained, the technical staff may be able to handle all the technical work quite well if the nontechnical work is not a responsibility. The availability of staff at the level needed must also be considered. A nontechnical employee will probably be easier to hire than a technical person because they are more easily obtainable. In the case study, it has been determined that the automated piece of equipment will be purchased and nontechnical staff will be added to the department. This decision was made after all costs and benefits were studied.

6. *Will the department need remodeling?*

On the flowchart, this question is represented by number 2. The physical layout should be efficient. Instruments or tasks should be grouped so that people can operate without either tripping over each other or having to do a lot of walking from one workstation to another. They should also be grouped so that one employee may be able to do multiple tasks. In the case study, remodeling is also dependent on two other considerations, the new equipment's size and shape and/or whether a new workstation will be created.

7. *When and how will the work get to the laboratory, and then to the microbiology department?*

On the flowchart, this question is represented by number 7. Will the work be received once a day or throughout the day, in batches or as single specimens? Will the work be brought to the hospital by a courier from the other hospital, or will our hospital send a courier to pick it up? There is a cost associated with the delivery whether their courier, ours or someone from the outside does the work. In addition to the cost of delivery, turnaround should be considered in this step. If the specimens are delivered only once a day this can add up to 24 hours to the turnaround time. This means if it would normally take 48 hours to report a result, it will now take 72 hours for a culture that is collected right after the courier has left. On the other hand, if every specimen is delivered as it is collected, this will add a significant cost to the process. A good compromise would be two deliveries a day, one in the morning and one late afternoon or early evening. Once the specimens are received who will deliver them to the department? Currently this is being done by nontechnical staff in a receiving area. Two deliveries a day will not add burden to the current workload, so this process will not change.

The preceding discussion shows that designing a process can be complicated. To make sure that everything is considered, it is helpful to produce either a paper product, or computer simulation similar to the flowchart in our illustration. Every process or step should be specific to the process that is being developed. It is a good guide for getting from point A to point B.

Workflow

Once the broad questions are identified and solutions are proposed, then setting up how the work transitions through the department—workflow—is the next step. The process design development is the overall plan or outline from which to work while workflow, although a part of the process design, is more detailed. Workflow (Figure 16-2) is the pathway the work follows from its beginning to its completion. Policies and procedures are developed at this stage.

Workflow can be divided into three phases: **preanalytical,** the **analytical,** and **postanalytical** (Table 16-1). The preanalytical phase consists of everything that occurs before actual testing. It is collecting the right specimen at the right time and under the right set of circumstances. The analytical phase is the actual testing of the sample. The postanalytical phase consists of everything that needs to be done; including reporting the results, after all testing is complete. It ties everything together and finishes the whole process. Of the three phases, the preanalytical is the hardest to control. The greatest number of errors occur in this phase because many more people are involved with it than in the other two. The people involved are more likely not to be laboratory employees. Communication and training are important if the right specimen is to be collected and delivered to the department at the right time. The analytical and postanalytical phases are much easier to control because they are performed by laboratory employees who are under the management of a laboratory supervisor or manager. Each of these workflow phases is further described in the following sections.

Preanalytical Phase
In the preanalytical phase, uniformity of procedures is important. If everyone is taught to do things the same way, errors can be reduced. The procedures should not be so complicated or cumbersome that no one wants to follow them; this causes an increase in errors. This especially applies to the collection process. If a specimen is improperly collected, it can affect the test results, which ultimately affects patient outcome. In any setting, well-written manuals with thorough training are vital.

The ordering process should use a standard language. Everyone should call the test by the same name and should use the same abbreviations. Deviations cause confusion and can lead to misinterpretations. The wrong specimen could be collected or the wrong test performed.

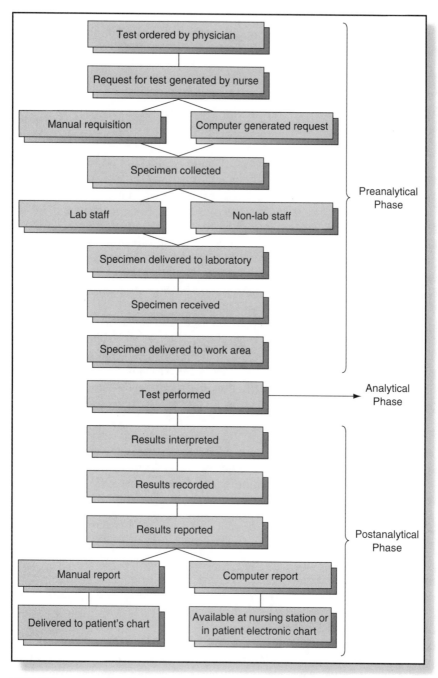

FIGURE 16-2.   **Flowchart of Workflow**

TABLE 16-1. Workflow Phases

Preanalytical	Analytical	Postanalytical
Ordering	Testing	Interpreting
Collecting		Recording
Transporting		Reporting
Processing		

After the specimen is collected, it must be transported to the laboratory. In a hospital, this may be as simple as walking down the hall. When specimens are delivered from an off-site location, the transportation process becomes more complicated. In the case study, the specimens are coming from a small hospital located an hour's drive away. Courier schedules will need to be established. Also before delivery, specimens must be stored so that specimen integrity is not compromised. The specimens need to be protected from such things as exposure to heat or cold. The specimens should not be too old to produce reliable results; hence, time frames must be established for "from time of collection to time of delivery." This will affect the courier schedule.

Once the specimen is ordered, collected, and transported, it must be received in the laboratory. This refers to the acceptance of the specimen, whether logging it in manually or in the computer. The receiving procedure should include what to do if the specimen is not acceptable, the wrong test has been ordered, or patient information is not complete. Then the specimen must be delivered to the work area. It does no good if it sits in the receiving area.

Analytical Phase

When the specimen arrives in the work area the testing is done. The physical layout of the area and how the test will be performed are important for efficiency. Will it be done by a manual method or will it be automated? What equipment should be used? These types of decisions are made during the process design development.

Postanalytical Phase

After the test is performed, the results must be interpreted (i.e., put into a format for reporting). Then it must be recorded and the results manually written on a log or placed in a computer log. The log is usually available only to laboratory staff.

From the log, the results are then reported; that is, they are made available to the person(s) that ordered the test or needs them to care for the patient. Until the final product is available to the people that need to know, the task or work is not complete. Many media, depending on the circumstances, are used to report tests such as the computer, paper, phone, mail, or fax. Remember, reports are not useful if they are hard to read and understand or if they are not easily accessible.

Workflow can be a complicated process. To help identify all the steps it is beneficial to draw a flowchart that is specific to the workflow being analyzed

(Figure 16-2). Each step should be specific to the work and department. It then serves as a guide for getting from the beginning to the end of a task.

PROCESS MANAGEMENT

The business of the laboratory is to provide information to the clinician to assist in patient care decisions. The clinical/hospital-based laboratory is integral to patient care and as such, integrated with the healthcare delivery system in which it resides. A reference or freestanding laboratory provides service in a different manner, yet is still a crucial part of patient care. In either case, the goals of the laboratory must be aligned with the overall goals of the healthcare system. It is then possible to analyze and define the current state, and all inherent processes, to determine if purposeful change can bring about measurable improvements that fit with the stated goals.

Process Management is defined as a systematic data based approach to monitoring and improving the performance of business. It is a management strategy that identifies opportunities for improvement using proven problem-solving methods. Process improvement has been around informally for thousands of years—theoretically ever since the caveman made the 2' wheel. Formal programs began in the 1940s and 1950s when Japanese businessmen discovered the methods taught by Drs. Deming, Juran, and Shewhart. The roots of process management have evolved from the basic Shewhart Cycle (see Chapter 5) popular in the 1950s to the more complex **Six Sigma** Methodology applied by modern businesses. Although a variety of names such as Total Quality Management and Continuous Quality Improvement have been used to individualize these methods, they all have a common goal: an efficient, effective process that produces highly satisfied customers. They also involve a number of quality—or process management—tools including PDSA *(Plan, Do, Study, Act)* (a.k.a. PDCA, Deming's Cycle, or Shewhart's Cycle). Many modern businesses have segued into the more complex Six Sigma methodology. Numerous models of process management, process improvement methods, and quality tools exist. Regardless of which quality management system is utilized, the expected results are the continuous monitoring of processes, looking for ways to make improvement without sacrificing quality.

Every organization can potentially improve its processes and the systems in which they operate. By mapping current processes, and defining a more efficient and smoother functioning future state, we can achieve measurable improvement in multiple areas: care delivery, cost effectiveness, and the work environment.

The team members actually performing the work become better informed about how their individual tasks contribute to the success of the entire organization.

How then can we, as laboratory managers, best serve the customer and ultimately achieve the best outcomes for the patient? How can we monitor and improve the performance of the laboratory to more resourcefully provide the delivery of services? How can we manage the process?

PROCESS MANAGEMENT TOOLS

Many businesses including health care organizations develop a Quality Philosophy or Quality Model based on a variety of process improvement methodologies. Time and money is invested in teaching the chosen methodology and some are groomed to be expert facilitators. If your organization does not offer this, you can still take advantage of these proven problem-solving methods. An example of a Process Management Tool called FOCUS-PDSA is shown here (See Figure 16-3). Each letter of the FOCUS-PDSA acronym stands for a phrase that describes a step in the order it needs to be taken to enact a process improvement. A Quality Improvement (QI) Review Form can be used to keep the team on track. (See Table 16-2.) Skipping steps can be tempting, but is discouraged as it usually calls for rework further along in the project.

The acronym **FOCUS-PDSA** stands for:

F – Find an Opportunity	**P** – Plan your Actions
O – Organize a Team	**D** – Do the Actions
C – Clarify Current Process	**S** – Study the Results
U – Understand Variation	**A** – Act on your Conclusions
S – Select Improvement	

The first step is often easy as the *Opportunity* finds you, perhaps as a recurrent customer complaint or a directive from administration. If the opportunity is not so clear, try surveying your customers and team members. You will find ideas that you may not have considered independently. *Organizing a Team* is not to be taken lightly. You must identify key players who are familiar with the process, have the ability to affect the process, are customers—internal or external, and have a stake in the outcome in order to select a lasting, meaningful change.

The next step—*Clarify the Current Process*—is done by gathering information from the users of the process so that a true picture of current operations can be mapped out. This stage consists of direct observation, measurement, and numeration. A process flow chart is often utilized at this point. If the climate of the organization is non-threatening and conducive to change, the team member whose tasks are being studied will welcome the analysis and participate by collecting data and providing frontline insight to the team. The accuracy and appropriateness of the information collected at this stage is important and every effort should be made to collect unbiased data. The participation of the individuals most affected by the proposed improvement should be emphasized and is crucial to its success.

The team member needs to understand that process improvement is a tool for positive change, and will result in innovation that better aligns the actions of an individual worker with objectives and visions of the organization.

Understanding Variation is the next step. This step is key to every Quality Management theory. It consists of determining which specific steps in the overall process need improvement. Quality is inversely proportional to variability. Questions to ask at this stage include: "How does this process vary from what the customer wants? What are the common causes of variation in the process? What are the special causes? What can be done to reduce variation?"

The options for improvement are then outlined and *Selected.* At this stage, the creative floodgates are opened and various ideas are entertained and analyzed for feasibility, practicality, cost, and effect on outcome. Once an idea is chosen, usually through a variety of quality tools (i.e., Brainstorming, Benchmarking, Multi-Voting, or a Selection Matrix) the change is introduced into the process flowchart and effects of the change on the future state are explored.

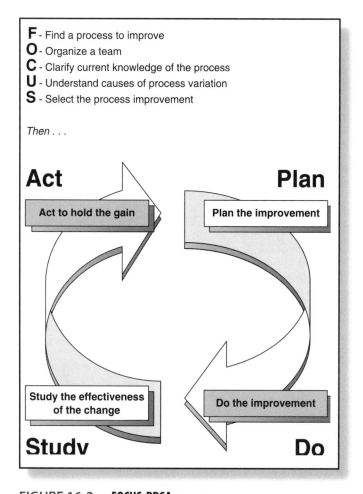

FIGURE 16-3.   **FOCUS-PDSA**

TABLE 16-2.   QI Review Form

Find an Opportunity

- Describe the data that quantifies the need: _____
- How can you narrow the scope? _____
- Opportunity Statement: *We have the opportunity to improve the _____ process. This process begins with _____ & ends with _____. If we meet our goal of _____, our key customers, _____ will benefit.*
- Describe the set of numbers that would tell you if the above process has changed: _____

Organize a Team

- Name key players & customers. (Which team members and customers are most familiar with the process?) _____
- Establish team ground rules: i.e. Meeting dates, team etiquette, etc. _____
- Review Opportunity Statement for clarity _____
- Establish timeline—write in projected completion date of each step: _____

F	O	C	U	S	P	D	S	A

Clarify Current Process

- Using input from the people listed above, make a flowchart of the current process.

  _____

- What are easy problems that could be solved immediately? _____
- Describe the data that quantifies the customer's expectations: _____

Understand Variation

- How does this process vary from what the customer wants? _____
- Why do special cause and common cause variations occur? _____

Select Improvements

- What are the root causes of the problem? _____
- List several ways that the process can be improved: _____
- What criteria will you use to evaluate the list of improvements? _____

Plan Your Actions

- Describe only one process improvement that will be piloted: _____
- Does your action plan describe who, what, when, and where? _____
- How long will you try the process before studying the data collected? _____

Do the Actions

- Are you following an Action Plan? _____
- Are you collecting data during this trial period? _____

Study the Results

- Did you make progress toward your goals? Why or why not? _____

Act on Your Conclusions

- Should the change be made permanent? _____
- Is another improvement needed? _____

If the change is doable, and not contraindicated by the outcome analysis, the change is *Planned* or incorporated into the future state map. The *Doing* stage translates to controlled implementation of the process change. Controlled in the foregoing sentence means that the effects of the change are observed, monitored, and measured. It is important that a measurable variable be defined prior to the implementation so that an objective assessment of the benefits of change can be made. Without empirical measurements of outcomes, we have no reliable way of *Studying the Results;* or in other words, of knowing if the change has brought about improvement. The final step of the FOCUS-PDSA method is to review the change by monitoring the effect it had on a measurable outcome. You will *Act on Your Conclusions* by determining if the change should be made permanent or if another improvement is needed. It is not unusual to have multiple cycles (often referred to as Rapid Cycle Changes) of the PDSA part of the formula. By introducing one small change at a time, studying what works and what does not, you can refine the process to relative perfection.

In recent years, efforts have been made to incorporate more sophisticated **process management tools** into the health care environment and specifically into the clinical laboratory. This is the methodology mentioned earlier and developed in manufacturing industries of *Lean Thinking, Lean Tooling,* and *Six Sigma.* What are Six Sigma and the Lean Philosophy? The term "Sigma" is from the world of mathematics and represents the statistical measure of variability within a selected process. In the manufacturing environment, it has been used to measure the number of products produced that do not meet quality control standards, or that simply do not function as intended. In service industries, it may be a measure of the number of transaction failures or an inordinate delay in the delivery of a service. The underlying assumption of the Sigma methodology is that the cause of a defect or failure is variation. If something works most of the time, then one can eliminate the reasons that create differences in the outcome of the process with the goal of eliminating failure. The number preceding Sigma, in this case Six, refers to the order of magnitude of the reduction in variation: Thus the higher the number, the fewer the failures. Six Sigma improvements mean that a process has been refined to reduce errors to 3.4 per one million opportunities. For practical purposes, an error rate at this level is virtually perfect.

The fundamental concepts of the Lean Philosophy are to define value by challenging traditional definitions, discovering what is of value to the customer, and then determining the value of each step leading to the delivery of the goods or service to the customer. This leads to mapping the "Value Stream" (the flow or movement [physical or informational] between processes) and redesigning the structure to respond to the needs of the customer. By adding value, and eliminating what does not add value, or even takes value away, the waste generated in the system is reduced or eliminated. Six Sigma uses a DMAIC (Define, Measure, Analyze, Improve, Control) tool similar to the FOCUS-PDSA tool for improving existing processes.

The full application of the Six Sigma methodology and Lean Tooling require extensive training and experience. A person achieving mastery of these system design methodologies are awarded certifications as "Black Belts," "Green Belts," and "Lean Tool Masters." As these technologies are applied even more broadly in the health care environment, improvements and efficiencies can be realized making the health care environment safer for everyone. Teaching Quality Improvement programs is an industry in itself. Much more information is available about the quality process, quality tools, and how to use them via literature and the Internet. Several websites offering more information include: *http://curiouscat. com/guides/* and *http://www.isixsigma.com/sixsigma/six_sigma.asp.*

STAFFING THE LABORATORY: HIRING, TRAINING, SCHEDULING, AND RETAINING

Staffing is defined as finding the right person to do the job at the time needed, that is, matching that person to the needs of the job. Staffing includes hiring, training, scheduling, and retaining, each of which is further discussed in the sections that follow. When a decision is made to hire a new employee, the level of staff needed must be determined. Will a person with or without a degree be needed? This is usually decided by the type of work to be done and regulatory issues associated with that work. Will the person need to be a specialist or a generalist? A specialist is someone with extensive knowledge in one area, while a generalist has knowledge of many. Will the person work full-time, part-time, or as needed (per diem)? Will there be shift work, weekend work, or holiday work? After deciding what is needed, the hiring process can start.

Hiring

The hiring process consists of two components, the application, and the interview. The application is a written document that lists the prospective employee's education, qualifications, and work experience. It can be used as an initial screening because if these do not meet the needs of the open position, no further action should be taken. If the applicant appears to meet your needs, then an interview should be scheduled. The interview is the oral process used to confirm the information in the application and to fill in any gaps. This is also an opportunity to explain to the applicant the job responsibilities, the hours/days/shifts that need to be worked, the benefits package that will be available, and the wages. If everything appears compatible for both parties, a job offer can be made and accepted.

Training

Once hired, the employee needs to be taught the procedures in the work area. If you expect an employee to do well in the position then that person must be thoroughly trained (see Chapter 9 for additional information regarding training). The initial training period is referred to as orientation. Having a complete, well-defined orientation helps everyone, the new hire and the trainer, because it defines the expectations and responsibilities of the position. It also helps the new employee to be productive and be able to operate independently.

Scheduling

When the training or orientation is complete, the employee must be scheduled to work. Scheduling is assigning the employee to work-specific hours, to a specific department, or to a specific task. The manager has the responsibility for scheduling to meet the needs of the department in the safest and most cost effective way possible. The number of hours that an employee is scheduled depends on their classification, full-time, part-time, or per diem. A full-time employee works 40 hours a week or 80 hours in two weeks depending on the work rule used. A part-time employee is regularly scheduled and works a defined number of hours that are less than the full-time employee's hours. This could be as little as 8 hours in a week or two week period to as much as 32 hours in a week or 72 hours in two weeks. The number of hours authorized often determines if the employee is qualified for benefits. In our case study, an employee must work at least 40 hours per 2-week pay period to be eligible to receive benefits. The employee can choose to work less than 40 hours but must be informed that they will not be eligible to receive benefits. These benefits often play a large role in the job search, but do not affect those who receive them elsewhere. A per diem employee (also known as PRN—as needed—or pool) is not regularly scheduled and has no set number of hours. This employee works when needed such as filling in for someone on vacation, someone absent due to illness, or during heavy workload periods. They help fill out the schedule as needed.

Two major scheduling formats are used to schedule employees. These are the **8/80 work rule** and the **40-hour workweek rule.** The 8/80 work rule has been used by hospitals for many years and they are the only employer allowed to use it, as defined by wage and hour regulations. Traditionally, in hospitals, employees have been scheduled to work 8-hour days. The day conveniently divides into three 8-hour periods. The 8/80 work rule covers a two-week time frame. During this time, the employee works an 8-hour day and any number of days up to 10 (80 hours) within the two weeks. Any time worked over eight hours in a day or 80 hours in two weeks is overtime and must be paid at the overtime rate. The 40-hour workweek rule means the employee is allowed to work any number of hours per shift, as long as the total hours worked in a week do not exceed 40.

Both scheduling models have their advantages and disadvantages. The 8/80 rule limits the number of hours in the day that can be worked, but more days in a row are allowed. The 40-hour workweek lets an employee work longer shifts but limits the number of days in a week to a maximum of five. This can save the organization overtime expenses when longer shifts are needed for covering the work. In today's environment, flexibility in scheduling has become an important issue to employees. Many managers are using both work rules to provide as much flexibility as possible. This does not mean the employee can use one work rule this week and the other next week, but it does give everyone more choices.

Depending on organizational needs, two employees working side by side could possibly work different types of schedules. No matter which work rule is used in developing a schedule, it should be impartial and based on organizational needs.

Scheduling begins with determining how many and what type of staff are needed to perform the average workload per shift. Workload and staffing information is usually based on historical data. This should include data for shift work, weekends, and holidays because laboratories are open 24/7 and must be staffed. This type of information needs to be used regardless of the size of the laboratory. In a large laboratory, the schedule is probably more departmentalized and complicated; a smaller laboratory would be simpler and include all areas, benches, and shifts.

The schedule should start out as a generic process; this would be the "ideal" schedule based on organizational needs. Once this has been developed, then individual employees and special requests can be plugged in. Schedules should also be determined far enough ahead so that everyone has advanced notice of when to work. A schedule is a dynamic process. It is continually changing based on the needs of both the organization and the employee. The schedule should be set up based on the pay period as the working unit. A pay period is usually two weeks no matter which work rule is used. At the end of each pay period the employee is paid for hours worked.

In any pay period, fourteen 24-hour days need to be staffed. No matter which work rule is used, a full-time employee cannot work more than the equivalent of ten days or 80 hours in the two weeks without incurring overtime. Part-time employees are hired to provide coverage when full-time employees are off work. In the case study, a generic schedule was developed for the entire laboratory using the 8/80 work rule. When using this rule, the day is divided into three shifts of eight hours each. These are called the day, evening, and night shifts. Historical data was used to determine workload, and levels of staffing for each shift, including both weekdays and weekends.

As an example of an 8/80 workweek schedule, Table 16-3 shows the staff required for each shift. Once the staffing levels are established, the number of employees needed to provide the staffing must be determined. An easy way to accomplish this is to establish the number of shifts needing to be worked for each job classification.

Remember, a shift using the 8/80 work rule is eight hours and in a 2-week period there are 14 days. A full-time employee works 10 of the 14 shifts. A part-time employee usually works the other four. Knowing this information, we can now calculate the number of people needed (Table 16-4). Once this information has been determined, a generic schedule can be developed (Table 16-5).

After the generic schedule is established, the names of the employees are filled in, taking into account special needs or requests such as vacations. If necessary, determine who will provide coverage for the special requests. Then add the work assignments. This can be done using numbers, colored dots, letters, or whatever works for this department (Table 16-6). Since most laboratories operate

24/7, military time is often used to show the start time of the shift in the scheduling process.

Return to the case study and the microbiology department. The current staffing consists of two full-time technical employees and one part-time technical employee. During the week, two people work days, and on weekends one person works. There are no evenings or night shifts worked in this area. The department is open from 0600 to 1700. Since most laboratories operate 24/7, military time is often used in the scheduling process. Thus, all times in this discussion are expressed in military time. One person reports at 0600 and the other at 0830 during the week, and one person works 0700 to 1530 on weekends (Table 16-7). If a stat Gram stain is needed at other times, the technical staff in the rest of the laboratory have been cross-trained to perform them. Cultures received during those other hours are set up by the same staff.

With the projected increase in work and with the addition of a new piece of equipment, it has been determined that nontechnical staff employees will also be needed. If the non-technical person is needed every day, that means there are 14 shifts to cover in the pay period. This means one full-time person and one part-time person will have to be hired to provide the coverage (Table 16-8). In addition, the hours the department must be staffed need to be adjusted. The cultures from the small rural hospital are scheduled to be delivered at 1100 and at 1700 during the week and at 1100 on weekends. Since workload usually decreases on weekends, it was felt that one delivery would be sufficient. This can be changed if needed. During the week, a delivery at 1700 will impact the evening shift if they are required to set up the cultures arriving at that time.

The generic schedule in Table 16-5 was developed using the 8/80 work rule. Some of the employees work six shifts in a row and others ten. If this schedule had been developed using the 40-hour workweek rule, the schedule could still look much the same as long as 8-hour shifts are still worked and the employee works every other weekend. When using the 40-hour workweek, the week is usually defined as Sunday to Saturday. It splits the weekend, which still allows employees to work six days in a row (or ten), but it must include the weekend.

In our case study in the generic example (Table 16-5) the 8/80 work rule is being used for scheduling. It has worked well for the department and will not be

TABLE 16-3.   Staffing for the Average Workload

	Day Shift	Evening Shift	Night Shift
Weekdays	3 technical 2 phlebotomy 1 secretary	2 technical 1 phlebotomy	1 technical
Weekends	2 technical 1 phlebotomy 1 secretary	1 technical 1 phlebotomy	1 technical

TABLE 16-4. Staffing

Day Shift

Weekdays   3 technical staff needed for 10 shifts = 30 shifts to cover
Weekends   2 technical staff needed for 4 shifts = 8 shifts to cover
                                        14 days   38 shifts to cover

If a full-time employee works 10 shifts, divide the 38 shifts by 10. This equals approximately four. Four full-time people are needed to provide this coverage.

Weekdays   2 phlebotomy staff needed for 10 shifts = 20 shifts to cover
Weekends   1 phlebotomy staff needed for 4 shifts = 4 shifts to cover
                                          14 days   24 shifts to cover

Divide the 24 shifts by 10. This equals 2.4, which means 2 full-time people and 1 part-time person is needed to provide this coverage.

Weekdays/ends   1 secretary needed for 14 shifts = 14 shifts to cover

Divide 14 shifts by 10. This equals 1.4, which means 1 full-time person and 1 part-time person is needed to provide this coverage.

Evening Shift

Weekdays   2 technical staff needed for 10 shifts = 20 shifts to cover
Weekends   1 technical staff needed for 4 shifts = 4 shifts to cover
                                        14 days   24 shifts to cover

Divide the 24 shifts by 10. This equals 2.4, which means 2 full-time people and 1 part-time person is needed to provide this coverage.

Weekdays/ends   1 phlebotomy staff needed for 14 shifts = 14 shifts to cover

Divide 14 shifts by 10. This equals 1.4, which means 1 full-time person and 1 part-time person is needed to provide this coverage.

Night Shift

Weekdays/ends   1 technical staff needed for 14 shifts = 14 shifts to cover
Divide 14 shifts by 10. This equals 1.4, which means 1 full-time person and 1 part-time person is needed to provide coverage.

changed. Suppose though that for some reason the workload does change in the general laboratory. The schedule will need to be adjusted to provide coverage. For this example, the workload has changed at two specific times of the day. The first time is from 2100 to 2400. The emergency room work has increased fourfold during this time and the evening shift is having trouble keeping up. To provide some relief it was decided that the night shift tech would start work two hours earlier at 2100 and work a 10-hour shift. The second time of the day that workload has significantly changed is from 1600 to 1500 because of blood arriving from off-site clinics. This occurs in the middle of the change of shift from days to evenings, and overtime is occurring because the day shift is unable to leave on time. An overlap is needed to provide coverage and reduce this expense. To reduce overtime, it was decided that one day-shift tech would start working 10-hour shifts from 0700 to 1700 (Table 16-9). Note the differences between Table 16-9 and Table 16-5. To work 10-hour shifts, a 40-hour workweek rule must be used when developing the schedule.

TABLE 16-5. 8/80* Generic Schedule

Day Shift	Sun	Mon	Tue	Wed	Thu	Fri	Sat
FT Tech	x	o	x	x	x	x	o
FT Tech	x	x	o	x	x	x	o
FT Tech	o	x	x	x	o	x	x
FT Tech	o	x	x	x	x	o	x
FT Phleb	x	o	x	x	x	x	o
FT Phleb	o	x	x	x	x	o	x
PT Phleb		x			x	x	
FT Sec	o	o	x	x	x	x	x
PT Sec	x	x					x
Evenings							
FT Tech	x	x	x	x	x	x	o
FT Tech	o	o	o	x	x	x	x
PT Tech		x	x	x			
FT Phleb	x	o	x	x	x	x	o
PT Phleb	x	x					x
Nights							
FT Tech	x	x	x	x	x	o	o
PT Tech	x					x	x

Note: * (8/80) refers to the 8/80 work rule, where 8 is eight hours in a day, and 80 is eighty hours in a work period.)

x = Working; FT = Full-Time; PT = Part-Time; o = Off; Tech = Technologist/Technician; Phleb = Phlebotomist; Sec = Secretary.

TABLE 16-6. Specific Schedule

Day Shift	Sun	Mon	Tue	Wed	Thu	Fri	Sat	Sun	Mon	Tue	Wed	Thu	Fri	Sat
Bob	C	o	C	C	C	C	o	o	H	H	H	o	H	H
Sally	H	H	o	H	H	H	o	o	BB	BB	BB	BB	o	C
Susan	o	BB	BB	BB	o	BB	C	H	o	C	F	H	C	o
Joan	o	C	H	F	BB	o	H	C	C	o	C	C	BB	o
Jessica	400	o	400	400	400	400	o	o	400	400	400	400	400	400
David	o	400	700	700	700	o	400	400	o	700	700	700	o	700
Cynthia		700				700	700	700	700				700	
Linda	o	o	700	700	700	700	700	700	o	700	700	700	700	o
Cathy	700	700	o	o	o	o	o	o	700	o	o	o	o	700
Evenings														
John	1430	1430	1430	1430	1430	1430	o	o	o	1430	1430	1430	1430	1430
Stephanie	o	o	1530	1530	1530	1530	1530	1530	1530	1530	1530	1530	1530	o
Amy	1530	1530	o	o	o	o	1430	o	1430	o	o	o	o	o
Dan	1500	o	1500	1500	1500	1500	o	o	o	1500	1500	1500	1500	1500
Mary	1500	1500	o	o	o	o	1500	1500	1500	o	o	o	o	o
Nights														
Judy	2300	2300	2300	2300	2300	o	o	o	2300	2300	2300	2300	o	2300
Jean						2300	2300	2300					2300	2300

Note: H = Hematology/Urinalysis/Coagulation; C = Chemistry; BB = Blood Bank; F = Float; o = Scheduled day off. Numbers indicate shift start time in military time.

TABLE 16-7. Current Microbiology Schedule

Micro	Sun	Mon	Tue	Wed	Thu	Fri	Sat
John	700	600	600	600	600	o	o
Karen	o	o	830	830	830	600	700
Larry		830				830	

Note: Numbers indicate shift start time in military time. o = Scheduled day off.

TABLE 16-8. Projected Microbiology Schedule

Micro	Sun	Mon	Tue	Wed	Thu	Fri	Sat
John	700	600	600	600	600	o	o
Karen	o	o	830	830	830	600	700
Larry		830				830	
FT New	800	o	1000	1000	1000	1000	o
PT New	800	1000				1000	800

Note: Numbers indicate start time (military time). In this projected schedule there are 2 employees working both Saturdays and Sundays. On these days, 1 employee works bench 1, the other works bench 2. The specific duties performed at specific hours are as follows: 600 = Bench 1 Special Cultures; 830 = Bench 2 Read Plates/Set Up Susceptibility Tests (MICs); 700/1000 = Set Ups/Gram Stains/Ordering.

o = Scheduled day off.

TABLE 16-9. 40-Hour Workweek Generic Schedule

Day Shift	Sun	Mon	Tue	Wed	Thu	Fri	Sat
FT Tech	o	o	*700	*700	*700	*0700	o
FT Tech	600	600	600	600	600	600	600
FT Tech	o	*700	900	700	o	900	o
FT Tech	o	700	600	700	700	700	o
PT Tech	700						700
FT Phleb	x	o	x	x	x	x	x
FT Phleb	o	x	x	x	x	o	x
PT Phleb		x	x	x		x	
FT Sec	o	o	x	x	x	x	o
PT Sec	x	x					x
Evenings							
FT Tech	x	x	x	x	x	x	x
FT Tech	o	o	x	x	x	o	o
PT Tech		x	x	x			
FT Phleb	x	o	x	x	x	x	o
PT Phleb		x				x	x
Nights							
FT Tech	o	o	*2100	*2100	*2100	*2100	o
PT Tech	*2100	*2100	*2100	*2100	*2100	*2100	*2100

Note: The full-time tech that works 2 ten-hour shifts will work 6 hours the next day so that overtime does not occur. Evening shift scheduling is not affected by the changes.

FT = Full-Time; PT = Part-Time; x = Scheduled work day; o = Scheduled day off; * = 10-hour shifts.

A third option for scheduling is called **self-scheduling.** Generational studies have shown that inflexible scheduling is considered poor working conditions by the newest to the work world. An increased number of younger workers willingly forego higher wages to achieve an agreeable work-life balance. Some companies have improved retention and recruitment by introducing such programs as self-scheduling into their organizations. Successful self-scheduling takes teamwork but the rewards for letting team members have some control over their schedules is well worth the effort.

Self-scheduling guidelines will need to be designed to meet the needs of the particular department. Two important points to remember as you create these guidelines are:

A. No one is guaranteed a specific schedule.

B. The needs of the department must be covered.

The following is an example of a successful self-scheduling plan:

1. Team members are divided into 2 groups, RED and BLUE. The groups alternate signing up first on the new blank schedule. Each group has 4 days to sign up. There is a maximum and minimum number of staff needed each shift. (The minimum number is the number of staff needed to perform the average daily workload and the maximum number is the most the budget affords working in one shift—these numbers are determined by the manager.) When the maximum number of staff is achieved, that date will be X'd out on the schedule. There is a week to make revisions after which the schedule is finalized and posted. Unbalanced schedules will not be finalized.

2. The second group to sign up should be the first group to make schedule changes. It is the responsibility of the second group to review the schedule at revision time and attempt to balance the schedule.

3. The manager tracks changes made to help balance the schedule. Changes to the schedule must be made in red ink to get credit for changing. (Pencil is used until revision time.)

4. If the schedule is not balanced after revisions, the manager will change staff according to the following guidelines:
   a. Staff not meeting their weekend commitment
   b. Per diem staff
   c. Staff in the second group who have not made changes to balance previous schedules according to past schedules
   d. Staff in the second group who have not made changes to balance the schedule in progress
   e. Staff in first group

5. If your schedule is changed without your approval, the manager will make every effort to notify you, and it will be your responsibility to either work the shift or find an even trade.

6. Each team member is required to work 4 weekend shifts per schedule. Day-shift and evening weekend shifts are Saturday and Sunday. Nightshift weekend shifts are Friday and Saturday.

7. During revision time, if you switch off a weekend shift, you must sign up for another weekend shift, if another weekend shift is low.

8. The manager may decrease the weekend commitment of a team member if it is in the best interest of the schedule.

9. Only an established number of team members may be granted PTO (paid time off) during the scheduling period.

10. All schedule change requests after the schedule is finalized must be approved by the manager. Every attempt must be made on the part of the team member to find an even trade for their request, if the request would reduce the number working that shift.

Retaining

Retention of team members is well worth putting forth a good effort. As the number of people entering the workforce decreases, people have more choice in the job market. Work-life balance, as mentioned earlier, is very important to workers in their 20s and 30s. This age group is not nearly as loyal to an employer as previous generations. The cost of recruiting, hiring, and orienting a new team member is approximately the cost of that position's annual salary. Remember, you will be paying two people to do one job for several weeks as they orient. If the person stayed long enough to accumulate benefits, they will be taking some of those benefits (PTO) with them when they leave. You may also be paying overtime to other team members to cover the vacated shifts while you recruit.

Retention may be as simple as recognizing each of your team members every day, giving praise where due, and treating the team fairly when making assignments or counseling them. Giving employees time for continuing education opportunities will also help. If an employee feels they have been recognized, treated fairly, and that they have an opinion that counts, they are more likely to stay with the organization.

SUMMARY

A process design serves as a blueprint for completing work or a task. It may be complicated or simple based on the size of the task and the setting for which it is being developed. Workflow and staffing are integral parts of process design development, providing the details of the blueprint. Further, the development of a process design is influenced by many other factors, each of which should be examined and analyzed.

As previously stated, workflow is an essential aspect of process design development. Three workflow phases must be considered: (1) preanalytical, (2) analytical, and (3) postanalytical. Of these phases, the preanalytical phase is the most difficult to control. The development of a workflow chart that identifies the specific points within each of these phases is indicated when performing workflow analysis.

Process Management is the management strategy of continuously monitoring the performance of processes and identifying opportunities for improvement using proven problem-solving methods. Many variations and methodologies are available in the literature and on the Internet. These may be dictated by your organization or you may research and choose the best approach for your department. Successful organizations continue to strive for perfection in processes without sacrificing quality.

Staffing is critical to process design development. Four components are involved in staffing. The first is hiring, which consists of two parts: (1) the written application and (2) the oral interview. Each part of the hiring phase provides specific information about the prospective candidate so that a good hiring decision can be made. Once an employee is hired, the second component, training, comes into play. Training consists of orientating the employee to the facility, the department, and to policies and procedures associated with performing the job. The third component is scheduling. The assignment of workers to jobs can be a complex task that consumes much of a laboratory manager's time. Two work rules may be used in scheduling employees in a hospital setting: the 8/80 work rule, or the 40-hour workweek rule. The development of a generic schedule will provide a basic plan from which a specific schedule may be designed and implemented. Self-scheduling is an option that offers flexibility and control to team members. Retention is the fourth stage of staffing. Once you have hired a good employee, effort should be made to retain that employee. Successful retention is cost effective and may improve outcomes as experienced employees become more proficient in their work.

The key to developing successful process designs is by approaching it carefully, one step at a time, addressing each appropriate issue. Along with the use of flowcharts, where appropriate, a successful process design may be developed.

SUMMARY CHART:
Important Points to Remember

➤ Process Management—Systematic approach to improving performance
  • Process Designs: Broad plans
    Things to consider: Size of Laboratory, Design of Laboratory, Equipment to Be Used, Test Methodology, Regulatory Standards, Staffing, Receipt of Work, Test Priority.
    Questions to be asked/answered: What task needs to be completed? What does it cost? How will the work be done? Will new equipment be needed? Who will do the work? Will remodeling be needed?

  • Workflow: How does the work go from the beginning to the end?

  Preanalytical: Everything that happens to the specimen or work before actual testing is completed.

  Analytical: The actual testing that is completed.

  Postanalytical: Everything that is done with test answers after the testing has been completed, including reporting of test results.

  • Tools: Use of Quality Management Model(s) to improve methodologies: FOCUS-PDSA, Six Sigma, and DMAIC.

➤ Staffing-Finding the right person at the right time to do the job.

  • Hiring: Written application lists education, qualifications, and work experience. Oral interview allows manager to confirm with applicant education, qualifications, and work experience.

  • Training: Orientation period that defines the expectations and responsibilities.

  • Scheduling: Two scheduling formats may be used as defined by the Wage and Hour Board.

  8/80 work rule—covers a two-week period and states that the co-worker may work no more than 80 hours in the period and eight hours in any given day. Any time exceeding these two rules incurs overtime.

  40-hour workweek rule—may work any amount in a given day, but may not work more than 40 hours in the week. Any hours worked over the 40 hours is considered overtime.

SUGGESTED PROBLEM-BASED LEARNING ACTIVITIES

Chapter 16: Process Designs—Workflow and Staffing

Instructions: Use Internet resources, books, articles, colleagues, etc., to present solutions to the problems listed below. There is no single correct solution to any problem.

Note to Instructor: Students in class may be divided into groups and given the problem-based learning activity to discuss and solve. Once the group has reached consensus as to a solution, the group may present it to the other students in the class. This activity will provide all students with information regarding solutions to the problem.

Problem #1

Choose a laboratory discipline, such as hematology or chemistry, and implement new technology/instrumentation for this discipline. How would this affect your current work processes?

Problem #2

Suppose your institution just contracted with a physician group to provide laboratory services. As laboratory manager, you must design a process to acquire samples, provide testing on the second shift, and produce results by the next morning.

Problem #3

Suppose your institution has merged with another institution and all redundant services will be eliminated. As laboratory manger, you must design an efficient laboratory operation to provide the necessary services at both institutions.

Problem #4

Using the projected microbiology schedule (Table 16-8) develop a schedule for the 40-hour workweek. Adjust the length of the shifts as needed to provide adequate coverage. See if less staff would be needed or if better coverage could be provided.

BIBLIOGRAPHY

Browne ED: "Workflow Modeling of Coordinated Inter-Health Provider Care Plan." Ph.D. Thesis. University of South Australia, 2005.

Chester E: *Getting Them to Give a Damn: How to Get Your Front Line to Care About Your Bottom Line.* Dearborn Trade Publishing, Chicago, IL, 2005.

Cornacchione KS, Forrest I, Harmon C, Hicks S, McLeay KL, Molas G, et al: *Revised MSICU Self-Scheduling Guidelines.* Self-Scheduling Committee Meeting, Morton Plant Hospital MSICU, Clearwater, FL, Feb. 2003.

George ML: *Lean Six Sigma for Service.* McGraw-Hill, New York, NY, 2003.

Gitlow H, Levine D: *Six Sigma for Green Belts and Champions: Foundations, DMAIC Tools,* *Cases, and Certification.* Pearson Prentice Hall, Upper Saddle River, NJ, 2005.

Jacobson J, Johnson M: Lean and Six Sigma: Not for Amateurs. *Lab Medicine* 2006: 37(3); 160-165.

Levoy B: *222 Secrets of Hiring, Managing, and Retaining Great Employees in Healthcare* Practices. Jones & Bartlett Sudbury, MA, 2007.

Lighter D: *Advanced Performance Improvement in Healthcare: Principles and Methods.* Jones & Bartlett Sudbury, MA, 2009.

Pande P, Neuman R, Cavanagh RR: *The Six Sigma Way Team Fieldbook: An Implementation Guide for Process Improvement Teams.* McGraw-Hill, New York, NY, 2002.

INTERNET RESOURCES

Baeyens T: *The State of Workflow.* Theserverside. com, May, 2004
http://www.theserverside.com/news/1365159/The-State-of-Workflow

Curious Cat Management Improvement Library–Dictionary. PDSA, PDCA, Deming Cycle, Shewhart Cycle. Curious Cat, 1996–2009
http://curiouscat.com/management/pdsa.cfm

Hospital Management: *Free Guide: Five Steps to Advance Quality Care Through Optimal Staffing.* Kronos, 2011
http://www.kronos.com

Prudent Practices in the Laboratory Handling and Disposal of Chemicals
http://www.nap.edu/readingroom/books/prudent

Six Sigma—What Is Six Sigma? iSix Sigma, 2000–2010
http://www.isixsigma.com/sixsigma/six_sigma.asp

Workflow Patterns Initiative, 2010
http://www.workflowpatterns.com

Laboratory Information Systems: Flexibility Is the Key to Modernization

Jane R. Semler, MS, MT(ASCP)

OBJECTIVES

Following successful completion of this chapter, the learner will be able to:

1. Describe the relationship between a laboratory information system and a computer network.
2. Describe the components of a computer terminal.
3. Describe the relationship between a laboratory information system and interface software.

4. Describe the relationship between discrete information stored in definition tables and how this information can be extracted into a report for use in patient care.
5. Describe the role of the electronic medical record in disease surveillance.
6. Describe the relationship between the laboratory information system and the hospital information system.
7. Give an example of how these data management systems can be used in decision making within the laboratory.
8. Give an example of increased workflow efficiency using electronic data management.
9. Give an example for employing the laboratory information system to improve quality.
10. Describe lean data management and how this concept relates to the implementation of a laboratory information system.
11. State the steps in acquiring a new laboratory information system.
12. Describe how data security impacts the laboratory.

KEY TERMS

Central Processing Unit (CPU)
Computer Network
Definition Tables
Disc Array
Electronic Health Record (EHR)
Electronic Medical Record (EMR)
Health Information Exchange (HIE)
Health Level 7 International (HL7)
Hospital Information System (HIS)
Laboratory Information System (LIS)

Lean Data Management
Local Area Network (LAN)
Mainframe Computer
Random Access Memory (RAM)
Redundancy
Request for Proposal (RFP)
Router
Standard Operating Procedures
  (SOPs)
Wide Area Network (WAN)

Case Study — Laboratory Information Systems

You are the manager of a clinical laboratory that serves the hospital in which it is housed, as well as a multispecialty clinic and more than 50 area long-term care facilities. Together, your laboratory serves approximately 8,000 patient beds, several physician practices, one research institution, and three food service industries in a large metropolitan area. Total yearly volume is about 250,000 tests. Your laboratory and its affiliates have been using the same laboratory information system for approximately 20 years. Three in-house computer specialists have been able to modify the current system to meet the changing needs of your facility. However, in the past year, two of these computer specialists have retired and the software provider is exiting the marketplace. Clearly, your laboratory will have to select a new laboratory information system. You are assigned the task of selecting and implementing a new system.

Issues and Questions to Consider:

1. *What tools will you use to assess the data management needs of your laboratory?*

2. *How will you ensure that the most important issue for your laboratory—flexibility—is addressed in the new system?*

3. *How will you facilitate the transition from the current system to the new one?*

4. *What specific components of the old system will you want to retain in the new system, in order to facilitate the transition?*

INTRODUCTION

In the age of laboratory and medical center restructuring, data management requires a high level of flexibility from a **laboratory information system (LIS)**. Increasingly, clinical laboratories are affiliated with research facilities, institutions involved in clinical trials, inpatient facilities, outpatient collection centers, and a network of hospitals. Bi-directional data management using the appropriate LIS is critical to maintaining these relationships in a cost-efficient manner. No longer are laboratory managers able to merely select a LIS from available prepackaged systems, and train staff in its use. Medical laboratory scientists must focus first on selecting a system that can be adapted to meet the ever-changing needs of a diagnostic center. They must be active participants in structuring the test parameters within the LIS. Laboratorians must continually work to customize the system according to changes in workflow and organization structure. Finally, laboratorians are responsible for maintaining the integrity of the data generated as it is transmitted to clients in-house or across regions, states, and countries. This chapter will provide a brief overview of the components of a laboratory information system, followed by a detailed discussion of the efficient application of this software.

SYSTEM COMPONENTS

All computer systems are composed of hardware, software, and tools for data entry and retrieval. A laboratory information system is a class of software used to handle information produced from laboratory testing. As such, all laboratory information systems function within the framework of a computer network.

Software and Networks

Computer networks are groups of connected computers, which share data by employing a standard set of specifications for the data transmitted. All computers within a network run the same software programs, which provide instructions for data management and manipulation. These networks can be connected by wires or through radio frequency (wireless), and are referred to as either a **local area network (LAN)**, indicating a geographically small area, or a **wide area network (WAN)**, indicating a large geographic area. **Routers** connect area networks to national networks that make up the Internet, or World Wide Web. An advantage of networks, is that they allow all connected computers to operate the same application software simultaneously. In the hospital setting, this allows nursing staff on patient floors to view test results, physicians to order tests from their offices, and technologists in the laboratory to enter patient results on the same patient. In an even broader example, physicians and nurses in an affiliated long-term care center can request tests; while technologists in the central lab facility enter results; and technologists at a reference lab enter newly received specimens. In each of the preceding examples, all access can occur simultaneously.

Hardware

All laboratory information systems function through computer terminals within each section of the laboratory. A computer consists of a **central processing unit (CPU)** (memory for storing data), and a system for entering and retrieving data. Data that is processed, or are waiting to be processed by the CPU, are stored in **random access memory (RAM)**. RAM has a very fast transfer rate, allowing rapid access to stored data. Data to be stored for long-term use is copied from the RAM to either an internal hard drive (magnetized metal discs), or to an external **disc array**, which consists of several linked hard discs. Long-term storage memory has a slower transfer rate but can accommodate large amounts of data. The CPU and RAM are mounted onto a motherboard that provides circuits for communication between computer components and connections for external devices, necessary for data input and output. These connections are standardized, and may be either a Universal Serial Bus (USB) or Firewire (IEEE 394) connection. Data entry and retrieval is accomplished through a keyboard, mouse, monitor, and printer.

In a hospital, individual computers operating data management systems within discrete areas, such as the laboratory, pathology, emergency room and pharmacy, are networked together and connected to a server, which processes data from each area. Servers from these areas are connected via an interface engine to the hospital **mainframe computer**, forming the **hospital information system (HIS)**. Computers functioning as servers and mainframes are constructed for durability and high volume data storage. They have **redundancy** of processors and other components so that downtime is minimized. In this type of networked hospital information system, individual, or embedded, computer systems can communicate with one another and can be replaced without loss of data or interruption to the other computers. Figure 17-1 illustrates a healthcare information system network.

Interface Software

Interface software allows communication between servers for different data management systems and between laboratory instruments and the LIS software. Interfaces also allow the hospital information system to communicate with off-site affiliates' data management software via the internet. Interfacing may be accomplished through software imbedded in the LIS or through a dedicated computer known as an interface engine. Often, the latter is required to manage the large volume of data transmitted by increasingly automated methods in laboratory testing. As medical centers increase their reach through satellite laboratories, outpatient collection centers, long-term care facilities, and regional reference laboratories, data management systems must be customized to accommodate these complex networks. For this reason, flexible interfaces are an important consideration when evaluating laboratory information systems.

Definition Tables

LIS software is structured around **definition tables** which contain the data entered by laboratorians, as well as other tables which manage technologist access, provide normal values, and record quality control data. Definition tables are probably the most apparent part of the LIS to laboratorians. The ease of use of any LIS is determined by the structure and completeness of these tables. Definition tables are essentially spreadsheets which are defined or customized by the laboratory. For example, a definition table may consist of the names of all the tests that could be ordered on a sputum sample. Another table may contain the reference ranges for these tests, while yet another table may provide possible

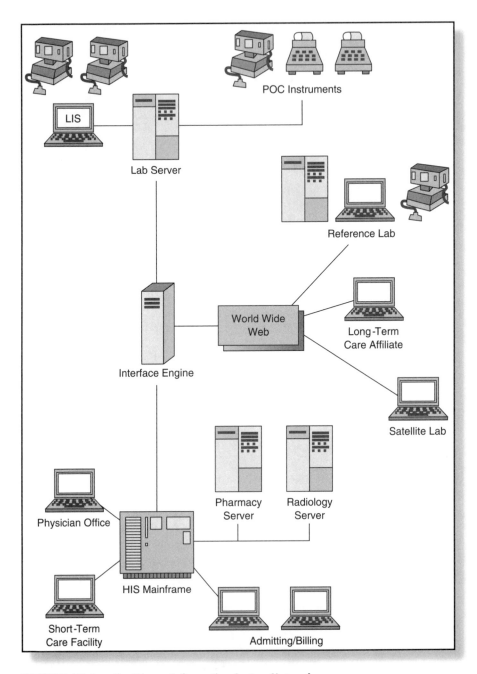

POC Instruments

LIS

Lab Server

Reference Lab

World Wide Web

Long-Term Care Affiliate

Interface Engine

Satellite Lab

Pharmacy Server

Radiology Server

Physician Office

HIS Mainframe

Short-Term Care Facility

Admitting/Billing

FIGURE 17-1.   **Healthcare Information System Network**

interpretations for result values. Other definition tables would contain patient information such as name and identification number. A table of users with assigned security access would also be required. Definition tables are organized into modules for each laboratory section and must be customized to meet the testing needs of each area. Figure 17-2 presents a sample module for the microbiology section.

Definition tables must contain at least one data item that is also present on another table. In this manner, definition tables are linked together; allowing data from different tables to be extracted and recombined into reports for a variety of uses by all members of the healthcare team. Figure 17-3 shows an example of data sets which are linked by matching data tables. During implementation of a new LIS, a system manager should be assigned to coordinate the development of definition tables. It is easy to see how the components of a laboratory information system function as part of the hospital information system to accomplish efficient transmission of patient test data. Data from the LIS can also be incorporated into the patient's electronic medical record, with the goal of employing electronic data management to improve laboratory efficiency, and reduce errors in patient care.

THE ELECTRONIC MEDICAL RECORD

The **electronic medical record (EMR)**, also referred to as the **electronic health record (EHR)**, is essentially an electronic form of the patient medical record. It contains information covering every aspect of patient care: demographics, physician notes on patient presentation and treatment progress, current and past prescriptions and other medications, vital signs, medical history, laboratory and pathology reports, radiology reports, and immunization records. Figure 17-4 shows an example of some of the healthcare entities whose data are incorporated into this record. This list will likely continue to expand as medical centers streamline laboratory testing to meet the increasing demands of declining budgets coupled with increased test volume and complexity. The electronic medical record operates under the **Health Level Seven International (HL7)** standards for compatibility of health information systems. HL7 is used in more than 55 countries, with the goal of creating widely used standards for healthcare data management. The EMR serves many functions including facilitating transportation of patient data to various health related service providers, enhancing communication regarding patient care, and aiding in administrative processing. Additionally, the EMR is becoming increasingly valuable to public health agencies to aid in disease reporting and statistical analyses. Table 17-1 lists the functions of the EMR.

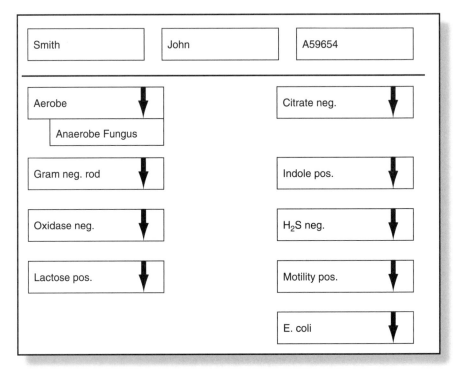

FIGURE 17-2.   **Example of LIS Module for Microbiology Section**

Note: pos = positive; neg = negative; H$_2$S = hydrogen sulfide.

Application to Public Health

With the increase in media and public attention to disease surveillance, the need for more rapid and accurate reporting of infectious diseases is evident. Concurrent shift toward the electronic medical record over paper records is filling this need. Until recently, public health departments have relied on physician or laboratory initiated manual report submission to track reportable diseases and outbreaks. Incomplete and slow reporting plagued this system, and resulted in inaccurate and delayed reporting to the public. Many public health labs still rely on this type of reporting. However, states are slowly switching to electronic reporting through direct networking with patient electronic medical records. This process can be viewed from the perspective of the clinical laboratory, which made similar transition years ago in switching to electronic reporting of patient results through the LIS. In the same way, the LIS is interfaced with the HIS and affiliate organizations via the internet; and public health departments are using interface software to access electronic medical records. Just as a decrease in laboratory reporting errors and shortened turnaround time resulted from the implementation of the LIS, public health labs hope to see

Admission Data

Patient ID#	Last Name	First Name	Age	Sex
A59643	Jones	Mary	59	F
A32976	Allen	Michael	37	M

Lab Test Requisition Data

Requisition#	Patient ID#	Test Name	Ordering Physician	Date
X593	A59643	Aerobic culture	Young, M	4/27/2010
X594	A32976	Glucose (fasting)	Sperry, J	4/27/2010

Lab Result Data

Requisition#	Test Result
X593	E. coli
X594	132 mg/dL

Reference Range Data

Test Name	Adult Male	Adult Female	Pediatric	Geriatric	Units
Aerobic culture	No growth/ normal flora	No growth/ normal flora	No growth/ normal flora	No growth/ normal flora	N/A
Glucose (fasting)	80-100	80-100	80-100	80-100	mg/dL

FIGURE 17-3.   Data Reports
Note: Matching data which link each data set are highlighted.

more accurate and timely reporting of disease outbreaks. Reports on the efficacy of employing the EMR in disease surveillance are on the rise and the results have generally been positive. One key factor in this outcome is that the reports contained in the EMR are coming directly from the clinical laboratory, rather than from direct care providers. Since laboratorians are already in the practice of generating standardized and accurate reports, it follows that use of these reports by public health agencies will improve overall reporting on public health

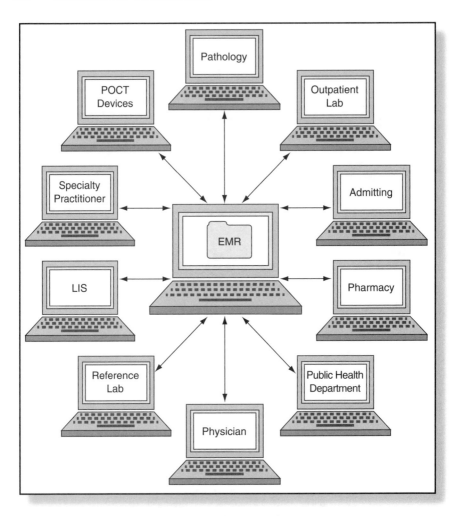

FIGURE 17-4. Input to Electronic Medical Record

threats. In fact, preliminary studies have shown that automatic reporting by laboratories is done much more frequently than spontaneous manual reporting by physicians. While laboratory reporting may lack the case data that can be provided by the practitioner, interfacing with the EMR allows further investigation of patient presentation and history. The use of integrating laboratory test data into the patient electronic medical record provides another example of the need for flexibility in LIS software.

Hospital Based Records

As demonstrated by the above discussion of disease surveillance, laboratory information systems must now communicate with many other information systems

TABLE 17-1. Functions of the Electronic Medical Record

- Maintain patient records
- Analyze patient demographics
- Compile data on errors in patient care
- Manage patient medications
- Organize patient history
- Manage physician notes
- Manage external reports from laboratory, radiology, physical therapy, etc.
- Record care plans and monitor progress
- Record patient instructions and patient mediated care plans
- Rapid and automatic reporting of infectious disease to public health agencies
- Tracking infectious diseases and nosocomial infections

both in house and at offsite facilities. Reports must be carefully standardized to maximize ease of data transfer and interpretation. Additionally, the electronic medical record (EMR) is quickly becoming the standard for patient recordkeeping. As laboratorians, we must adjust to having test results included in these patient records rather than separated by a standalone LIS. The laboratory's goal is to ensure that clinicians who read these reports will not misinterpret them due to poor report formatting or content. We must remember that the electronic laboratory report will include not only results from the in-house lab but must also integrate reports from any reference labs or specialty testing facilities that are contracted by the facility. Consistency in report formatting and result generation is key to producing a report that is accurately interpreted. Increasingly, the need to integrate electronic data management systems into the EMR is met by an additional piece of software known as the **health information exchange (HIE)** hub. This technology provides an additional interface which allows users to view a consolidated electronic medical record including all lab and pathology test results. The following scenario illustrates how laboratory professionals can benefit from implementation of electronic medical records.

Jacob Mosley, MS, MT(ASCP) at Memorial Hospital in Charleston, West Virginia, is reviewing cases for release in the LIS. He notices that patient (X) has a cerebrospinal fluid culture that is pending release (positive for N. meningitis); and also, a positive blood culture which is still in progress. He knows that all positive blood culture bottles are sent to a reference lab for identification. Checking the LIS, which is interfaced with the reference lab, he notes that this result is still incomplete. Mosley then checks the HIS to see if patient X is in-house or at one of the several regional medical centers with which Memorial is affiliated. Noticing that the location for patient X is listed as "outpatient," Mosley becomes concerned, and considers placing a call to the patient's physician due to the serious nature of these results. However, remembering that the hospital has recently transitioned to the electronic medical record, Mosley checks this information and realizes that patient X is a resident at one of the long-term care facilities affiliated with Memorial Hospital. Satisfied that this patient is being properly cared for as an inpatient at this facility, Mosley releases the CSF culture result.Within the hour, the West Virginia Bureau for Public Health receives a report of the invasive Meningococcal infection, and phones the patient's physician to advise her on the protocol for isolating infected patients.

This case illustrates how the laboratory can use information provided to the LIS from the HIS, and the EMR when making decisions regarding patient results. Ultimately, the integration of these information systems will improve the quality of patient care, by allowing all healthcare professionals to access a greater amount of patient information than was possible with paper records.

IMPROVED LABORATORY EFFICIENCY AND REDUCING ERRORS THROUGH THE LIS

In addition to providing healthcare workers with a broader scope of patient information, electronic data management will also result in a more rapid turnaround time for result reporting, and a decrease in clerical errors which result when manual data management is employed. Many patients have noticed that physicians no longer take notes on a paper chart, but rather bring a laptop into the patient examination room. The information gathered from the patient exam is entered directly into the electronic medical record, reducing the possibility of lost or erroneously recorded information. Physicians can order laboratory tests from the exam room, and instruct patients on where to go for the outpatient testing. This process minimizes errors such as ordering tests for the wrong patient. When testing is completed, results are easily accessed by the physician in his practice. Then the physician can prescribe treatment or request that the patient return for a follow-up visit. Electronic data management offers a quicker turnaround time, and reduces errors associated with filing faxed paper reports. This all results in an improved patient outcome. Medical centers that do not offer LIS interfacing with various data management systems are at a disadvantage in recruiting physician clients. With the development of HL7 standards, physicians expect to easily access all reports for their patients; whether the physician is in their office, doing hospital rounds, or on-call from their home. Patients realize the impact of laboratory information systems as well. Although patients may not be aware of the complexities of data management in the laboratory, they are acutely aware of test turnaround time, and accurate and timely transmission of laboratory results to their physician. In order for medical centers to compete on the regional and national level, they must employ flexible data management systems capable of interfacing with a variety of healthcare information systems. Clinical laboratory data usually makes up the largest portion of the electronic medical record, underscoring the importance of the LIS in the healthcare marketplace.

Information Processing and Workflow

If the goal of implementing a new LIS is to improve efficiency, workflow within the laboratory must be considered when evaluating LIS software. Maximizing laboratory efficiency is increasingly important in light of the increasing shortage of medical laboratory scientists, demand for more rapid turnaround time, and increasing regulatory requirements. The LIS is one way to increase this efficiency by incorporating interfaces for instruments and external electronic data management systems which will streamline laboratory workflow. Further, the LIS allows for easy scalability as test volume increases. Finally, laboratory information systems provide automation for some of the workflow steps, freeing valuable technologist time for more vital steps, such as review of critical result values.

Since multiple instruments in all sections of the laboratory will be interfaced with the LIS, it is important to consider the movement of specimens and test requests through the laboratory as a model for structuring the LIS. Figure 17-5 is a simple workflow diagram, which illustrates the increased efficiency of instrument interfacing with a LIS.

Quality Initiatives

Quality initiatives continue to be of interest to laboratory managers and hospital administrators. Increased quality (and decreased error) translates into increased efficiency and profit. Increased quality often means increased patient satisfaction, and a positive reputation for the facility. Because of these factors, laboratorians continually strive to improve quality. Most sources of laboratory error are either pre-analytical or post-analytical. Analytical errors are less common due to well-trained laboratory staff, and improvements in laboratory instrumentation and automation. Common pre-analytical errors include incorrect specimen labeling and incorrect manual entry of information onto paper forms. A common post-analytical error is incorrectly reporting results from one patient on a different patient with a similar name or identification number. With the exception of incorrect specimen labeling, these errors can be virtually eliminated through the use of an interfaced LIS. Communication with the electronic medical record further reduces pre- and post-analytical errors.

One function of the LIS, that should be utilized more often, is generating quality control reports. Although different laboratory information systems offer diverse reporting options, most can be set up to generate a variety of reports useful in correcting pre- and post-analytical errors. As an example, a laboratory manager may want a report to identify errors in result reporting. The lab manager can create a definition table for "amended reports," indicating that a correction was issued to rectify a previously erroneous result. The manager can then set the LIS to search daily, or weekly, for reports that have been amended; and can monitor these errors to discern details, such as what was reported incorrectly and for what reason. LIS searches can be set up to further identify recurring patterns; such as those occurring with a particular analytical method, or during a particular time of day. The LIS can even assist managers with the problem of incorrect specimen labeling. Consider a LIS "test" entry called "Patient Issue:" specimen processing technicians could use this test to enter problems related to specimen collection, such as incorrect or missing wrist identification band, hemolyzed sample, IV line, etc. By monitoring this test log, the laboratory manager can recognize recurring problems, and work with the phlebotomy staff to resolve these issues.

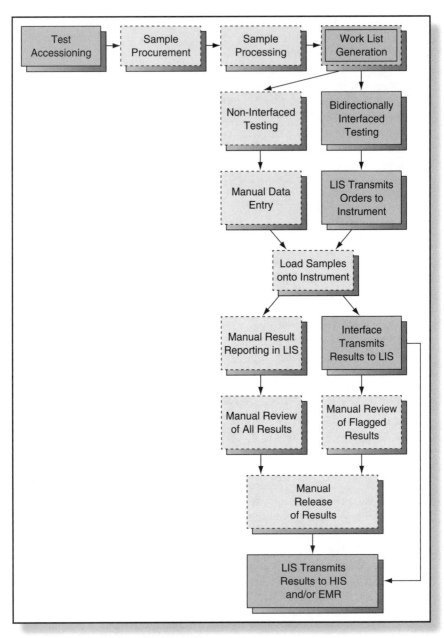

FIGURE 17-5.   **Workflow Diagram**

Note: Manual steps are represented by dashed boxes, and solid boxes represent electronic steps.

Lean Data Management

Another improvement to laboratory operations, made possible through implementation of a functional LIS, is **lean data management**. Lean management refers to a generic idea of improving efficiency through eliminating wasteful practices. In a tangible product-based operation, wasteful practices are easy to detect; but when the product is data, waste is more difficult to define. Consider the amount of technologist time spent in sending out amended reports for errors in patient results caused by manual data entry. Also consider the time spent by physicians searching for reports that are not visible in the electronic medical record, and must be accessed by a computer within the hospital information system. Consider the time a phlebotomist spends consulting with the nursing and laboratory staff to determine the time a specimen was collected when no electronic record is available, and the tube is not labeled with this information. In each of these instances, and many others, waste is present. Lean data management cannot only assist in identifying this waste, but can prevent it, resulting in more efficient laboratory operations, higher quality patient care, and a positive bottom line. The key principles in lean data management are: value, flow, pull, and improvement. Table 17-2 lists the principles of lean data management.

The concept of value in data management means that the LIS must support the work of the laboratory. All of the steps involved in data management must, ultimately, produce a better quality product for the end user, typically another member of the healthcare team. A better quality data product is one that is more accurate, timely, and easily interpreted. The flow principle refers to the many steps involved in data management. Refer to the data tables in Figure 17-3 to see how data from one part of the LIS flows into another table and will ultimately form the report that is part of the electronic medical record. It is rare in data management to find a single "flow;" rather, most processes are complex and depend on many steps to produce a complete product (data report).

The pull principle of lean data management mandates that manufacturers of laboratory information systems (or any data management system) should only design and produce systems that are desirable to consumers during the appropriate time period. Thus, the "pull" which drives development of new functions and processes comes from user demand, eliminating wasteful implementation and

TABLE 17-2. Principles of Lean Data Management

- Value
- Flow
- Pull
- Improvement

training for products that are not needed. In order to accomplish the goals of lean data management, regular review by laboratory staff and vendors is necessary to keep pace with changes in workflow, instrumentation, regulations, and facility agreements. Thus, "Continuous Improvement" is the final component in lean data management.

LIS ACQUISITION

Acquiring and implementing a new laboratory information system is a huge process which takes several months to a year or more to complete. This is often a stressful time for laboratorians as they transition from the old, comfortable LIS to a new and more complex, albeit more functional system. Due to the inconvenience and risk in changing to a new LIS, most laboratories make the switch only every 10–20 years. Typical reasons for seeking a new LIS include: outgrowing the capabilities of the current system; increased need for flexibility that cannot be accommodated through an older system; termination of support for the old system; and a medical center merger which requires a change to a common LIS. There are several steps in completing the process of LIS acquisition; from choosing a system, to ensuring the security of patient data. Table 17-3 lists the steps in LIS acquisition.

Define System Requirements

This step involves construction of a workflow diagram and consideration of the data management requirements for each step in the workflow. Laboratory managers should assemble a selection team of lead technologists who can provide insight into any particular needs or constraints in their section. Of particular concern are instrument interfaces and workload, deficiencies in the current system, need for customization, and budget.

TABLE 17-3.   Steps in LIS Acquisition

- Define system Requirements
- Request Bids
- Request Demonstrations
- Assign Staffing Roles
- Implementation
- Standard Operating Procedures
- Data Security
- Data Retention

Request Bids

Laboratory managers and the LIS selection team evaluate several vendors with systems that may meet the requirements detailed in the acquisition process. Laboratories may solicit bids from various vendors using a **Request for Proposal (RFP)**. This document includes specific requirements and questions concerning each vendor's product capabilities. Vendors may include in their bids proposed solutions to certain problems outlined in the RFP. It is important to ask whether these solutions are currently in use in other laboratories or whether they would need to be developed and, if this is the case, whether development costs are included in the bid.

Request Demonstrations

Laboratory managers will want to see the top two to four products in action before making a decision. This may be in the form of an in-house demonstration, or a visit to other facilities currently using the LIS, or both. The laboratory manager will also contact other sites using the LIS to ascertain details such as: how the implementation process was handled; whether vendor support was available and timely; the type of pitfalls encountered; and the overall satisfaction with the product. Generally, vendors will provide a list of sites currently using their LIS, but this list may include only "satisfied" customers. The manager may want to ask for a complete list of users in order to get a more accurate assessment.

Assign Staffing Roles

Once a LIS is selected, the laboratory manager should devise a plan to allocate technologists' time during training and implementation of the new system. A major challenge during the transition from old to new software is proper staffing to maintain regular laboratory operations. Additional staff may be required to handle testing responsibilities, while other laboratorians are in training. Managers should also expect data management tasks to take longer during the transition period, until staff become accustomed to the new system. The additional staff should be able to prevent any serious delays in turnaround time. Special roles during implementation include the system manager, who will coordinate development of definition tables, receive input from other laboratory staff, and work with the LIS vendor to resolve any problems. Additionally, each lab section should designate a "super user," who will receive extra training and will coordinate LIS implementation within his or her section. This individual should also compile a list of problems which need to be resolved by the system manager or vendor. The staff designated as super users will be virtually unavailable for regular laboratory duties during the implementation period.

Implementation

This is the process of putting the new LIS into use. Although seemingly simple, there are several considerations before changing to the new LIS. First, it is prudent to consider the problems likely to occur as the lab switches to the new LIS. There will be some downtime, increased turnaround time for most tests, increased technologist frustration, and time lost to training and re-training. Plans should be made to accommodate as many of these "planned" risks as possible because other problems will certainly arise that had not been previously considered. Second, there is usually a period of system duplication during which the new system is "tested" for performance; and if problems arise, patient testing can be handled by the old LIS. Third, adequate training must also be conducted in an organized manner. All laboratorians will be trained in the use of the new system; and this will necessitate restructuring shifts and possibly requiring overtime pay, in order to ensure that all laboratory operations are adequately staffed during the training process. Vendors may be contracted to provide various forms of support to laboratory staff during and after implementation. This support should be clearly defined in terms of scope and cost in the bid, so that no questions arise after the system is implemented, should re-training be required. The specific day and time when the new LIS is officially implemented for routine use is referred to as the "Go-live" date. This date should be carefully chosen. For example, a laboratory manager may wish to avoid the early morning when test volume is at its peak. Conversely, the decision may be made that this is the opportune time to make the switch, because the LIS will be fully tested by the high test volume, and the most experienced staff will likely be present. A backup plan should be in place to define the circumstances under which implementation would be halted, and the lab would return to the old LIS should the new LIS fail. Extra staff will be needed during implementation to overcome the loss of productivity as staff adjust to the new LIS.

Standard Operating Procedures

Changes in protocol related to the new LIS will require evaluation and updating of the laboratory **standard operating procedures (SOPs).** These procedures will be useful in training staff to use the new system. Additionally, procedures should be in place to handle required maintenance of the LIS as well as unscheduled downtime. Scheduled maintenance should be carried out at times that are least disruptive to laboratory operations. Scheduled maintenance includes items listed in Table 17-4. Proper maintenance and updating of hardware and software components will minimize the occurrence of unplanned downtime; however, unforeseen downtime will occur due to natural disasters, extended power interruption, or system malfunction. During periods of LIS unavailability, manual record keeping will be required. When the LIS regains function, all manual records must be entered into the LIS.

Data Security

Whenever electronic data management is employed, care must be taken to guard against inappropriate release of information, access by unauthorized individuals

TABLE 17-4.   Scheduled Maintenance

- Hardware repair or replacement
- Software updates
- Backup of data
- Restoration of lost data
- Data retrieval
- Security updates

or groups, and excessive system unavailability. In the context of healthcare, these security breaches are even more significant. Federal regulations, under the Health Insurance Portability and Accountability Act (HIPAA), mandate that patient health records must be kept confidential. Security breaches, whether apparent or actual, undermine patient confidence. Furthermore, system downtime causes significant disruption to patient care, resulting in decreased patient satisfaction. Most security failures inadvertently occur through actions by data management system users. This inappropriate disclosure may be intentional or unintentional, and may follow an attempt by a patient or other individual to deceptively gain access to information. Whatever the circumstances, the consequences of security breaches are the same and users must always strive to avoid these costly disruptions. Laboratory information systems maintain an electronic record of user actions so it is easy to discern where a breach has occurred. Other systems in place within LIS software help to maintain data security and minimize downtime. These include: secure locations for system hardware which are at lower risk for damage by fire or flood; password protected access by registered users only; antivirus/malware software; and good computing practice which includes regular data backups to a secure, off-site location. In general, it is best to restrict user access to job-related LIS functions and to limit the number of users authorized to modify the LIS database.

Data Retention

Archives of all laboratory data must be kept for a period of time determined by applicable regulatory agencies and facility protocol. These archives are typically stored on tape cartridges/external hard drives or backup computers. Care must be taken to ensure that data can be retrieved when adopting a new LIS.

SUMMARY

Selection and successful implementation of a laboratory information system requires advanced planning and detailed customization. This is necessary to achieve the flexibility needed to accommodate the complex networks in which medical centers operate. Laboratory information systems must interface efficiently with the hospital information system and electronic medical record to facilitate efficient, accurate, and cost-effective patient care.

SUMMARY CHART:
Important Points to Remember

- ➤ Flexibility is the key to an efficient laboratory information system.
- ➤ A laboratory information system is a class of software used to handle information produced from laboratory testing.
- ➤ Laboratory information systems function within a system of networked computers.
- ➤ Interface software allows communication between instruments, the LIS, and other data management systems, including the electronic medical record.
- ➤ Definition tables are spreadsheets containing data generated in all aspects of patient care.
- ➤ The electronic medical record facilitates transfer of patient information to health care providers.
- ➤ Use of a LIS will result in cost and time savings over manual paper reporting.
- ➤ Use of a LIS will result in fewer pre- and post-analytical errors when compared to manual paper recording.
- ➤ A LIS can be used to assess quality assurance deficiencies.
- ➤ Acquiring a LIS requires careful consideration and will take many months to complete.

SUGGESTED PROBLEM-BASED LEARNING ACTIVITIES

Chapter 17: Laboratory Information Systems: Flexibility Is the Key to Modernization

Instructions: Use Internet resources, books, articles, colleagues, etc., to present solutions to the problems listed below. There is no one correct solution to any problem, and these should provide excellent discussion topics.

Note to Instructor: Students in class may be divided into groups and given the problem-based learning activity to discuss and solve. Once the group has reached consensus as to a solution, the group may present it to the other students in the class. This activity will provide all students with information regarding solutions to the problem.

Problem #1

Research LIS vendors and prepare a chart detailing the pro's and con's of each system. How would you decide which system to choose?

Problem #2

Pathology staff at your medical center are reluctant to implement an electronic medical record. As laboratory manager, explain how you would work with other members of the health care team to present the pro's and con's of making the switch from paper medical records. Would your group ultimately recommend to keep using paper medical records, or to implement the EMR?

Problem #3

Suppose your laboratory is experiencing a high percentage of post-analytical errors related to reporting, releasing, and/or interpreting patient results. Suggest methods for elucidating where these errors are occurring and how to change standard operating procedures to decrease the number of errors in the future.

BIBLIOGRAPHY

Aller RD: Pathology's Contributions to Disease Surveillance: Sending Our Data to Public Health Officials and Encouraging Our Clinical Colleagues to Do So. *Arch Pathol Lab Med* 2009: 133; 926-932.

Bersch C, DiRamio D: *Lab's HIE Solution Connects LIS to EMR and HIS.* MLO-Online, 2009.

Bordowitz R: Electronic Health Records: A Primer. *LabMedicine* 2008: 39(5);301-306.

Hicks BJ: Lean Information Management: Understanding and Eliminating Waste. *International J of Information Management* 2007: 27; 233-249.

Jackson BR, Harrison JH: Clinical Laboratory Informatics. In Burtis CA, Ashwood ER, Bruns DE: *Tietz Fundamentals of Clinical Chemistry.* Elsevier-Mosby-Saunders, St. Louis, MO, 2008.

Lifshitz MS, et al: Clinical Laboratory Informatics. In McPherson RA: *Henry's Clinical Diagnosis and Management by Laboratory Methods,* ed 22. Elsevier-Mosby-Saunders, Philadelphia, PA, 2012.

Overhage MJ: A Comparison of the Completeness and Timeliness of Automated Electronic Laboratory Reporting and Spontaneous Reporting of Notifiable Conditions. *American J of Public Health* 2008: 98(2); 344-350.

Ovretveit J, et al: Implementation of Electronic Medical Records in Hospitals: Two Case Studies. *Health Policy* 2007: 84; 181-190.

Pantanowitz L, et al: Laboratory Reports in the Electronic Medical Record. *LabMedicine* 2007: 38(6); 339-340.

Welder AM, et al: *Lab Replaces Homegrown Laboratory Information System.* MLO-Online, 2008.

Wooster G: *An LIS Supports Quality Initiatives.* MLO-Online, 2008.

INTERNET RESOURCES

Health Level Seven International (HL7)
http://www.hl7.org

Interactive Laboratory Information Management System (LIMS) Magazine, Laboratory Informatics Institute, Inc.
http://www.limsfinder.com

Lab InfoTech Summit
http://www.labinfotech.org

LIS and LIMS Resource, Patent Safe Electronic Lab Notebook, Amphora Research Systems
http://amphora-research.com

The Office of the National Coordinator for Health Information Technology. U.S. Department of Health & Human Services, 2011
http://healthit.hhs.gov/portal/server.pt/community/healthit_hhs_gov_home/1204

LIS Vendor Websites

Antek Healthware, LLC.
http://www.antekhealthware.com

CIMScan—Wireless Monitoring System, CIMTechniques, Inc.
http://www.cimtechniques.com

CLIN1—Clinical Software Solutions
http://clin1.net

Data Innovations Middleware Solutions: Instrument Manager™, Data Innovations, Inc.
http://www.datainnovations.com/Products/InstrumentManagertrade/tabid/53/Default.aspx

Fletcher-Flora Health Care Systems, Inc.
http://www.fletcher-flora.com/clinics-and-reference-labs.html

Michael E. Kurtz, MS, MBA
Susan L. Conforti, EdD, MT(ASCP)SBB

CHAPTER OUTLINE

OBJECTIVES

Following successful completion of this chapter, the learner will be able to:

1. Define marketing and explain its role in the clinical laboratory.
2. List the elements of the marketing mix.
3. Identify and explain the elements of the marketing environment.
4. Identify steps in the marketing analysis process.
5. Analyze effective business strategies for a laboratory operation.
6. Develop and implement a marketing plan.
7. Describe the regulatory restrictions on marketing in the health care setting.

KEY TERMS

Five Forces Analysis	Marketing Mix
Market Analysis	Marketing Plan
Market Demand	Marketing Research
Market Segmentation	Niching
Marketing	SWOT Analysis
Marketing Concept	Telehealth
Marketing Environment	Telemedicine

Case Study   Marketing Concepts

Laboratory Services, LLC, is a provider of specialty laboratory services to the medical, diagnostic, and pharmaceutical industry. As a result of an aggressive local marketing campaign, the laboratory has experienced double-digit growth in each of the last 5 years. The rate of growth has begun to slow, and the number of potential new clients is limited. Your hospital administration expects a 15% increase in laboratory revenue during the next year. The laboratory manager and staff agree that there is excess capacity of labor and technology. The planning team decides to expand from a local laboratory operation to a national operation. As marketing manager you must develop a marketing plan to achieve the organizational goals.

Issues and Questions to Consider:

1. List possible causes of the market decline experienced by the laboratory.
2. What would you use to determine the root cause of the market decline?
3. What kind of pricing strategy would you use?
4. What promotional activities may assist you in reaching your goals?
5. What limitations must be considered?

INTRODUCTION

In this age of information, consumers of healthcare have exceptionally high expectations. If we are sick, we go to the doctor, expect him/her to make a diagnosis, and provide treatment. If the doctor cannot, we expect him/her to send us to a specialist that can determine a diagnosis. In addition, we want the full range of medical services available to us regardless of our ability to pay. Thus, the clinical laboratory is a far different place, as a result of the changes in the needs and expectations of patients and physicians. Driven by economic necessity and technologic advances, the physician demands a higher level of accuracy from laboratory tests, and better efficiency than in the past. Patients subjected to advertising, media blitzes, and the Internet, are more aware of laboratory capabilities, and are more demanding in their expectations.

The current healthcare market environment, including the regulatory environment, the development of large integrated delivery networks, and the advent of managed care organizations, has placed additional cost pressures on laboratories. The hospital laboratory, once a significant source of revenue for the institution, is now faced with consumers and physicians demanding higher quality, while the government is reimbursing laboratories less for Medicare patients. The large integrated delivery networks are increasingly demanding cost reductions; and managed care organizations are pressuring laboratories to lower fees for service.

Hospital laboratories that attempt to exist on inpatient revenues alone are doomed to a downward spiral of reducing staff and services. At the same time, physicians and patients are demanding more and better services. Because laboratories have a high fixed cost structure and are capital intensive, the result is operational losses. Faced with these pressures, laboratories have to increase revenues or face being downsized, out-sourced, or shutdown completely. In fact, many large integrated delivery networks have outsourced this function.To lower costs, hospital administrators are shortening the length of stay. As a result, more illnesses are being treated on an outpatient basis. Thus, the only source of increased testing volumes comes from outside the hospital.

Because of this new paradigm in healthcare, laboratory managers must be skilled practitioners in marketing and business planning. These skills can assist managers in increasing volume, controlling costs, and increasing profit. Managers with these skills can improve quality and add value, because they know how to provide superior service and develop innovative strategies.This chapter covers basic marketing concepts and explores ways to incorporate them into strategic business planning in the laboratory.

MARKETING CONCEPTS

Businesses today operate using different philosophies or tenets. What philosophy or tenet they choose may be directly related to their industry, market, or product. A business philosophy held by many modern companies is called the **marketing concept**. This philosophy holds as its central tenet the following: the key to achieving the goals of the organization consists of being more effective than the competition in satisfying the needs, wants, and demands of the customer. Thus, the primary focus of a market-oriented organization is the customer. Successful companies applying this marketing concept integrate customer needs into their marketing program, and increase profit by improving customer satisfaction. Every aspect of their operation has as its single purpose, value delivery to the customer. The structure of this type of organization would appear as a triangle with the customer at the top (Figure 18-1). This type of organization is exemplified in the mission statement of Southwest Airlines, "The mission of Southwest Airlines is dedication to the highest quality of Customer Service delivered with a sense of warmth, friendliness, individual pride, and Company Spirit."

In a marketing oriented laboratory, customers are represented at the top of an organizational chart represented by a triangle. All marketing decisions flow from the customer rather than the product or sales teams. Employees that directly interact with the customer are higher on the chart than upper management who may have no direct contact with the customer.

Another business philosophy is the **production concept**. According to this concept, customers will buy goods produced in adequate volume at a low enough price. An example of this is the Texas Instrument Company that sells calculators. The **sales concept** entails factory products sold by aggressive selling and promotion. These types of companies such as General Motors profit by selling high volumes of cars. They frequently use sales incentives such as rebates and premiums.

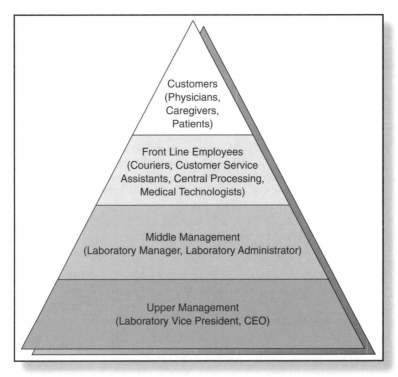

FIGURE 18-1.   Organizational Structure of a Marketing Oriented Laboratory Business

Marketing in a company employing the marketing concept can be defined as a process by which individuals and groups obtain what they want, through creating, offering, and exchanging products or services of value with others. All the activities, associated with providing the means by which buyers can purchase a product or service, and the process of inducing them to do so, are marketing activities. Even though marketing is a business function, as is financing, human resources, or research and development, it does not take place within the confines of a marketing department. Rather, it entails every activity a company does, from product conception until the product wears out, or is consumed. This exchange of goods and services for something of value takes place in a **market**. A market is a web of interactions among those who have commercial relationships or the potential for such relationships with other buyers and sellers of similar commodities.

All the potential customers sharing a particular need or want, who might be willing and able to exchange something of value to satisfy that need or want, make up a market. A market may be defined mathematically as $M = qnp$; where q equals the average quantity purchased, n equals the number of consumers, and p equals the average price paid for a product or service. A market does not belong to the company, but is external. Abundant markets exist: Californians, teenagers, homemakers, outdoorsman, women, teachers, train hobbyists, hospitals, and laboratories are all examples of markets. People over 50 years old make up one of the fastest growing markets. Markets exist for goods and services, for money and credit, for communication and technology services, and for information.

Market segmentation allows the marketing manager to break up markets into smaller, more manageable pieces. This is possible because occupants of the market have similar wants, needs, and demands. They also respond similarly to market stimuli, such as advertising and distribution. A plastic surgeon and a neurosurgeon are both surgeons; but the plastic surgeon's preferences may not be shared by the neurosurgeon. Teenagers and senior citizens both share a need for clothing; however, their preferences for certain styles may be quite different. Market segmentation is a legitimate business strategy used by companies to create a competitive advantage. Focusing on a specific subsection of a market is a strategy called **"niching."** For example, Saint Louis University Coagulation Consultants is a specialty laboratory that only provides testing for the diagnosis and management of patients with bleeding and thrombotic disorders. Another more common example is a teenager who is more likely to shop at Old Navy, rather than at Lord and Taylor's department store.

THE MARKETING MIX

The role of marketing in an organization is to achieve its strategic objective by deciding who will sell what, where, to whom, in what quantity, and how. The set of tools that the firm uses to pursue their marketing objectives is referred to as the **marketing mix**. This includes product, price, place, and promotion (Table 18-1).

TABLE 18-1.   The Marketing Mix

Product: *what the firm offers to the public for sale.* Includes product quality, brand, packaging, features or service options, delivery, training, warranty, repair and other value-added product or service options which would provide a competitive advantage to the firm.

Price: *the amount of money a customer pays for a product or service.* Pricing options include selling wholesale or retail, offering discounts, sales, and credit.

Place: *how and where the product is offered to the buying public.* Includes warehousing, distribution, and retail or wholesale outlets and the Internet.

Promotion: *the means by which a company communicates and promotes its products to its target market.* Includes sales and marketing personnel, advertising, public relations, direct marketing, telemarketing, and online marketing.

Product

Product is what the firm offers to the public for sale. This would include the product quality, brand, packaging, features, or service options. It also includes delivery, training, warranty, repair, and other value-added product or service options, which would provide a competitive advantage to the firm. Product or service is the cornerstone of the marketing mix. Companies using this marketing concept, view product as a solution to a customer's need. Different laboratories may emphasize different products. A specialty laboratory may only offer microbiology, coagulation, blood banking, or toxicology. Another may emphasize routine testing, requiring a fast turn-around-time. Still others may concentrate on services that provide interpretation of laboratory results and advice on the medical management of patients that receive laboratory testing.

Price

Critical to the marketing mix is **price**. This is the amount of money a customer pays, for a product or service. Pricing options include selling wholesale or retail, offering discounts, sales, and credit. Price is part of the total marketing package offered to the customer referred to as **value**. If a customer perceives the price as higher than the value received in purchasing the service or product, the customer will either buy a substitute product from another supplier, or will forego purchase of the product. Laboratories may offer discounts to client accounts because they do not incur the cost of billing the patient. The laboratory market environment today is almost totally cost-driven, and may dictate a pricing strategy based on matching the competition's price. Products or services that are purchased strictly on the basis of price are called commodities. As healthcare becomes more cost-driven, laboratory testing becomes viewed as a commodity or basic material or good, instead of something of higher value, by hospital administrators who search for low-cost solutions, with little consideration to the value of laboratory testing.

Pricing strategy may also be determined by the profit margin imposed on the laboratory by hospital administration. Other laboratories may determine price on a cost plus basis. They determine how much it costs to perform the test, and add a percentage to cover overhead expenses and profit. Using price as a competitive weapon is risky because it could lead to a price war. The purchase of a product or service may be value driven rather than price driven. A department store such as Neiman Marcus may offer the same quality product of another department store, but the name and personal service provide the perception of increased value to the customer who is willing to pay a higher price.

Place

Place is how and where the product is offered to the buying public. It is difficult to walk in any building and not encounter either a Coca-Cola or a Pepsi vending machine.

Most companies now offer their products via the Internet. Place also includes the use of marketing to make its product available to its customers. This comprises warehousing, distribution and retail, or wholesale outlets. Many hospital laboratories will choose to market only in their local area, whereas others may have regional, national, or even global market interests. Most large commercial laboratories have located phlebotomy stations in physician offices for the convenience of the patient, and some physician's offices have even placed laboratories in their office suites. Place includes how laboratory results are transmitted to the customers. Many laboratories have direct electronic or web-based computer links to their client's laboratory information systems (LIS), or physician office practice management systems. These links allow the electronic exchange of patient demographic information, test orders, and results between information systems. This benefits the client by eliminating duplicate and manual data entry, decreasing transcription errors and personnel time involved with reference laboratory/client transactions. Most reference laboratories also have their test directories and other user information available online or on compact discs.

Promotion

The means by which a company communicates and promotes its products to its target market is called **promotion**. This includes sales and marketing personnel, advertising, public relations, direct marketing, telemarketing, and online marketing. Many promotional channels exist for laboratory services. Numerous national publications such as the *Clinical Leadership and Management Review, Medical Laboratory Observer, CAP Today,* or *Advance for Laboratory Administrators* are available. This kind of exposure requires an ample marketing budget. Less expensive solutions for laboratories serving only a local market include local business newspapers or publications of the local medical society. A web page provides ample market coverage, can be changed rapidly, and is relatively inexpensive. Desktop software, such as Microsoft Expression Web 4 or Adobe Contribute CS5, can help the novice produce an informational website for around three hundred dollars. A professional website design company can produce a site that includes client functionality and interactivity for under four thousand dollars. Client communiqués, such as test updates, new test announcements, or laboratory service brochures can often be produced on the desktop inexpensively, and can be directly mailed or e-mailed to the customer. These same documents can double as a marketing tool by laboratory sales staff during client visits.

An excellent and inexpensive way to promote laboratory services is to provide customers with continuing education opportunities. Because travel and education budgets in laboratories are disappearing, a laboratory can add value to its product by solving this problem for clients. This can be in the form of local seminars, providing speakers to client hospitals or laboratories, producing an educational newsletter, or posting educational material online. Many professional organizations such as the Clinical Laboratory Management Association (CLMA), the American Society for Clinical Pathology (ASCP), or the American Society for Clinical Laboratory Science (ASCLS) offer onsite-continuing education and teleconferences that can be offered to clientele.

Promotional approaches should be linked to the products and the approach that is the most consistent with the total marketing strategy. The laboratory-marketing manager should interact with the marketing personnel from the hospital to make sure that the laboratory strategy does not conflict with the overall strategy. To meet business objectives each element of the marketing mix must be consistent and complement the overall business strategy of the organization.

THE MARKETING ENVIRONMENT

Markets exist in a **marketing environment**. A successful company recognizes the needs and wants of its customers. It keeps a close eye on trends that may provide the company with opportunities to expand its markets. John Naisbit refers to these opportunities as megatrends or economic, social, political, and environmental changes that influence the environment for a long time. Factors that influence the marketing and business planning of a company include: demographics of the market; the existing economic climate; political, legal, and societal structures; available technologies; and natural resources.

Demographic Environment

People make up markets. Therefore, demographic information is vital to the success of any marketing program. Population numbers stratified by age and gender, educational levels, ethnic backgrounds, and growth rates are all aspects of the **demographic environment**. The graying of American baby boomers has created healthcare market demands as well as significant opportunities. Marketers design and promote their products to attract different age groups. For example, the marketing of toothpaste is specific for adults and children. The travel and leisure industry has also responded to this market demand. The promotional approach for a weekend getaway is more sedate for people over 50, than it is for young adults.

Economic Environment

The people that make up a market cannot buy products or services without purchasing power. This can be affected by elements of the **economic environment**. The housing market, savings rate, debt load, interest rates, money supply, inflation, availability of credit, bank lending, and employment levels all can have tremendous impact on the amount of disposable income, or money available to purchase products. If interest rates are high, sales of automobiles, boats, and houses all decrease. If interest rates are low and credit is available, sales of these items increase.

The recent global economic crisis has reduced purchasing power and lowered consumer confidence in buying new products and services. In a downturn economic environment, consumers actively seek out services that yield the greatest value, and use products that last longer. Luxury items are no longer a priority. Marketing strategies must adapt to the more basic priorities that surface in a downturn economic environment by promoting value, trust and reaching out directly to target groups. Although healthcare services are needed, regardless of economic climate, healthcare organizations must use more cost effective marketing strategies, and be proactive in attracting new potential clients to offset the loss of revenue from fewer requests for "elective" type procedures and services.

Political and Regulatory Environment

The **political** and **regulatory environment** can dramatically and quickly affect business. Legislation regulating business has steadily increased. Laws governing advertising, business practices, pollutants, and employer-employee relations continue to proliferate. Larger companies employ full-time lobbyists to favorably impact legislation in their favor. Rulings by regulatory bodies such as the Food and Drug Administration and the Federal Trade Commission can significantly impact the way companies conduct business.

Lawsuits against tobacco companies and gun manufacturers have produced large product liability settlements. The threat of legislation requiring small businesses to offer healthcare to all employees, along with other burdensome regulations, threatens their well-being and discourages entrepreneurs from venturing into the marketplace. The government has not ignored the laboratory industry. The Clinical Laboratory Improvement Act of 1988 (CLIA '88), administered by the Department of Health and Human Services, mandated laboratory practice changes. Its purpose, which was to ensure quality laboratory testing, has placed demands on clinical laboratories. These regulations can be found in the Code of Federal Regulations Section 353 of Chapter 42. The Occupational Health and Safety Administration (OSHA) implemented new blood-borne pathogen standards in 1993. In 1996, the Centers for Medicare and Medicaid Services (formerly the Health Care Financing Administration) issued guidelines requiring medical necessity documentation for laboratory tests billed to Medicare. These guidelines continue to evolve and impact laboratory management functions. The Stark Ban, named after Peter Stark, chair of the Subcommittee on Health of the House Ways and Means Committee, prohibits self-referral of laboratory testing to physician-owned laboratories.

More recently, the Health Information Technology for Economic and Clinical Health Act (HITECH) was signed into law as part of the economic stimulus package and the American Recovery and Reinvestment Act of 2009 (ARRA). HITECH requires significant changes to the privacy and security of health information that is included in the Health Insurance Portability and Accountability Act (HIPAA) of 1996. HITECH also specifies changes with respect to how the HIPAA regulations and penalties are enforced. Under HITECH, if a patient pays in full for a service or treatment, the patient may request that his or her medical information be restricted. HITECH places limitations on both the delivery and content of marketing messages, how personal health information can be used for marketing purposes, and prohibits the sale of personal health information without authorization. The Office of Inspector General (OIG) has recently developed a set of essential elements to guide clinical laboratory managers with the development of mandatory compliance plans that protect against fraud and abuse in national health care programs. Compliance plans should be implemented and enforced. OIG recommends that laboratory compliance plans incorporate honest, fully informative, and non-deceptive marketing practices, and that marketing information with respect to laboratory services is clear, correct, and non-deceptive.

Technological Environment

Today's firms spend a large percentage of their revenues on research and development. The rapid pace by which technology changes has necessitated large expenditures to gain or maintain the competitive advantage. Success in the **technological environment** plays a key role in the success of a firm. New markets exist in communications for **telehealth**, **telemedicine**, cellular phones, satellite television, and global positioning devices. The advent of DNA technology has opened markets in agriculture for genetically modified seeds, and in the pharmaceutical industry in the development of new drugs. This has expanded product lines in laboratories with new test development to diagnose and monitor genetic abnormalities. It is estimated that, as a result of the mapping of the human genome, tens of thousands of new drugs may be marketed in the next five to ten years.

Natural Environment

The **natural environment** affects companies. Natural resources, including oil and water, are obtained from a single source. Companies need access to these raw materials and available energy supplies to manufacture their products. The market is negatively affected when the costs of natural resources rise as a result of inflation. For example, oil prices increased from $2.23 a barrel in 1970, to $34.00 a barrel in 1982. The big three American automakers, with their gas guzzling big cars, lost significant market share to Japanese automakers that responded to the market with smaller more fuel-efficient automobiles. A shortage of wood has caused prices of new homes to rise, resulting in a decrease in new home sales.

The market must continually adjust to fluctuations of both the availability and cost of natural resources.

MARKETING RESEARCH

Marketing research is a crucial part of a marketing program. It is a technical and systematic approach to obtain data relevant to a specific market. It may be defined as a systematic design, collection, analysis, and reporting of data and findings relevant to a specific marketing situation. For example, a community hospital located in a metropolitan area wants to place a billboard along a highway leading into town. It hires a market research firm to investigate whether or not the cost of placing the billboard will exceed the benefits. The marketing research firm will determine what market to target, what services to advertise, where and when to place the billboard, and what the results of the advertising campaign achieved.

Sources of market research information are abundant. Syndicated research firms, such as A.C. Nielsen, gather consumer and trade information, and make this information available for a fee. Marketing research firms such as Maritz Market Research operate on a contract basis and participate in the design, collection, and reporting of data to a firm's marketing department. Market researchers can provide specialized research such as going into the field and collecting data through interviews, focus groups, and market surveys. The laboratory diagnostic equipment manufacturers conduct numerous focus groups as part of their design and build process. A typical company may budget 1% to 2% of annual sales to market research. For smaller companies, this may be much less. For a typical hospital laboratory, a budget line for market research may be nonexistent.

However, it is possible to collect useful information from a variety of alternate sources. Internal publications such as the balance sheet, income statement, customer lists, and other hospital or laboratory records are sources of marketing information. Government publications such as the *U.S. Industrial Outlook, Statistical Abstracts*, and *County and City Data Book* are available at any public library. Other government organizations including the U.S. Chamber of Commerce can provide useful information. Trade associations or professional organizations such as the College of American Pathologists, American Society of Clinical Chemistry, American Clinical Laboratory Association, American Hospital Association, and the Medical Group Practice Management Association conduct studies and make them available without cost to their membership. *The Washington G-2 Report, Modern Healthcare*, and the *Healthcare Trends Report* provide updates on trends and current opportunities in healthcare. The marketing research process begins by identifying a problem and developing the research plan and methodology. Data are then collected and analyzed. The process culminates with a final report and presentation describing the findings. An example of this process is the following: the laboratory outreach business in a hospital laboratory has declined by 25% over the last 6 months. The hospital vice president in charge of the laboratory asks the laboratory administrator to explain the variance for budgeted revenue. The laboratory administrator, in turn, assigns the laboratory-marketing manager to look into this situation. The laboratory-marketing manager develops a market research plan. A customer survey is constructed, and mailed to all laboratory customers who have sent specimens for testing to the laboratory within the past two years. The survey reveals that a price increase at the beginning of the current fiscal year has changed the market positioning of the laboratory. This revealed that they are no longer the low-cost supplier in this market. The results are presented to the laboratory administrator who decides to lower testing prices to maintain the laboratory's competitive position. Three months after prices are lowered, 5% of the lost market share has been regained.

MARKET ANALYSIS

The basic marketing concepts discussed here must be integrated into a marketing plan developed in the context of the organization's overall business strategy. This is accomplished by a continuous process of analyzing market opportunities, known as **market analysis**. This also includes developing a marketing strategy, planning and implementing the plan, as well as revising the plan by responding to market forces. This cycle, if successful, leads to improved products, added value to the customer, and higher sales and profits for the company (Figure 18-2).

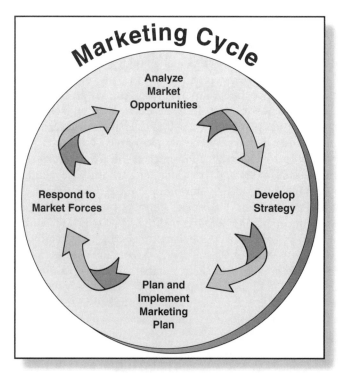

FIGURE 18-2.   The Marketing Cycle

Note: The marketing process is a continuous cycle because market forces and the market environment are changing continually. Revisions to the marketing plan are made in response to these changes.

Market Demand

An analysis of market opportunities should begin by an assessment of the **market demand**. For a laboratory, this would be the total number of laboratory tests performed in a particular market. For example, the number of physician offices plus the average number of tests performed per patient visit, plus the number of patient visits, constitutes the market demand for laboratory testing from physician offices. Other market segments may include nursing homes, skilled nursing facilities, hospital laboratories, industrial clients, or government facilities. The total market demand would represent the sum of these individual market segments.

If sufficient demand is present, assessment must be made of how much of this total market demand the organization desires to capture. If the market demand is 1 million laboratory tests, and a 30% share of the market is desired, you must have the capacity to do 300,000 laboratory tests. How much you capture may be a direct result of how many resources the organization is willing to expend, and how aggressively this market opportunity is pursued.

SWOT Analysis

Decisions to pursue marketing opportunities are determined by analyzing factors internal and external to the company. Internal factors include identification of the company specific (**S**)trengths and (**W**)eaknesses and external factors include identification of industry specific (**O**)pportunities and (**T**)hreats. This process is often referred to as a **SWOT analysis**. Marketers perform SWOT analysis of their competitors to evaluate their potential in the marketplace. Refer to Chapter 10 for more details.

Five Forces Analysis

Michael Porter has expanded this model to include the personal values of the key implementers as an internal factor. For example, in a laboratory that is trying to start an outreach program, it is important to establish that hospital management, key in the implementation of a marketing program, understands the goals and objectives of the marketing plan. The hospital management buy-in is essential to the program's success.

Porter also developed the **five forces analysis** model as a framework for analyzing external opportunities and threats. These five forces are the bargaining power of suppliers, the bargaining power of buyers, the threat of new entrants, the threat of substitute products, and the rivalry among existing firms (Figure 18-3).

For example, in a particular local market there may be five community hospitals with laboratories, two of which have outreach programs. In addition, there are three commercial laboratories conducting business there. Now suppose a community hospital without an outreach program desires to share in this market. The business or marketing manager analyzes the five forces. In this case, the threat of substitute products is a strong force, because the physician's office has several choices of laboratory testing suppliers. This weakens the laboratory testing

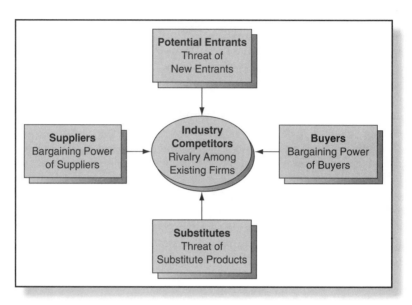

FIGURE 18-3.   Porter's Five Forces Model

Note: Michael Porter, of the Harvard Business School, developed this model to analyze the competitive environment that exists external to a company by considering five forces depicted above.

supplier's ability to raise prices. The threat of new entrants is probably low, owing to the large number of suppliers already in this particular market, and the bargaining power of buyers is strong, because of the number of suppliers. The business manager concludes that the ability of an outreach program to control pricing and earn profits is limited in this market. He, therefore, decides not to invest in an outreach program.

DEVELOPING MARKETING STRATEGIES

Porter identified three generic business strategies for dealing with the five forces: cost leadership, product differentiation, and focus. Cost leadership requires tight cost control, efficiencies of scale, and a structured organization. Product or service differentiation requires a strong research and development function, skilled marketing, and highly skilled labor. The focus strategy is a combination of both cost leadership and differentiation.

Other models of industry and competitor analysis have been developed. A well-known model is the growth share matrix developed by the Boston Consulting Group. This model describes a scenario in which an industry's growth and a firm's market share are proxies for competitive position and cash flow required for operating. The matrix is divided into stars (modest growth/positive cash flow), question marks (high growth/negative cash flow), cash cows (low growth/large positive cash flow), and dogs (low growth/negative cash flow). This model has

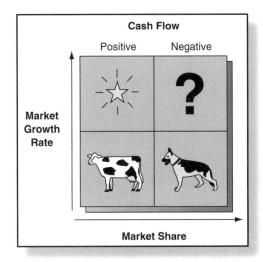

FIGURE 18-4.   Boston Consulting Group Market Model

Note: The Boston Consulting Group Model was developed to assist business to analyze their competitive position in the market.

limitations because of many underlying assumptions and conditions imposed on the model (Figure 18-4).

Regardless of the model, a competitive strategy that fails to produce a competitive advantage is a failure. The Gap has broadly outperformed JCPenney on a consistent basis. What resources, capabilities, or distinct competencies does the Gap have that JCPenney does not? Should JCPenney reengineer their competitive strategy? The Gap has built a competitive advantage and created more customer value that is positively reflected in profit and growth. Michael Porter described the process of creating customer value as a chain. (See Figure 18-5.) This **value chain** has four levels of support activity represented by the vertical links in the chain, and five primary activities of a firm, represented by the horizontal links of the chain. The support activities include: firm infrastructure, human resource function, technology, and materials management. Primary activities include inbound and outbound logistics, operations, marketing/sales, and customer service. Both vertical and horizontal links in the chain lead to increasing profit margin. Laboratory inbound logistics include all the steps of getting the specimen into the laboratory. For example, the decision to contract courier service or provide that as an in-house function can have an effect on customer-perceived value. Are the couriers polite? Do they provide excellent service? Are they on time? Are they professional?

Operational activities are all the preanalytical and analytical variables intrinsic in laboratory testing. Attention to detail in your quality assurance (QA) program, selection of instrumentation, methodology, or suppliers can add or detract value to the product or service.

Outbound logistics or putting the results in the hands of the customer is where many laboratories fall short. The processing department and medical technologist/clinical laboratory scientist can turn out a result, but it means nothing

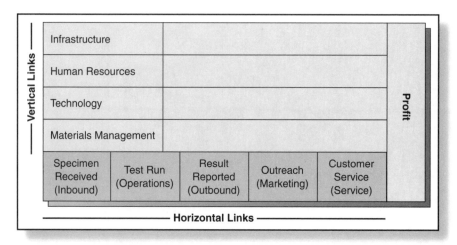

FIGURE 18-5.   The Customer Value Chain

Note: Horizontal links represent primary activities of a company. Vertical links represent companywide support activities.

until a physician reads the result. Creating value is a team effort. Marketing/sales and customer service are vital links in the chain. Most laboratories are proficient at finding new business, but are not proficient at providing good customer service.

Value creation can also be defined mathematically as Value minus Cost (V–C). A company is profitable if the value of a product or service to a customer is greater than the cost. Companies can create greater profit by lowering costs or increasing value. Laboratory tests account for more than 50% of the objective data used to diagnose and treat disease. However, they represent only 3% to 5% of the average total charge for inpatient admissions. Laboratory tests represent less than 3% of the average total charge for patients admitted for surgery, invasive procedures, or those treated in the ICU. Thus, laboratory tests are the most cost-efficient source of objective medical data. The value of a laboratory test to a hospital or patient is greater than the cost to them. Results of inexpensive clinical laboratory tests are frequently used to determine the need for more expensive diagnostic procedures, or to guide the selection of expensive therapeutic options. Accordingly, the costs for performing clinical laboratory tests are more than offset by the savings generated by efficient resource allocation. For example, a patient presents in the emergency room with chest pain and a cardiac troponin is ordered. The result is negative. The patient is given a consult for risk factor modification such as diet and exercise. The total cost of the consult was $200. Without the negative test result, the patient may have undergone a stress test and/or cardiac ECHO (cost $800 to $1800). The price of the troponin assay was $25. The value, therefore, was above $800. The total value to the hospital of the cardiac troponin assay was $775 ($800 – $25). This number, however, is not accounted for in the hospital accounting system.

The basic building blocks of competitive advantage are elements that either raise value (RV) or lower costs (LC). These are superior quality (RV), superior efficiency (LC), superior customer service (RV), or superior innovation (RV).

Healthcare consumers today consider superior quality a given. A physician with a laboratory result that does not match a clinical picture will begin to question the integrity of the laboratory result. Mislabeled, lost, or damaged specimens and errors in reporting results are among the common errors that separate high-quality laboratories from laboratories that provide "superior" quality. Superior efficiency can lower costs and increase profit. Being able to provide batch testing, while maintaining competitive turnaround time, is an example of superior efficiency. Expanding test menus; keeping up with the latest available technology; and finding new and innovative ways to meet the customer's needs, wants, and demands; increase value. When value exceeds price, the customer is more likely to buy. When price exceeds value, the customer will find a substitute product.

PUTTING IT ALL TOGETHER: THE MARKETING PLAN

The market analysis and strategic plan are synthesized into a written marketing plan. A **marketing plan** is an action plan or a road map to guide the company from one place to the next. It describes products or services and their benefits and features. It targets markets and its buying habits, defines competing products or services, and the customer problem that the product or service solves. The plan contains the goals and objectives of the program. Goals specify the necessary levels of achievement; objectives are the specific actions taken to achieve the goals. The marketing objectives should lead to sales. They should be distinct and measurable and have a time limit for accomplishment. If the plan has multiple objectives, the objectives should be consistent and not in conflict with each other. All parts of your marketing plan should support these objectives.

In addition to the market analysis and product or business strategy, the plan should include the marketing and sales strategy, distribution channels, and advertising and promotional plans using the concepts of the marketing mix. Marketing restrictions, if they exist, must be included in the plan. It should also contain a realistic budget detailing the cost of implementing the plan. It is important to remember that market fundamentals which were in place when the plan was written may change. A contingency planning component based on assumptions may be important in the volatile healthcare atmosphere that exists today.

Finally, the plan should contain or reference the mission and vision of the organization. Vision describes where the business is headed, and mission refers to the way business will get there. Mission statements should be shared with managers, employees, and customers, and should provide a shared sense of purpose and direction.

SUMMARY

Today's healthcare environment demands a new skill set among laboratory professionals. Successful managers will need to understand basic business concepts such as marketing and finance. Knowledge and expertise in analyzing marketing opportunities and developing business strategies is essential to adding value for purchasers of laboratory services. Quantitating this value, in terms of increased business, lower operating costs, increased revenue and higher profit, is essential to create buy-in from hospital administrators, managed care companies, and third-party payers, whose buying power you are trying to attract.

SUMMARY CHART:
Important Points to Remember

➤ The primary focus of a market-oriented organization is the customer.

➤ Marketing is defined as a process by which individuals and groups obtain what they want, through creating, offering, and exchanging products or services of value with others.

➤ The marketing mix includes product, price, place, and promotion.

➤ Factors that influence the marketing and business planning of a company include demographics, economic climate, political and regulatory structures, technologies, and natural resources.

➤ The Health Information Technology for Economic and Clinical Health Act (HITECH) strengthens the privacy and security of health information that is part of the Health Insurance Portability and Accountability Act (HIPAA) of 1996.

➤ HITECH places limitations on both the delivery and content of marketing messages, how personal health information can be used for marketing purposes, and prohibits the sale of personal health information without authorization.

➤ Laboratory compliance plans should be implemented and enforced.

➤ Marketing practices and information with respect to laboratory services must be clear, correct, and non-deceptive.

➤ The five forces analysis model is a framework for analyzing both the external opportunities and threats of any organization.

➤ Regardless of the model, a competitive strategy that fails to produce a competitive advantage is a failure.

➤ Creating value is a team effort. Marketing, sales, and customer service are important links in the value chain.

➤ A marketing plan guides the company. The plan contains goals and objectives. The objectives should be measurable and have a time frame for accomplishment. The plan should include a marketing strategy, advertising strategy, and contain a realistic budget for implementation.

SUGGESTED PROBLEM-BASED LEARNING ACTIVITIES

Chapter 18: Marketing Concepts

Instructions: Use Internet resources, books, articles, colleagues, etc., present solutions to the problems listed below. There is no one correct solution to any problem.

Note to Instructor: Students in class may be divided into groups and given the problem-based learning activity to discuss and solve. Once the group has reached consensus as to a solution, the group may present it to the other students in the class. This activity will provide all students with information regarding solutions to the problem.

Problem #1

Suppose your administrator instructed you to provide him/her with alternatives for acquiring additional revenue by eliminating the excess capacity.

Problem #2

Develop a marketing plan for providing services to a long-term healthcare facility.

Problem #3

Develop a marketing plan for providing services to a government-supported dialysis center.

BIBLIOGRAPHY

Baker M, Hart S: *The Marketing Book.* Butterworth-Heinemann, An imprint of Elsevier, Burlington, MA, 2007.

Drozdenko RG, Drake PD: *Optimal Database Marketing Strategy, Development, and Data Mining.* Sage Publications, Thousand Oaks, CA, 2002.

Evans R, Berman B: *Marketing: Marketing in the 21st Century,* ed 10. Atomic Dog Publishing, Cincinnati, OH, 2007.

Kalb IS: *E-Marketing: What Went Wrong and How to Do It Right.* K&A Press, 2004.

Kotler P: *According to Kotler: The World's Foremost Authority on Marketing Answers Your Questions.* Amacom, a division of the American Management Association, New York, NY, 2005.

Kotler P: *Marketing Insights from A to Z. Concepts Every Manager Needs to Know.* John Wiley and Sons, Inc., Hoboken, NJ, 2003.

Lamb CW, Hair JF, McDaniel C: *Marketing With Infotrac.* Thompson South-Western, Mason, OH, 2010.

INTERNET RESOURCES

The American Recovery and Reinvestment Act of 2009: Information Center. Internal Revenue Service, 22 Mar 2011
http://www.irs.gov/newsroom/article/0,,id=204335,00.html

American Society for Clinical Pathology (ASCP), 2011
http://www.ascp.org/

ARUP Laboratories: National Reference Laboratory. University of Utah, Salt Lake City, UT, 2011
http://www.arup-lab.com

Clinical Laboratory Management Association (CLMA), 2011
http://www.clma.org/

Comparative Effectiveness Research Funding, American Recovery and Reinvestment Act of 2009: United States Department of Health & Human Services, 2011
http://www.hhs.gov/recovery/programs/cer/index.html

Health Information Policy: U.S. Department of Health & Human Services
http://www.hhs.gov/ocr/privacy/hipaa/administrative/enforcementrule/hitechenforcementifr.html

Model Compliance Plan for Clinical Laboratories: Office of Inspector General (OIG) of the Department of Health & Human Services, 2010
http://oig.hhs.gov/fraud/docs/complianceguidance/cpcl.html

Notice of Proposed Rulemaking to Implement HITECH Act Modifications. United States Department of Health & Human Services, 2011
http://www.hhs.gov/ocr/privacy/hipaa/understanding/coveredentities/hitechnprm.html

Recovery.Gov: *Track the Money.* United States Government, 2011
http://www.recovery.gov/

Saint Louis University Coagulation Consultants: SLU*Care*—The Physicians of Saint Louis University, St. Louis, MO, 2011
http://www.slu.edu/x26597.xml

Strategies for Career Success

Laboratory managers encounter daily some of the issues related to personnel, training and education, finance, marketing, standards and regulations. Ethical conduct plays a role in these daily activities. Success in your career is also dependent on incorporating values of ethics and morality into the ethics of management.

Section V consists of two chapters, one that focuses on ethics and one that discusses career planning. Chapter 19 discusses ethical issues in laboratory management. Chapter 20 presents strategies for career planning, networking, and professional development. It is imperative that laboratory managers not only prepare themselves for career enhancement, but also groom their employees for a successful career in laboratory medicine. Developing a career plan, creating opportunities, and promoting professional development, provide the basis for career success.

Section V Contents:

Ethical Issues in Laboratory Management

Adil E. Shamoo, PhD, CIP

CHAPTER OUTLINE

OBJECTIVES

Following successful completion of this chapter, the learner will be able to:

1. Discuss the importance of ethical issues in laboratory management.
2. Identify the ethical principles at stake when faced with a moral dilemma.
3. Identify areas of laboratory management that may face ethical issues.
4. Recognize boundaries of ethical laboratory management and its value.
5. Delineate and discuss the ethical decision-making process for laboratory management.

Case Study Ethical Issues in Laboratory Management

A colleague asks his friend, a technologist, for the results of his girlfriend's pregnancy test. The technologist obliged after telling his friend that he is doing him a big favor, and that he should not tell anyone that he told him. The test was positive. The laboratory manager was told about it through another employee.

Issues and Questions to Consider:

1. Evaluate the information and the problem.
2. Identify the stakeholders.
3. What are the values at risk?
4. What are the moral responsibilities of the laboratory technologist?
5. What are the moral responsibilities of the laboratory manager?
6. How should the laboratory manager proceed?

INTRODUCTION

In order to achieve a task (small or large) that requires a group of individuals with the same or complementary skills, management of the group or the organization is an essential component of a successful organization charged with completing a task. Even though modern management principles of an organization are relatively recent phenomena, nevertheless the management practices have been in existence for thousands of years. The Romans were great engineers whose management skills allowed them to achieve complex and large tasks such as building roads, bridges, and aqueducts. Effective management requires knowledge, leadership, competence, and moral authority. Managers of organizations operate in a community and the society. Therefore, our human values of ethics and morality must be incorporated into the ethics of management. This is because management ethics involves management activities that can encompass all of the good or bad of our humanity. Managers, by virtue of their job, are leaders. Therefore, the ethical or unethical behavior of a leader clearly would heavily influence the effectiveness of the leader on the outcome of the organization.

On a daily basis, laboratory managers encounter issues related to personnel, education and training, finance, marketing, standards and regulations. Ethical conduct plays a role in the daily activities of the laboratory manager.

Some of these activities, as they relate to ethical laboratory management, may involve the following:

1. Confidentiality of the information
2. Fraud and abuse of charges
3. Fraud and misconduct of data
4. Marketing and advertising
5. Quality of services
6. Profits
7. Human resource issues: workers' salaries, working conditions, drug testing, etc.
8. Conflict of interest
9. Regulatory compliance

Our individual and society's ethical values will have a crucial impact on all of these activities, as well as on our society at large, when these managerial issues are addressed.

This chapter will explore ethical theories, ethical decision-making, and potential ethical issues in some of the items listed above. In addition, some case examples will be presented.

ETHICAL THEORIES

Most ethical theories, concepts, and principles deal with one or more of the three most important parameters: 1) Actor, 2) Act, and 3) Outcome. The theories that deal with the Actor and his/her character traits are called virtue ethics. Ethical conduct, therefore, is determined by the person's virtuous characteristics such as honesty, honor, courage, humanity, benevolence, fairness, and temperance. Aristotle was a strong proponent of virtue ethics. The virtue of integrity is the consistency of virtuous behavior such as honesty and fairness. Ethical behavior requires learning good behavior and practicing it. This is similar to playing an instrument or learning mathematics; it requires learning the theory and a lot of practice, as Aristotle stated. Moreover, these characteristics are developed within the context of community. The individual influences the community and certainly, the community influences the individual. Ethical leadership greatly depends on virtue ethics. The leadership sets the tone for the organizational culture in terms of honesty, courage, fairness, and wisdom of decisions. Members of the organization emulate, in large part, their leaders.

The theories that deal with the Act itself by the moral agent (Actor) are within the second category of "Act." The moral agent ought to know the difference between right and wrong action. The eighteenth century German Enlightenment philosopher, Immanuel Kant, was a proponent of this approach. Kant emphasized that the reasons for action (i.e. motives of the agent) matter a great deal.

Therefore, he advocated doing the right thing for the right reason. He introduced the concept of categorical imperative (CI) of "what if everyone does it." This is basically a restatement of the "Golden Rule" which requires that you treat others as you want them to treat you. In addition, proponents of the natural law also have advocated that life, health, happiness, and pleasure are naturally good; whereas, death, suffering, disease, and pain are bad. Furthermore, advocates of natural rights may fall into this category since they contend that certain rights are endowed to us. These rights may include life, liberty, prosperity, freedom of thought, and freedom of religion, without any duties or obligations to others. The seventeenth century British philosopher, John Locke, was the champion of natural rights.

The theories that deal with outcomes (third category) are concerned with the consequence of the action by the "actor." The individual's motive is less important than the outcome. The eighteenth century philosopher, Jeremy Bentham, and the nineteenth century philosopher, John Stuart Mill, developed the theory of utilitarianism. The basic tenet of the theory is that our actions should have the best overall consequences for the largest number of people. For example, the political system of socialism is derived from this theory. Cost/Benefit analysis is a derivative of this theory. The social contract theory also falls within the outcome domain, since people living in a society have obligations to the society by the very nature of accepting to live in a community and society.

APPLIED ETHICAL PRINCIPLES

Let us imagine a very large circle representing the domain of ethical conduct in life. Ethical conduct governs societies in all areas of life from family, community and education, to business and government. Imagine a small concentric circle within this large circle representing the domain governed by laws and related legal structures. Laws are areas in which society has decided to make unethical behaviors illegal and has provided remedies including punishment. The remaining area between the two circles are the ethical norms by which society expects us to abide. (See Figure 19-1.) These are the norms all societies utilize to enforce social controls. Usually, societies enact laws to govern a specific area where a continuous and flagrant infringement on the societal expectation of ethical norms occurs. If a society abides only by what is legal, the civil society will cease to exist. This is not to say that all laws in every society are ethical. The best example is that slavery was legal but yet unethical. The more the society is free, the greater the

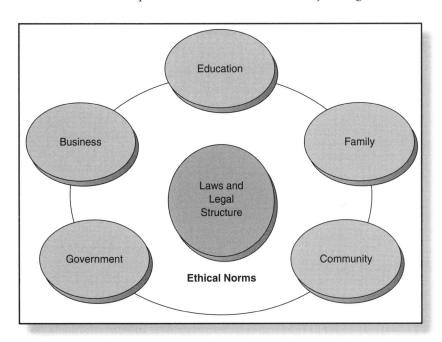

FIGURE 19-1.   Ethical Conduct in Life

likelihood that its laws are ethical. There is always a tension between increasing the legal circle and reducing it in order to lessen the regulatory compliance burden on the society. It is also important to note that, when we discuss unethical behavior, one may erroneously get the impression that everyone is unethical. Most individuals are noble people and well intentioned. Discussing pathology in ethical behavior is no different from discussing and studying pathology in medicine. Pathology in medicine affects only a very small percentage of the population. Nevertheless, studying pathology helps us to learn how to prevent and treat the pathology.

Moreover, we like to have the best possible treatment to prevent pathology. In ethics, this is no different; we study ethical conduct in order to prevent the pathology of unethical behavior, and remedy it in the most ethical manner.

It is important to derive simple ethical principles. The following ethical principles can be deduced from the above brief discussion of ethical theories and from the fact that they can be considered to be prima fade principles (See Table 19-1). These principles are not absolute rules. It is recommended to use these principles; but when they come in conflict with each other, we should choose which ethical principle will have a higher priority than the others. In fact, one can find a case whereby each of these ethical principles falls apart.

We will list the three broad categories of ethical principles with few sub-categories. We will only discuss a limited number of the most important sub-categories.

TABLE 19-1.   Categories of Ethical Principles

Integrity of Conduct	Honesty
	Objectivity
	Openness
Respect for Persons	Fairness
	Loyalty
	Respect for subordinators/colleagues
Social Responsibility	Do good; Do no harm
	Public responsibility
	Obeying laws and regulations
	Efficiency

1. Integrity of Conduct

This is an area of ethical duties for managers that involves multiple specific areas such as:

a) Honesty,

b) Objectivity, and

c) Openness.

Honesty is a crucial characteristic for managers in acquiring, recording, and manipulating the data. Trust among subordinates for honest leadership is important to promulgate good practices. Objectivity in reporting the information to patients, subordinates, or upper management is at the heart of the truthfulness of the data. Openness engenders public trust in the system. For example, if conflict of interest exists, then transparency and managing the conflict of interest become an important part of good management practices.

2. Respect for Persons

This is an area of ethical duties for managers that involves issues of:

a) Respect and the protection of autonomy;

b) Fairness;

c) Loyalty; and

d) Respect for subordinators and colleagues.

In the area of respect and the protection of **autonomy**, each individual should have free and full rights for decision-making. We should all respect the rights of each individual to exercise his/her rights. Assuming a rational individual, then the individual should be able to make an informed and responsible choice. Even if the choice is not a responsible one and it does not infringe on someone else's rights, we must respect it and the individual will bear its consequences.

However, none of us in a position of management are left alone to make decisions. Managers have to comply with numerous directives from upper management, as well as inside policies and outside regulatory agencies. Therefore, autonomy can be limited because other forces come into play, such as issues of justice and serving the public good.

In the area of fairness, Aristotle said "equals should be treated equally and unequals unequally." In a society, we should allocate resources fairly. In addition, we should distribute the risks and benefits to the largest number of population (i.e. the greatest good). This is what is called "social justice." We should not have a segment of society reaping benefits, while another segment of society takes all the risks that brought the benefit. There should be justifications as to why people are treated differently.

Respect for subordinates and colleagues is an extension of respect for others, and gives deference to others to make their own free choice.

In the area of loyalty, one should be loyal to his/her organization, and to his colleagues as long as it is ethical.

3. Social Responsibility

This is an area of ethical duties for managers that involves issues of:

a) Do good and do no harm;

b) Public responsibility;

c) Obeying the laws and regulation; and

d) Efficiency.

In the area of "do good and do no harm," the two concepts are interrelated principles of doing good and preventing, or not inflicting, harm. "Doing good" denotes a positive action; whereas, "do no harm" is a passive state of refraining from harm. However, preventing harm could be a positive act. This is why these two principles are so interrelated. Some argue that beneficence should be optional on the individual rather than mandatory. I think in some cases beneficence can be optional, like giving financial aid to the needy; but it is obligatory when you see a car accident, and you are the only one who can stop and help.

In short, these ethical principles are summarized in relation to three broad principles: **Autonomy**; **Beneficence/Nonmaleficence** (do good/do no harm); and **Justice**. One usually can remember these three broad principles more easily than the detailed ones.

It is of interest to note that the American Society for Clinical Laboratory Science (ASCLS) has a Code of Ethics for its members on its website. Among the ethical principles they enunciate are: a) duty to the patient requiring competence and strict confidentiality; b) duty to colleagues and the profession with respect to all involved; and c) duty to society to adhere to laws and regulations.

ETHICAL DECISION-MAKING PROCESS

Now that we have discussed the ethical theories and principles, we can utilize them to guide us to make an ethical decision. An ethical decision is usually needed when there is a moral dilemma. In other words, there are moral choices one has to make. For example, when shopping for a car, selecting what color you should choose is not an ethical dilemma. However, an individual trying to decide whether or not to ask his brother to write his term paper for him is a moral dilemma. In a moral dilemma, you have two choices or more. What is the right thing to do? How do you arrive at an optimal ethical decision? What values are involved and which ones have priority and why? These are all factors involved in an ethical decision-making process (See Table 19-2).

Let us discuss the process of ethical decision-making (See Figure 19-2). As we mentioned earlier, there has to be a moral dilemma first in order to go through the process.

1. State the Problem
For the case study at the beginning of the chapter, the problem is that the technologist revealed confidential information, and the moral dilemma for the manager is what to do about it.

Let us take the case study and analyze it. The manager clearly has a moral dilemma of what to do with the employee and other related issues within the laboratory. Moreover, the manager has to deal with the situation in a fair and just manner, in order to set the moral standards and to maintain or increase the morality of the laboratory. Furthermore, resolving the issue will reflect a great deal of the manager's skills.

2. Collect and Verify the Information
Did we verify that the technologist gave the information regarding the pregnancy test? Let us assume the answer is yes. How much information was disclosed? The employee is a valuable staff member with five years of excellent working habits. Apparently, several other employees learned of the incident. Let us assume we have all of the information.

TABLE 19-2.   Steps of the Ethical Decision-Making Process

1. State the Problem.
2. Collect and Verify the Information.
3. Identification of the Primary Stakeholders.
4. Determine Any Violation of Laws.
5. Delineate Harm.
6. Delineate Options.
7. Make a Decision.
8. Defend the Decision.

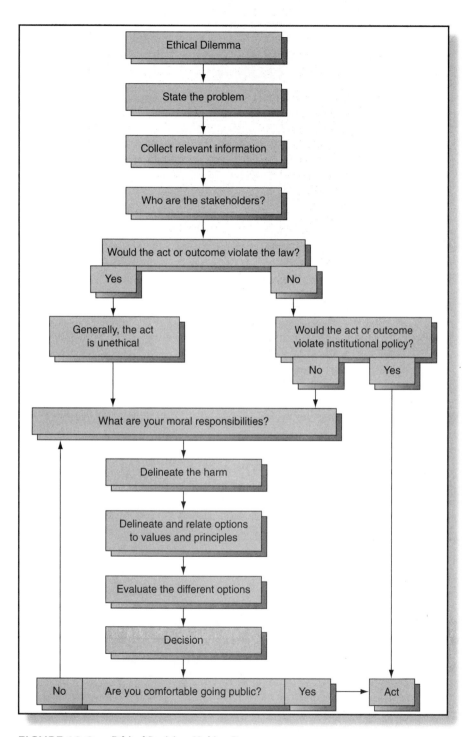

FIGURE 19-2. Ethical Decision-Making Process

Adapted from: Shamoo AD, Resnik DB. Ethical Issues for Clinical Research Managers. *Drug Information Journal* 2006: 40; 371-383.

3. Identification of the Primary Stakeholders

The stakeholders are: the friend, girlfriend, technologist, and the manager. The secondary stakeholders who will be affected by this problem are the other employees and the organization. The tertiary stakeholders are the profession and the society at large.

4. Determine Any Violation of Laws

Has anyone violated the law? Since confidential information has been revealed, the answer is, "yes." There are state and federal laws prohibiting such disclosure. The manager can take action according to the law. However, legal actions are not usually prescribed to deal with the individual in such cases. In this case, the act or its outcome of revealing confidential information is unethical. You will need to go to the next step of delineating options. If the act (unlike this case) was legal, then the question ought to be, "Does it violate any organizational policies?" At this stage, the manager can take action.

5. Delineate Harm

We can all agree that the primary harm from this infringement can occur to the girlfriend. Her confidential information has been revealed; and thus, her autonomy has been violated. The girlfriend may even suffer dignitary harm from being embarrassed that others have such private information on her, and so on. Harm may occur to her by the possible loss of her boyfriend or her job. Once the information has been leaked, some employers under the guise of competence may not want a pregnant person employed for various reasons. Harm could also occur to the technologist himself since he may be fired or reprimanded. In addition, harm could occur to the manager since he/she will have to spend valuable time and energy handling the incident. Secondary harm could affect other employees since they are coworkers in the laboratory, and the manager and upper management may provide more oversight. Tertiary harm could come to the profession by casting doubt on the integrity of the profession. Finally, society may be harmed since no one would like to see such unethical behavior become the common norm.

6. Delineate Options

In part, the following options are available:

a) Do nothing.

b) Fire the technologist.

c) Suspend the technologist for a short period of time with or without pay.

d) Reprimand the technologist and require education and training.

e) Inform the girlfriend and apologize.

f) Require all laboratory personnel to undergo education and training.

g) Institute a new policy for the laboratory in order to protect confidentiality.

We can choose to do one or more of the listed options, and there are many more options in addition to these. For every suggested resolution, we need to discuss the risks and benefits.

The option of doing nothing is unethical since harm has occurred without accountability and responsibility. Doing nothing sends the wrong message to all involved. Some may recommend firing the technologist. However, firing a valued technologist for a first offense may be an over-reaction and not commensurate with the infringement. Firing the individual may inhibit others in the future from coming forward. Firing could cause a hardship to the technologist and his family way over and above the harm done to others due to infringement. Therefore, it can be argued that using the other four options listed above or their combination depends on more detailed information. Honest individuals can differ in the proposed solution within the ethical boundaries. It is important to note that option (a) is unethical, and option (b) may be unethical. One cannot simply make all options as ethically equivalent because they are not. More detailed information may even eliminate other options as unethical. We have in this section related and evaluated the options to different values and principles.

7. Make a Decision
Let us assume we chose options (d), (e), (f), and (g). This is probably the most comprehensive resolution.

8. Defend the Decision
Now we have to address the final step of whether we are comfortable if this information becomes public, and we must determine if our decision can be defended. The reason for this final question is to eliminate the factor that we may be hiding something unethical. If the answer is yes, in that we are comfortable with the decision if everyone knows about it, then we should act. Otherwise, we should start the evaluation all over again. However, there are unique circumstances that may render going public as inappropriate, and could cause even more harm to the individual. This is one of these cases; because going public would bring greater harm to the girlfriend. The girlfriend could be subjected to more embarrassment, as well as to loss of potential jobs (unlikely), since we do not know the circumstance and implications of her positive pregnancy test, and this may invite speculation.

ETHICAL CHALLENGES IN LABORATORY MANAGEMENT

As we have mentioned earlier, societies determine which ethical issues, if violated, will result in punishment. The area of laboratory management is a good example of how the legal circle was widened at least twice in the past twenty years in order to provide legal remedies for violators of the ethical norms. There are billions of public dollars spent annually by the federal government on government-supported health care such as Medicare and Medicaid. Prior to 1988, various laboratories set their own standards for quality of their tests (for example, for cholesterol and Pap smear evaluation). Due to serious violations and concerns, in 1988 the federal government enacted into law the Clinical Laboratory Improvement Amendment

(CLIA) (Public Law, 1988). CLIA established quality standards for all laboratory tests to ensure accuracy and reliability. Society was no longer willing to risk the public good on the ethical and professional standards of those in the field.

The second example is the passage in 1995 of the final rule for "Medicare Program; Physician Financial Relationship" (42 CFR Part 411) which addressed the issue known as self-referral. A good number of laboratories were owned by physicians or members of their families. In some cases, physicians would order tests (or unnecessary tests) for their patients to be conducted in the laboratory in which they, or members of their family, had a financial interest. There was clearly a conflict of interest issue and a great opportunity for abuse of public money. This practice was clearly unacceptable to the public and the government. This was the reason the Health Care Financing Administration (HCFA), now called the Center for Medicare and Medicaid Services (CMS), issued in 1995 the final rule forbidding self-referral, "except under specified circumstances."

Nine categories of potential areas of questionable ethical conduct in laboratory management are listed in the introduction. We will not be able to discuss all of these areas. However, we would like to expand on several of them. In our case study, we discussed the importance of confidentiality of the information. One of the most important ethical areas in this field is the area of fraud of charges, and fraud and misconduct of data. There are literally hundreds of millions of dollars lost annually due to fraud and abuse. In part, because the federal government is paying the bill, patients do not check what they were billed for; thus making it easy to commit fraud. The most prominent areas of fraud and abuse are: charges for services not performed; unnecessary testing (i.e. not medically necessary); waiver of co-payments and deductibles; fraudulent or inaccurate data; and unbundling of laboratory tests so that the laboratory charges are higher than if the charges were all part of one service. Another area of concern as we mentioned earlier, is marketing and advertising. In some fraudulent practices, the laboratory advertises for free testing for a particular disorder; however, the laboratory requires all patients fill out a form that in essence is used for billing purposes.

Another example of an ethically troubling issue in a laboratory occurred in 2004 in Maryland General Hospital in Baltimore, Maryland. The allegations are that in over a year, hundreds of patients received incorrect HIV and hepatitis test results, and the patients were not notified. Some patients were HIV positive and were told the test was negative, and some the reverse. The laboratory personnel overrode the results from the controls. Moreover, a former laboratory worker complained to the management about the quality of tests without any results. A state official, once he learned of the laboratory practice, was quoted as saying: "I think this is unconscionable behavior; people not being told about the status of their test."

In brief, the laboratory manager must comply with: 1. Continuous training and education; 2. Apply standards of performance and quality; and 3. Provide sufficient resources for the performance of the task. In addition to these three standards, the International Union of Pure and Applied Chemistry (IUPAC), in its 1988 guidelines for training in clinical laboratory management, requires a detailed set of knowledge and skill to fulfill the highest ethical and quality laboratory product (IUPAC, 1990).

SUMMARY

Training and education in ethical issues in laboratory management is an essential component of a student's education. Students, as potential laboratory managers, need to be aware of potential ethical problems they will face. Not only do managers need to deal with a particular problem, but they also need to set the standard for ethical managerial competence and to set an example for others. In order for laboratory managers to be effective, they need to understand the ethical decision-making process to be able to analyze the particular moral dilemma with which he/she is faced. Ethical managerial leadership provides a setting for all to work in a cooperative and successful manner, which is part of being a true professional.

SUMMARY CHART:
Important Points to Remember

➤ Effective management requires knowledge, leadership, competence, and moral authority.

➤ Our human values of ethics and morality must be incorporated into the ethics of management.

➤ Ethical leadership greatly depends on virtue ethics.

➤ The leadership sets the tone for the organizational culture in terms of honesty, courage, fairness, and wisdom of decisions.

➤ Most ethical theories, concepts, and principles deal with the most important three parameters: 1) Actor, 2) Act, and 3) Outcome.

➤ The theories that deal with the Actor and his/her character traits are called virtue ethics.

➤ Theories that deal with outcomes are concerned with the consequence of the action by the "actor."

➤ The basic tenet of the theory of utilitarianism is that our actions should have the best overall consequences for the largest number of people.

➤ The ethical conduct governs societies in all areas of life from family, community, and education to business and government.

➤ These ethical principles are summarized in relation to three broad principles: Autonomy; Beneficence/Nonmaleficence (do good/do no harm); and Justice.

➤ Laboratory managers should: 1. Provide continuous training and education; 2. Apply standards of performance and quality; and 3. Provide sufficient resources for the performance of the task.

SUGGESTED PROBLEM-BASED LEARNING ACTIVITIES

Chapter 19: Ethical Issues in Laboratory Management

Instructions: Use Internet resources, articles, textbooks, colleagues, etc., to present solutions to the problems listed below. There is no one correct solution to any problem.

Note to Instructor: Group activities in order to provide division of labor as well as discussions are encouraged. Students in class may be divided into groups and given the problem-based learning activity to discuss and solve. Once the group has reached consensus as to a solution, the group may present it to the other students in the class. This activity will provide all students with information regarding solutions to the problem.

Problem #1

Develop a code of conduct for the laboratory for employees and managers.

Problem #2

Develop a case study of an ethical issue in the laboratory. List ethical and unethical solutions, and reasons why they are ethical/unethical.

Problem #3

Develop an educational program that you may require for all employees of the laboratory in ethics.

BIBLIOGRAPHY

American Society for Clinical Laboratory Science (ASCLS). *ASCLS Code of Ethics.* Accessed 8 April 2011, at: http://www.ascls.org/?pag e=Code&hhSearchTerms=CODE+and+OF +and+ETHICS

Informational Sheet Guidance for Institutional Review Boards (IRBs), Clinical Investigators, and Sponsors. FDA U.S. Food and Drug Administration, Science & Research, United States Department of Health & Human Services. Last updated: 5 April 2011. http://www.fda.gov/oc/ohrt/irbs/belmont.html

International Union of Pure and Applied Chemistry (IUPAC). Clinical Chemistry Division, Commission on Teaching of Clinical Chemistry and International Federation of Clinical Chemistry Education Committee. *Training in Clinical Laboratory Management (Guidelines 1988). Pure & Appl. Chem* 1990: 62(2); 365-372. Available at: http://www.iupac.org/publications/pac/1990/pdf/6202x0365.pdf

National Commission for the Protection of Human Subjects of Biomedical and Behavioral Research. *The Belmont Report: Ethical Principles and Guidelines for the Protection of Human Subjects of Research.* Department of Health, Education, and Welfare, 18 April 1979. Accessed 8 April 2011, at: http://ohsr.od.nih.gov/guidelines/belmont.html

Shamoo AD, Resnik DB: *Ethical Issues for Clinical Research Managers, Drug Information Journal* 2006: 40; 371-383.

Shamoo AD, Resnik DB: *Responsible Conduct of Research,* ed 2. Oxford University Press, New York, NY, 2009.

U.S. Department of Health and Human Services. Centers for Disease Control and Prevention. *Current CLIA Regulations (including all changes through 01/24/2004).* Accessed 8 April 2011, at: http://wwwn.cdc.gov/clia/regs/toc.aspx

INTERNET RESOURCES

Applied Ethics Resources on the World Wide Web
http://www.ethicsweb.ca/resources/

Colero L: A Framework for Universal Principles of Ethics. U.B.C. Centre for Applied Ethics
http://www.ethics.ubc.ca/papers/invited/colero.html

DHS Division of Aging and Adult Services, Arkansas Department of Human Services
http://www.daas.ar.gov/

EthicsWeb
http://www.ethicsweb.ca/

MacDonald C: Moral Decision Making—An Analysis
http://www.ethicsweb.ca/guide/moral-decision.html

Procedural Ethics: Chronological Site
http://www.cs.bgsu.edu/maner/heuristics/toc.htm

United States Department of Justice (USDOJ): Deputy Attorney General: Publications and Documents. Health Care Fraud Report Fiscal Year 1998. United States Department of Justice, 2011
http://www.usdoj.gov/dag/pubdoc/health98.htm

United States Government Printing Office. Code of Federal Regulations, HCFA: 42 CFR Part 411, HCFA. United States Government Printing Office, 6 April 2011
http://www.access.gpo.gov/nara/cfr/waisidx_02/42cfr411_02.html

ACKNOWLEDGMENT

This paper was supported in-part by a grant from: Fogarty International Center/NIH 1R25TW007090-01.

Career Planning & Professional Development

Denise M. Harmening, PhD, MT(ASCP), CLS(NCA)
Anastasiya O. Sepikova, BA

CHAPTER OUTLINE

OBJECTIVES

Following successful completion of this chapter, the learner will be able to:

1. Define the responsibilities of professional life.
2. List the elements of a successful career.
3. Describe several skills related to the planning and implementation of a professional development plan.
4. Describe a unified view of a professional career in light of the professional community, the workplace, personal needs and interests, and collaboration with colleagues.
5. Outline a customized plan for professional development and identify the main skills needed to make that plan succeed.

KEY TERMS

Curriculum Vitae (CV)
Dedication
Flexibility
Networking

Positive Attitude
Professional
Resume
Subspecialties

"There are no secrets to success. It is the result of preparation, hard work, and learning from failure."

—Colin Powell

INTRODUCTION

The necessity of career planning and management is one of the many challenges facing the laboratory scientist today. These challenges come to us from all directions: new regulations and technologies, the relocation and restructuring of the workplace, the reorganization of institutions in response to changing national perspectives and priorities, economic pressures from government and the private sector, and the need for a lifelong process of continuing education in the aftermath of the "knowledge explosion."

These issues are the product of larger concerns: the healthcare crisis, the information explosion, quantum leaps in technologic innovation, and economic shifts keenly felt inside and outside the workplace. The long-term effects are just starting to surface and be identified; the short-term effects, dictating the way we conduct our day-to-day lives, are what we must all cope with—and somehow adjust to.

This chapter explores the elements of successful career planning by describing career priorities and **professional** development programs. Strategies for creating opportunities, networking, and using a strategic development plan are presented. Suggested problem-based learning activities related to the material presented in this chapter are located after the summary chart.

THE SUCCESSFUL CAREER PLAN

The time is past when we could operate on a safe routine within a narrow specialty with set procedures, feeling confident that nothing dramatic would change from year to year. No longer can we afford to be out of touch with political, economic, social, and scientific developments, or to ignore our connection with related disciplines within the layer context of medicine. The pressure is on to determine our own destiny in our institutions, professional associations, and work environments. Vital to any successful career is a plan. Success is the outcome of the ability to create a custom-designed, multifaceted professional development program that facilitates lifelong learning. A personal commitment to professional development should be made in at least one of the following areas: expansion of the applied body of knowledge, growth through professional activities, scholarship, teaching, research, and/or community service.

A philosophy of life that focuses on attaining and maintaining high standards of practice in educational, professional, and/or research activities should be developed. Professionals are obligated to share knowledge and expertise with co-workers and colleagues at all levels of practice: local, state, and national. Each has the responsibility to contribute to and expand the overall body of knowledge within the profession. Exchanges through networking play a key role in professional development, providing an immeasurably valuable range of advantages and benefits.

NETWORKING

Networking is essential to your professional and personal development. Learn to network and capitalize on the knowledge and expertise of colleagues. Learn to extract information from peers, encouraging and partaking in collaborative efforts. You are not alone. Cooperation and the "team approach" are the keys to any successful career whether in nonprofit, service-oriented organizations or industry. Knowledge and resources in the field are not a zero-sum issue—they expand when shared.

In today's job market and economy, many professionals have difficulty finding employment, especially in a position or industry they desire. According to the Federal Bureau of Labor Statistics, approximately 7 out of 10 jobs are found through networking. By capitalizing on the relationships you have with people, and cultivating your network, you have a higher chance of getting a job. Posted jobs are highly competitive and "sticking out in the crowd" is unlikely. When you use networking to find a personal connection to your preferred organization, you have instantly found a way to stand out from the crowd. Networking does not happen naturally for everyone and requires consistent effort. When beginning to network, start with the resources you already have. Make a list of contacts. List people you know, your family knows, friends, relatives, colleagues, and acquaintances. This may provide you with a list of people in various industries and professions. Expand your network by visiting the career resources center, or alumni office at your educational institution. Try to gather information about job shadowing opportunities, internships, or alumni that could become part of your network. Attending networking events such as career fairs, seminars, and professional meetings are good ways to begin expanding your network. Similar events

TABLE 20-1.   Advantages and Benefits of Networking in the Profession

- Exchange of research and teaching techniques and technologies
- Extension of professional contacts and networks for departments and staffs
- Opportunities for joint ventures and collaborative development of grants, scholarships, and other support and subsidies
- Productive matching and complementary working between and among facilities, administrative systems, and operations, leading to interaction, enrichment, and resource sharing for faculty, staff, and administrations of all participants

are held by local employment agencies and professional societies. After establishing your network, it is important to stay in touch with these individuals, and help other people by becoming one of their contacts.

There are several ways to network, and today networking is easier than it has ever been in the past. The numerous professional and/or social networks on the Internet make it easy to communicate and stay in contact with people you already know, as well as find or meet new people, exchange information, gather information, or even find a job. Internet social media sites, such as LinkedIn and Facebook, are increasingly being used by employees and employers alike. Utilizing social and professional networking sites provides opportunities for expanding your network; sharing knowledge and expertise, locally, nationally, or even internationally; and marketing yourself to find the best job. Table 20-1 lists the advantages and benefits of networking in the profession.

PROFESSIONAL DEVELOPMENT PROGRAMS

Professional development can be defined as the establishment of activities and procedures to assist acquisition of the knowledge, expertise, and attitudes that enable increased effectiveness in performing all functions related to professional life.

Personalized professional development programs should seek to prepare competent practitioners while developing professional attitudes, attributes, and values. Specifically, the programs should be designed to accomplish one or more of the following goals:

1. Develop personal attributes to enhance scholarship, productivity, and exchange of ideas.
2. Promote contributions to the profession and community.
3. Cultivate awareness of professional issues and responsibilities for enhancement of the scope of practice.
4. Serve as a catalyst to fulfill goals and maintain high standards of practice as set out in both our philosophy of life and professional philosophy.

Figure 20-1 outlines some of the self-directed professional development aspects that could be activated to accomplish these goals.

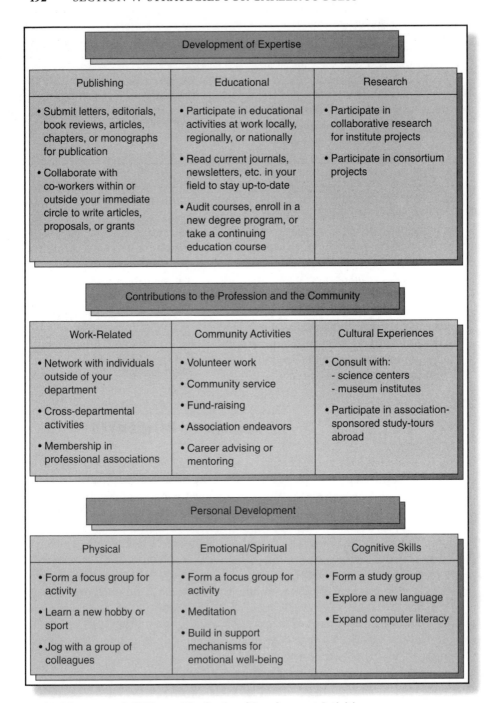

FIGURE 20-1.   **Self-Directed Professional Development Activities**

The development of expertise is achieved in several ways, some of which include publishing works, educating yourself, and participation in professional projects or research. Publishing works may include submitting letters, editorials, book reviews, articles, chapters, and monographs. This demonstrates your contribution to the field while building an audience. Collaboration with coworkers on publishing articles, proposals, and grants broadens your knowledge base by introducing and sharing new ideas, information, technology, etc.

It is important to further your education and stay up-to-date with changes and advancements in your field, or specialty. Participating in educational activities at work, locally, regionally, or nationally facilitates this process. Reading current journals, newsletters, and other publications is an essential supplement. In addition, enrolling in a new degree program, taking continuing education courses, or simply auditing courses are good ways to expand your knowledge base. Developing expertise can also be accomplished by participating in collaborative research, institute, and/or consortium projects. Working with experienced professionals or peers also expands your knowledge base and network.

Contributions to the profession and the community can be work-related, community activities, and/or cultural experiences. Work-related professional and community contributions may include activities such as networking with individuals outside of your department, participating in cross-departmental activities, as well as having a membership in a professional association. Volunteer work, community service/activities, fund-raising, association endeavors, and career advising or mentoring are more examples of methods of contributing to the profession and the community, while providing opportunity to cultivate your network. Moreover, contributions to the profession and the community through cultural experiences, such as consulting with science centers, museum institutes, and participating in association-sponsored study-tours abroad, are also valuable to developing expertise.

Personal development, including physical, emotional or spiritual, and cognitive skills, is fundamental to an individual's professional development. Activities to promote personal development significantly depend on the individual and his/her interests, abilities, and needs. Forming an interest group may be beneficial for physical, emotional, spiritual, and cognitive development. Other examples of physical activities include learning a new hobby or sport, or jogging with a group of colleagues. Building support mechanisms for emotional well-being such as meditating is just one example of activity that contributes to emotional or spiritual development. Exploring new languages or expanding computer literacy are just a couple of examples of methods for developing cognitive skills.

Three elements are critical to this basic approach:

1. **Flexibility:** Flexibility is the capability to adapt to new, different, or changing requirements. It is the ability to take new directions and opportunities as they emerge. This often means looking at crises and obstacles as an invitation to redefine, rethink, and respond with enthusiasm and energy,

rather than with pessimism and anxiety. Creative problem solving will be called into play. Implicit is open-mindedness about who we are, what we can do, where we are headed, and our growing roles and potential power as part of the healthcare team.

2. **Dedication** to the profession: The term reflects a profession broader and more demanding than the traditions of **subspecialties** alone. The concept of dedication as "self-sacrificing devotion" is timely and appropriate.

3. **Positive attitude**: Optimism, and the vitality it generates, independent of changing circumstances, are essential for personal and professional advancement and achievement. We are being asked to think beyond the problems of today, and create momentum, which can carry us into a new era of competence, pride, and influence. This is a task we must take upon ourselves; its rewards will not be conferred from the outside. Power is born from within. We must learn to take control of our profession and determine our own destiny. As practitioners, we are steadily becoming more assertive and creating our own opportunities, rather than complacently waiting for them to be handed to us.

Professional development must become a new part of the career process for all laboratory scientists—practitioners, faculty, and students. It cannot remain an optional activity to be considered only if and when time and funds permit. More importantly, it is an investment in yourself. The benefits are many; ranging from job security to the satisfaction of contributing to society, and the joy of personal and professional growth—both collective and personal.

CREATING OPPORTUNITIES

We must learn to foster the growth and development of our own careers. This entails expanding our general knowledge base and cultivating skills such as quantitative reasoning, problem solving, decision-making, and communication skills. Identifying strengths and weaknesses is helpful as part of the process of getting to the answer of WHO you are, and who you want to become. One plan for professional development consists of capitalizing on strengths while addressing weaknesses to neutralize or make assets of them. Assessing your personality in terms of work ethic, principles, values, personal style, and preference in the work environment is a worthwhile investment to begin the process (see Keirsey Temperament Sorter and other self-assessment tools discussed in Chapter 3). Always be prepared for any opportunity by knowing what your strengths and weaknesses are; how you can use your strengths to your advantage; and develop your weaknesses into strengths.

Throughout your professional career, it is important to have an updated **resume** and **curriculum vitae (CV)**. Resumes are typically one or two pages in length, although this may vary depending on your experience, or the position you are applying for (employers may have their own requirements). Resumes are short and meant to be persuasive, listing only the most relevant experiences, qualifications, skills, certifications, and other information relevant to the job. Resumes should also highlight your strengths, and provide proof of how your potential employer will benefit from hiring you.

There are several different resume styles. Some of the common types are the chronological, targeted, and functional resume. Each one is slightly different from another, primarily dependent on its purpose, or what you are trying to achieve with your resume. In a chronological resume, everything is listed in order of importance, depending on the job or skills required. It can be listed from past to present or the reverse, dependent on the requirements of the employer. In a targeted resume, you match your experiences to the qualifications and requirements of the job description as much as possible. The content of your resume should be customized to the position you are applying for in the institution or company.

Curriculum vitae are used mostly in the academic and scientific professions, instead of a resume, as well as when applying for a position internationally. A curriculum vitae (CV) is like a resume, except it is long, comprehensive, and informative. A curriculum vitae is useful for keeping track of all previous experiences: educational, professional, international, volunteer, etc. It includes all positions and duties performed education, qualifications, certifications, publications, association memberships, awards, honors, etc. However, when applying for a job, it is beneficial to create a new version of your curriculum vitae and omit any unnecessary information.

A cover letter is another important part of the job application. It is almost always required, and is considered proper etiquette to include when sending a resume or curriculum vitae for a job application. Cover letters are simple and straightforward, and should reflect and act as an introduction to your resume/curriculum vitae. This is your chance to show the potential employer why you are the right person for the position, by explaining how your qualifications fit the employer's requirements, and how the employer could benefit from having you as an employee. It also highlights your accomplishments that are relevant to the position without the employer searching for this information in a comprehensive and lengthy CV.

Another important step in creating your opportunities is interview preparation.

Be sure to research the company you are interviewing with beforehand, and learn about what the company does, how the company is organized/structured where it stands among its competitors, and how the company is doing business-wise. Study the resume you submitted and think about questions you may be asked, such as: "How does this (previous experience listed in resume) relate to the position you are applying for?" There are numerous possibilities for questions you may be asked during an interview. Several Internet resources provide other samples of common interview questions and can be located on websites, such as *Monster.com*.

Below are a few sample interview questions:

- "Tell me about yourself."
- "Describe your ideal boss."
- "How would your previous employers describe you or what would they say about you?"
- "What is your greatest weakness?"
- "What are some of your strengths?"
- "What are you most proud of?"
- "Why do want to work here? Why do you want this job?"
- "Tell me about a time when you faced adversity in the workplace and how you dealt with it."
- "Where do you see yourself in one year? Where do you see yourself five years from now?"

There are several strategies that can be used to answer questions during an interview. One method is to think about the question for a moment, and directly answer the question in a concise manner. When thinking about the interview questions, always try to relate your answer to the job to which you have applied. Do not trail off at the end of making a statement; this may show a lack of confidence. In addition, it is also a good idea to make a list of questions to ask the interviewer.

Even though you have already sent your resume to the interviewer, always bring extra copies of your resume with you, including one for yourself. Dress professionally and never under-dress for an interview; it is always better to be over-dressed. To ease anxiety, make sure to eat a light snack before the interview. This will keep your blood sugar and energy levels up. Be confident, polite, assertive, and honest. After an interview, it is proper etiquette to always send a thank you letter or card, via e-mail or mail — as soon as possible, whether you receive any feedback or not. Even if you do not receive any feedback or a job offer, thanking the person or company for their time and giving you the opportunity to interview with them will leave a good impression. However, it is also important to follow up with the interviewer within the next week.

STRATEGIC DEVELOPMENT PLAN

After learning to create your own opportunities and knowing how to capitalize on them, it is important to formulate a strategic development plan based on answers to the following "Who, Where, What, How, and When" questions.

1. Who am I as a professional and as a person?
2. Where do I want to be in 1 year, 3 years, 5 years, 10 years and by the close of my career?

3. What are the steps to get there?
4. How do I make opportunities happen?
5. When do I start?

Table 20-2 consists of a suggested timetable for creating your own opportunities. The strategic plan must include a way to acquire the requisite knowledge, skills, and attitudes for approaching your primary goal. There must be built-in mechanisms for maintaining your effectiveness, improving your approach to fulfilling responsibilities, and making satisfying adjustments to changes in your environment and circumstances. You can expect your overall goal to bring about improvements in the overall quality of your life.

CONTINUING DEVELOPMENT

It is your responsibility to facilitate your continuing development in order to meet your own needs, as well as those of your employer and others important in your life. You must be prepared to meet the demands for new knowledge, skills, and attitudes inherent in a changing society and workplace. This includes learning to be intuitive and anticipating change.

You must learn to increase your capabilities to effectively clarify your goals and values, in order to relate to others, and choose among competitive alternatives you have created and discovered for yourself. For this planning process, problem solving and decision-making are crucial processes. Both require the development, fine-tuning, and polishing of a range of abilities. Table 20-3 lists the basic abilities pivotal to effective problem solving and decision-making.

SUMMARY

A strategic development plan, using the techniques of opportunity creation, including utilizing your network and resources, can clarify and even plot your professional goals. It will put your planning into perspective for immediate visualization. By this process, the "perfect" job can suddenly become a reality, replacing anxiety and anticipation of a new position. Having "seen" this shining future image, you can then advance confidently, creating excellence as you go forward. Personally or professionally, there is no more satisfying venture.

TABLE 20-2.   Timetable for Creating Your Own Opportunities

	YEAR 1	YEAR 3	YEAR 5	YEAR 10
WHO				
WHERE				
WHAT				
HOW				
WHEN				

TABLE 20-3.   Key Problem-Solving and Decision-Making Skills

- Ability to analyze, store, and retrieve theoretical knowledge.
- Ability to coordinate or modify human behavior in complicated structures.
- Ability to engage in participatory decision-making.
- Ability to regulate and modify individual and group behavior.
- Ability to resolve conflicts in a professional and productive manner.
- Ability to respond to change and adapt creatively.

SUMMARY CHART:
Important Points to Remember

➤ Attaining and maintaining high standards of practice; sharing knowledge and expertise; contributing to and expanding overall body of knowledge are the responsibilities of a professional life.

➤ Flexibility, dedication to the profession, and a positive attitude are three elements that are basic to achieving the goals of professional development.

➤ Three abilities essential to effective decision-making are:

1. Ability to analyze, store, and retrieve theoretical knowledge.
2. Ability to coordinate or modify human behavior in complicated structures.
3. Ability to engage in participatory decision-making.

➤ Three abilities essential to effective problem-solving are:

1. Ability to regulate and modify individual and group behavior.
2. Ability to resolve conflicts in a professional and productive manner.
3. Ability to respond to change and adapt creatively.

➤ Expansion of the body of knowledge, growth in professional activities, scholarship, teaching, community service, professional activities, and research are all areas of professional development.

➤ Professional development in terms of operative skills is establishing activities and procedures to assist acquisition of the knowledge, skills, and attitudes that enable increased effectiveness in performing all functions related to professional life.

➤ The Five-Question Strategy for Creating Your Own Opportunities:

1. Who am I?
2. Where do I want to be in _____ years?
3. What are the steps to get there?
4. How do I make the opportunities happen?
5. When do I start?

➤ Professional development has become very important to laboratory science due to: new challenges, new regulations and technologies, the knowledge explosion, restructuring of the workplace, reorganization of institutions to respond to changing perspectives and priorities, economic pressures, and the growing need for continuing education.

SUGGESTED PROBLEM-BASED LEARNING ACTIVITIES

Chapter 20: Career Planning & Professional Development

Instructions: Use Internet resources, books, articles, colleagues, etc. to present solutions to the problems listed below. There is no one correct solution to any problem.

Note to Instructor: Students may be divided into groups and given the problem-based learning activity to discuss and solve. Once the group has reached consensus on a solution, the group may present it to other students in the class, thus providing all students with information about potential solutions.

Problem #1

Use the information in this chapter to identify methods of expanding your network.

Problem #2

Spend some time thinking about your goals and where you see yourself in the future. Utilize the suggested Timetable for Creating Your Own Opportunities (Table 20-2) and list your answers to the following "Who, Where, What, How, and When" questions and the corresponding years: 1) Who am I as a professional and as a person? 2) Where do I want to be in ___ years? 3) What are the steps to get there? 4) How do I make opportunities happen? 5) When do I start?

Problem #3

Find a job posting for a position you are interested in and create a targeted resume. Share your resume with colleagues, relatives, and professionals in your network, and request feedback. Use the suggestions to edit your resume and send it back out to your contacts.

BIBLIOGRAPHY

Bureau of Labor Statistics, U.S. Department of Labor: *Occupational Outlook Handbook, 2010–11 Edition*, Clinical Laboratory Technologists and Technicians. Last modified 29 Sept 2010. Accessed 17 Feb 2011, from: http://www.bls.gov/oco/ocos096.htm

Bureau of Labor Statistics, U.S. Department of Labor: *Occupational Outlook Handbook, 2010–11 Edition*, Medical and Health Services Managers. Last modified 29 Sept 2010. Accessed 17 Feb 2011, from: http://www.bls.gov/oco/ocos014.htm

Chappelow C, Leslie J: *Keeping Your Career on Track: Twenty Success Strategies*. Center for Creative Leadership, Greensboro, NC, 2005.

Hering B: *7 Questions That Make Interviewers Cringe*. CareerBuilder, 15 Sept 2010. http://msn.careerbuilder.com/custom/msn/careeradvice/viewarticle.aspx?articleid=2347

Kelly A: *Decision-Making Using Game Theory: An Introduction for Managers*. Cambridge University Press, Cambridge, England, 2003.

Marion P: *Career Tune Up*. Artemis Arts Library, San Francisco, CA, 2005.

McConnell C: *Umiker's Management Skills for the New Health Care Supervisor*, ed 4. Aspen Books, Denver, CO, 2005.

Pearce C, Maciariello J, Yamawaki H: *The Drucker Difference: What the World's Greatest Management Thinker Means to Today's Business Leaders*. McGraw-Hill, New York, NY, 2009.

Powell C: *Career Planning Strategies*, ed 5. Kendall/Hunt Publishing Company, Dubuque, IA, 2004.

Simmers L: *Health Science Career Exploration*. Delmar Learning, Clifton Park, NY, 2004.

Tracy B, Fraser C: *TurboCoach: A Powerful System for Achieving Breakthrough Career Success*. AMACOM Div American Management Association, New York, NY, 2005.

Warner J: *Problem Solving & Decision-Making Profile Facilitator's Guide*. HRD Press, Amherst, MA, 2003.

Yeung R: *The Ultimate Career Success Workbook: Tests & Exercises to Assess Skills & Potential!* Kogan Page Limited, Sterling, VA, 2004.

INTERNET RESOURCES

American Society for Clinical Laboratory Science (ASCLS)
http://www.ascls.org/

American Society for Clinical Pathologist (ASCP), Career Center
http://www.ascp.org/MainMenu/About ASCP/ASCP-Career-Center.aspx

Career Planning
http://careerplanning.about.com/

Career Resources Toolkit for Job-Seekers. Quintessentials Careers
http://www.quintcareers.com/career_resources.html

Clinical Laboratory Managers Association (CLMA), Career Center
http://careers.clma.org/home/index.cfm?site_id=131

Clinical Laboratory Scientist/Medical Technologist (CLS/MT) Accreditation Information. National Accrediting Agency for Clinical Laboratory Science (NAACLS)
http://www.naacls.org/accreditation/cls-mt/

E-Span Career Companion
http://www.careercompanion.com

Farrell B: *Preparing Your Resume Packet*. American Society for Clinical Laboratory Science, Washington, D.C., Accessed 19 Apr 2011, at: http://www.ascls.org/?page=Grad_Res

Focus V2. Career & Education Planning, Copyright 2009: Career Dimensions®, Inc.
http://www.focuscareer.com/

Harvard University, Office of Career Services. *Resumes* http://www.ocs.fas.harvard.edu/students/materials/resumes.htm

LinkedIn http://www.LinkedIn.com

Mapping Your Future http://mappingyourfuture.org/

Occupational Information Network (O*NET) http://online.onetcenter.org

Princeton Review. Career Quiz http://www.princetonreview.com/careerquiz.aspx

The Art of Career and Job-Search Networking: Critical career networking tools and resources for all job-seekers http://www.quintcareers.com/networking.html

The Importance of Networking and Relationship Building. Special Counsel, 2011 http://www.specialcounsel.com/legal-jobs/articles/importance-of-networking/

Glossary

This alphabetized glossary contains definitions of the bolded terms found throughout the text as well as select related terms pertaining to the principles of laboratory management.

40-Hour Workweek: A work rule consisting of varying hours worked per shift with a maximum of 40 hours per week. Overtime is defined as any time worked over 40 hours in one week.

8/80 Work Rule: A work rule consisting of ten 8-hour work shifts for a total of 80 hours worked within a two-week period. Overtime is defined as any time worked over 8 hours in one day or 80 hours in two weeks.

Accountability: Acceptance for success or failure.

Accreditation Standards: Guidelines used by various professional organizations in the voluntary accreditation process of laboratories and hospitals.

Affective Domain: A category of learning that is focused on attitudes, feelings, and behaviors. It also includes professional development issues, in this case pertinent to laboratory work, such as ethics, initiative, interpersonal skills with others, patient confidentiality of laboratory results, and professional interaction with other members of the health care team.

Affirmative Action: A duty imposed on certain federal contractors and subcontractors to not discriminate and take proactive measures in employment

decisions on the basis of race, color, sex, and national origin.

Age Discrimination in Employment Act of 1967 (ADEA): A federal law passed in 1967 that prohibits discrimination in employment against persons aged 40 years and older.

Ambulatory Payment Categories (APCs): A prospective payment system for hospital-based outpatient services. Services that are similar in terms of resource consumption are grouped into categories and a payment rate is calculated for each category. Patients may have more than one APC per visit.

Americans with Disabilities Act (ADA): A federal law that prohibits employers from discriminating against qualified individuals with a disability in employment decisions.

Analytical Phase: The phase of workflow consisting of actual testing of the sample.

Anchoring Trap: A decision-making trap in which the mind gives disproportionate weight in favor of the first information it receives.

Application: A written document that details a perspective employee's education, qualifications, and work experience.

503

Appraisal Cost: Represent the costs of laboratory activities associated with measuring, evaluating, or auditing products or services to assure conformance to regulatory, accreditation, and customer requirements. Considered "good" quality costs because the related activities help the laboratory catch and correct nonconformances before they adversely affect the quality of laboratory service or patient safety.

Appropriation Budget: A type of budget commonly associated with government agencies and characterized by an authorized spending level for a specific period.

Assets: The resources owned by the organization. Assets can have a physical form, such as a building, or may be intangible and have economic value.

At-Will Employment Doctrine: A common law employment standard that defines the employment relationship as terminable at the will of either party, at any time, for any reason.

Authority: The right to make decisions.

Autocratic Style: A group-decision making technique in which the leader of a group makes a decision without consulting with the others in the group.

Autonomy: Allows rational individuals to make their own decisions and act on them.

Balance Sheet: A financial statement that represents the financial position of an organization at a particular point in time, or (usually) at the end of an accounting period.

Behavioral Approach: An approach to leadership that is focused on what a leader "does" rather than what a leader "is." The behavioral approach took the position that leadership can be learned through education, training, life, and work experience.

Benchmarking: The process of determining a standard (i.e., best practices) used in measuring and/or judging quality to achieve superior customer results and business performance.

Beneficence: An ethical principle that entails an obligation to protect persons from harm. The principle of beneficence can be expressed in two general rules: (1) do not harm; and (2) protect from harm by maximizing possible benefits and minimizing possible risks of harm.

Billable Procedure: A laboratory test that is billed to a payer (the payer may be an individual or a private or government insurer).

Blake-Mouton Managerial Grid: A leadership model proposed by Robert Blake and Jane Mouton who visualized leadership styles in terms of a balance between concerns for getting the job done and the working relationships that must be integrated to achieve effective leadership.

Bona Fide Occupational Qualifications (BFOQ): Requirements that are essential for successful performance of the job, despite the fact that they may be related to a legally protected classification such as age, sex, or religion. Race can never be a BFOQ.

Brainstorming: A method for developing creative solutions to problems by focusing on a problem, and then deliberately coming up with as many unbounded solutions as possible and then pushing for ideas as far as possible. In this phase, "the sky is the limit."

Break-Even Analysis: A process performed using the costing information to determine if the total of all fixed and variable costs equals the amount of revenue generated (the break-even point). One of the uses for this method is to help determine the best alternative between several possibilities (i.e., decisions about providing in-house testing versus using a reference laboratory).

Break-Even Point: The point at which there is no profit or loss from performing a test, but that the total of all fixed and variable costs, equals the amount of revenue generated by the test. Used to determine the number of tests needed to be performed to generate enough revenue to cover the expenses incurred.

Browser-Server Model: A computer model, fundamental to Internet interactions, from which end-users may directly access (browse) specialized information that is available on demand from powerful server computers, thus creating a user-friendly interface for navigating the network.

Budget: A financial plan for allocating funds to cover the expenditures such as supplies, salaries, and overhead involved in the operation of the laboratory.

Budget Justification: A report that compares the budget to actual events (particularly actual expense). The report highlights any variances present and should propose concrete solutions for any encountered.

Budgeting: A system for formalizing in writing a quantitative financial plan supportive of the institution's financial mission, for a given period.

Budget—Performance Report: A document that provides forward looking financial information for a given time period based on past performance and analysis of the future. It compares budget expectations with actual performance.

Bureaucracy: A form of organization with functional specialization, clear delineation of authority, and decision-making based on rules developed to pursue organizational goals consistently and efficiently.

CAP: College of American Pathologists.

Capital Budget: A plan that identifies anticipated purchases of capital assets and the expected source of funds required to make the purchases.

Capitation: A payment methodology used to reimburse managed care plans whereby a provider is paid a set amount per member per month for contracted services regardless of the number of services used by the patient.

Carve Out (Carved Out): A type of payment plan in which the reimbursement rate is based on the type of care being provided. For example, a hospital room rate may be at a set reimbursement rate unless the patient is in a special care unit (such as ICU). These special care unit days are "carved out" of the set reimbursement rate and may have a separate per diem rate, or they may be reimbursed on a fee-for-service basis.

Case Mix: The mix of patients seen by the provider based on diagnosis, severity of illness and utilization of services. The higher the case mix, the more costly the care.

Cash Flow Projection: A projection of all changes affecting cash in the categories of operations, financing, and investments.

Cash Flow Statement: A financial statement that reflects the flow of cash through an organization over a period and is segmented in three distinct categories: cash flow from operating activities, cash flow from investing activities, and cash flow from financing activities.

CDC: Centers for Disease Control and Prevention.

Centers for Medicare and Medicaid Services (CMS): A federal agency who partnered with the Centers for Disease Control and Prevention (CDC) to develop the CLIA'88 regulations. The CMS, formerly known as the Health Care Financing Administration (HCFA), is responsible for the following activities: registering laboratories for CLIA certificates, collecting fees, on-site and self-inspection surveys, survey or guidelines and training (for enforcement actions when needed), approving proficiency testing providers, accrediting professional organizations, and exempting states.

Central Processing Unit (CPU): The core piece of hardware in a computer system. It controls the interpretation and execution of instructions provided by the software.

Character: A suggested leadership quality that refers to a person who promotes ethical decision-making and expects ethical behaviors from others.

Charge Description Master (CDM): A list of all billable services, their associated CPT (billing) codes, and the price that is charged to the patient or insurance carrier.

Clinical Laboratory Improvement Amendments of 1988 (CLIA'88 or CLIA): A set of quality standards mandated by the federal government to ensure accuracy, reliability, and timeliness of patient test results.

Closed System: An organization that is internally focused (less considerate of external forces), in which top-down authority and reliance on policy and procedures are typical. In a relatively stable, slow changing environment, the closed, mechanistic approach may be appropriate.

Coercive Power: The capacity to apply punishment to those who refuse to comply with requests or demands.

Cognitive Domain: A category of learning that is focused on acquiring and applying knowledge.

COLA (Formerly known as the Commission of Office on Laboratory Accreditation): A voluntary organization that initially accredited only physician office laboratories. Today, COLA also accredits other test sites including those located in small hospitals.

Collaboration: The act of working together with other individuals to achieve a common end.

Collaborative Management: A scenario in which individuals feel appreciated and understood; they are not forced to comply by a mandate from their supervisor. Individuals work with their supervisors to make decisions and to solve problems. The four basic principles of collaborative management are trust, understanding, independence, and solutions.

Communication: The act of disseminating and receiving information using either written or oral transmission; may be formal or informal in nature.

Competency: The knowledge, skills, abilities, or characteristics associated with high performance on a job such as problem solving; definitions of a competency include motives, beliefs, and values.

Competency-Based Performance Evaluation: An evaluation based on a limited number of specifically defined tasks that are taught and assessed by direct observation during orientation and then periodically thereafter.

Competency Modeling (Model): A performance evaluation design that uses core competencies (organizational capabilities or strengths—what an organization does best).

Compliance: The adherence to applicable requirements, rules, standards, regulations, and guidelines to maintain licensure and accreditation.

Computer Network: A group of computers connected via wires or through radio frequency (wireless), which share data by employing a standard set of specifications for the data transmitted.

Confirming-Evidence Trap: A decision-making trap in which there is a mental bias that leads managers to seek out information to support their existing point of view while avoiding information that contradicts it.

Congruence Model: An organizational model that shows detailed elements of an open system and the dynamics involved; used to analyze environmental relationships of an organization and to assess the relationships of its constituent parts.

Consensus: General agreement of an issue/solution reached by more than one individual; individuals may not like the decision made but are willing to "live with it."

Consultative Style: A group decision-making technique in which the leader obtains suggestions and ideas from group members and then makes a decision that may or may not reflect the group members' influence.

Continual Improvement: Constantly striving to improve services, products, or processes. Often achieved by using quality improvement methods (i.e., Plan-Do-Check-Act (PDCA) cycle, Shewhart Cycle, Six Sigma, etc.).

Contribution Margin: The amount remaining from sales revenue after variable expenses have been deducted.

Controlling: A performance measurement of implementation whereby adjustments and corrective actions can be taken to ensure that organizational goals are achieved.

Coordination: The blending of functions so that they are intertwined and build on each other thereby minimizing the risk of duplication or redundancy.

Co-Payments: A dollar amount representing a predetermined proportion of total medical costs that the insured has to pay out of pocket (that is, self-pay) each time health services are received after the deductible has been paid.

Core Competency: A term that refers to organizational capabilities or strengths—what an organization does best.

Corrective Action: Taking action to make changes in the process to conform to established protocols and/or procedures.

Cost: The charge (in dollars) associated with providing a billable procedure; also known as an expense; assets that have been purchased such as inventories of lab supplies that have yet to be used, or equipment whose cost has not been expensed through depreciation.

Cost Accounting: A system for providing analysis or forecast of information to be used in financial decision-making.

Cost-Benefit Analysis: One approach for determining and comparing the forward looking, incremental costs, benefits, and values of solution alternatives. It is designed to determine if the results are of significant benefit to justify the cost of taking the action.

Cost Center: An organizational unit for which revenue and expenses are accumulated separately in the accounts.

Cost per Reportable: The cost of the reagents and the equipment used to run the test is a set, pre-determined amount contracted with the vendor for each test reported.

Cost-per-Test: The sum of the expenses required to perform one laboratory test. Also referred to as *microcosting*.

Cost-Volume-Profit (CVP) Analysis: More commonly called *Breakeven*.

Courage: A suggested leadership quality that refers to the willingness to make change and accept challenges to the status quo.

Credibility: A suggested leadership quality that refers to excellent credentials, substantive knowledge, and sound practical experience that a successful leader possesses.

Criteria-Based Performance Evaluation: An evaluation based on rating the performance of the employee on specifically defined criteria such as knowledge, judgment, attendance, and reliability.

Cultural Intelligence: A person's ability to function effectively in situations characterized by cultural diversity.

Culture: Basic assumptions, values, and norms shared by members of the organization.

Current Value of Money: The value of money today versus its value at a point further in the future.

Curriculum Vitae (CV): A document used primarily in the academic and scientific professions, as well as internationally when applying for a job; similar to a resume, except it is long, comprehensive, and informative.

Database: A set of data organized into tables. The rows of the tables are made up of records, and the columns of the tables are fields that contain the same kind of data elements.

Debt Ratios: Ratios used to determine the organization's ability to meet long-term debt obligations.

Decision Making: The process of choosing among several alternatives.

Decision Tree: A graphic diagram consisting of nodes and branches used for visualizing alternative choices facing managers in a given situation or problem. The nodes represent decisions to be made. The branches are alternative choices.

Dedication: Devotion to the job or profession.

Deductibles: Dollar amounts that insured individuals must pay first (usually annually) before benefits of an insurance plan are payable.

Definition Tables: A collection of records arranged in rows that define the procedures and terminology of a computer-based information system. In a laboratory information system (LIS), these tables contain such information as test definitions, patient ward locations, and physician demographics.

Delegation: A group decision-making technique in which a leader turns over a problem to the group and lets them generate and evaluate alternatives and attempt to reach agreement on a solution without any leader involvement.

Demographic Environment: An aspect of the marketing environment that is focused on the people who make up the market; consists of population numbers stratified by age and gender, educational levels, ethnic backgrounds, and growth rates.

Department: A cost center or group of cost centers with one person given responsibility for operations.

Dependency Theory: A theory based on where power comes from. According to this theory, individual/group A will have power over an individual/group B, if B is dependent on A.

Depreciation: A dollar amount determined by the number of years over-which a piece of equipment is accounted for on the general ledger; typically, the dollar amount that is "written off" is the same over the useful lifetime of the equipment.

Descriptive Database Table: A collection of records arranged in rows that contain the historical events that have occurred in a database. In a laboratory information system (LIS), these tables contain such information as patient demographics, test orders, and test results.

Diagnostic Related Groups (DRGs): A patient classification system, initially developed to evaluate quality and resource consumption in a hospital setting, used in the Prospective Payment System (PPS) for inpatient care for Medicare patients. Services that are similar in terms of resource consumption are grouped into categories and a payment rate is calculated for each category.

Direct Expense (Cost): All of the charges (in dollars) directly related to performing a laboratory test. It includes the reagents, consumables, labor, and benefits, etc.

Directing: The use of leadership skills to obtain unified action through issuing directives, building participation, and achieving consensus. Also known as leading.

Disc Array: A disk storage system that consists of several linked hard discs.

Document Control: A structured document control system links a laboratory's policies to respective processes and procedures and ensures that only the latest approved versions of documents are available for use.

Economic Environment: An aspect of the marketing environment that focuses on the purchasing power of the people in the market; this environment may be affected by many factors including the savings rate, interest rates, money supply, and inflation.

Economies of Scale: Increased cost efficiencies achieved when producing or performing a larger quantity of goods or services.

Electronic Health Record (EHR): Individual patient data or medical record kept in an electronic form.

Electronic Medical Record (EMR): Individual patient data or medical record kept in an electronic form.

Emotional Intelligence: A concept proposed by Daniel Goleman, which consists of basic emotional competencies that describe the abilities needed to manage our relationships and ourselves effectively. These include self-awareness, self-management, social awareness, and social skills. A suggested leadership quality that refers to the basic emotional competencies that allow leaders to manage themselves as well as their relationships with others effectively.

Empower: A suggested leadership quality that refers to the ability and willingness of a leader to share power/authority. This may be done by delegating responsibility to others whenever possible.

Environment: External forces that affect an organization's ability to achieve its objectives and goals. Environment may include suppliers, customers, competitors, and regulators and encompasses economic, political, cultural, and technological driving forces.

Equal Employment Opportunity Commission (EEOC): A federal agency with the duty of administering a variety of federal laws including Title VII of the Civil Rights Act of 1964, the Americans with Disabilities Act (ADA), the Age Discrimination in Employment Act (ADEA), and the Equal Pay Act (EPA).

Equal Pay Act (EPA): A provision of the federal Fair Labor Standards Act of 1938 that prohibits discrimination in the payment of wages based on gender.

Essential Functions: Those duties and responsibilities that are critical for successful performance of the job.

Expense: The charge (in dollars) of providing a billable procedure; also known as cost.

Expense Budget: A document that identifies planned expenditures based on forecasted units of service.

Expert Power: The type of power derived from power holders' superior knowledge, skills, and abilities.

External Failure Costs: Occur after release of laboratory test results or reports and during or after the furnishing of a laboratory service to a customer (e.g., blood collection, pathology consultation, etc.). Considered "bad" quality costs.

Failure Costs: The price the laboratory pays for nonconformance (resulting from products or services not conforming to requirements or customer/user needs, they are the costs resulting from bad quality), and are considered losses.

Fair Labor Standards Act of 1938 (FLSA): A federal law that defines how and when employees shall be paid and setting standards for minimum wage, wage classification such as exempt or nonexempt status, hours of work, and overtime payments.

Family and Medical Leave Act of 1993 (FMLA): A federal law that provides eligible employees with up to 12 weeks of unpaid leave for the employee's own serious health condition, to care for an immediate family member who has a serious health condition, after the birth of a child, or placement of a child in the employee's home for adoption or foster care.

Fee-for-Service: A payment method whereby a provider is paid a specific amount for a specific service. Fees charged will increase if the corresponding costs increase.

Feedback Skills: Skills that supervisors find necessary to effectively communicate with their employees about things such as work performance. Such skills include communicating clear goals and objectives, listening, praising the positive aspects, and diplomatically identifying situations in which corrections may be necessary to make before they become a problem.

Financial Accounting: The process of generating financial records and forecasts and performing strategic planning for an entire entity; often produced by the department of finance in the institution.

Financial Management: The process of planning, organizing, directing, controlling, and evaluating available monetary resources. The primary goal of financial management is to ensure the profitability and survival of the organization.

Financial Ratios: A tool consisting of ratios that managers use to manage finances and thus maintain internal control of these finances. It is based on the premise that ratios mean nothing unless it can be compared to something else.

Financial Ratios and Analysis: Used to evaluate financial statements.

Fishbone Diagram: A diagram that systematically analyzes cause and effect relationships and identifies potential root causes of a problem.

Five Forces Analysis: A marketing analysis model that serves as a framework for analyzing external opportunities and

threats. The five forces are the bargaining power of suppliers, the bargaining power of buyers, the threat of new entrants, the threat of substitute products, and the rivalry among existing firms.

Fixed or Static Budget: A type of budget that contains estimates for a single level of activity.

Fixed Costs: Expenses that do not change over a given period regardless of testing volume. Examples include administrative salaries and rent.

Flexibility: The capability to adapt to new, different, or changing requirements. It is the ability to take new directions and opportunities as they emerge.

Flexible or Variable Budget: A budget that takes into account the fact that certain costs vary with the level of activity, and other costs remain fixed over a relevant range of activity. Flexible budgets are designed to anticipate the possibility of change and show planned revenues and expenses at various levels of activity.

Flowchart: A picture or diagram of a process used to graphically represent the sequence of activities in a process and shows where instructions are needed.

FOCUS-PDSA: An acronym for a process management tool, which stands for: **F**ind an opportunity, **O**rganize a team, **C**larify current process, **U**nderstand variation, **S**elect improvement, **P**lan your actions, **D**o the actions, **S**tudy the results, **A**ct on your conclusions.

Food and Drug Administration (FDA): A federal agency of the United States Department of Health & Human Services (USDHHS). One of the FDA's responsibilities includes categorizing test methods for complexity.

For-Profit Entity: A privately held company (i.e., a corporation), whose profits are taxed by the government and distributed to the owners (individuals or shareholders). Its primary purpose is to generate adequate revenue to be profitable.

Framing Trap: A decision-making trap that deals with how one views his/her own choices or how one frames the questions around the problem. A frame may lead individuals into other decision-making traps such as anchoring.

Full-Time Equivalent: The equivalent of one employee working full-time; that is, 2080 hours per year.

Functional Structure: An organizational model that is hierarchical and bureaucratic in nature; specialized units within the model report in an upward chain of command; responsibility and authority within the organization are clearly understood.

Functions: A management term referring to a process and strategy for dealing with issues of change.

Global Transformational Leadership: Transformational leadership in the international or global setting.

Goals: Outcomes that one strives to achieve.

Governmental Payers: Public sources of funding (such as Medicare and Medicaid) that pay for the care of a patient.

Hardware: The physical pieces of equipment that make up a computer system such as the central processing unit, display monitors, keyboards, and printers.

Health Care Financing Administration (HCFA): See Centers for Medicare and Medicaid Services (CMS).

Health Information Exchange (HIE): A piece of software, which integrates electronic data management systems into the Electronic Medical Record (EMR) and provides an additional interface that allows users to view a consolidated electronic medical record including all lab and pathology test results.

Health Insurance Portability and Accountability Act of 1996 (HIPPA): A federal statute that requires most patient information to be considered protected and confidential.

Health Level Seven International (HL7): Standards set by the HL7 organization, for compatibility of health information systems, with the goal of creating widely used standards for health care data management, which are used in more than 55 countries.

Health Maintenance Organization (HMO): The most common type of managed care organization. See *Managed Care* for further details.

Hierarchical Database: A structured set of data organized into tables that link records together like a company organizational chart. Records can be retrieved only through the top level of the structure.

High Complexity Testing: The most difficult laboratory testing determined by examining seven criteria among which are test system, troubleshooting, test interpretation, and judgment.

High-Low Analysis: Shows how to determine the relationship between two related variables and derive a cost formula or function that determines the levels of fixed and variable costs. The function can then be used to estimate or budget future costs.

Hiring: Choosing the person who will be doing the work.

Historical-Based Budgeting: Budgeting above 100% of the previous year. To budget in this way, the total spent in the previous year is divided by 12. The number obtained plus a percentage for inflation is used to budget for the upcoming year.

Hospital Information System (HIS): A computer system consisting of servers from different areas in the hospital connected via an interface engine. Designed to manage the hospital's medical and administrative information in order to enable health professionals to perform their jobs effectively and efficiently.

Human Resource Management (HRM): The overall management of the people within an organization as resources including activities related to recruitment, selection, development, staffing, scheduling, and performance.

Humility: A suggested leadership quality that refers to the ability of a leader to realize that others may also have good ideas and accept the fact that one may be wrong.

Implementing: The act of putting a plan into operation by carrying out the steps and activities designated to achieve the goal.

Income Forecasting: An estimation of future revenues used to set goals.

Income Statement: A financial document indicating what has transpired financially within an organization over a period, usually monthly or yearly; a document that represents the financial outcome of an organization over a period.

Incremental Budget: Addresses only changes like new equipment, new positions, and new programs. It assumes that all current operations are essential to the process and working at its peak performance. The advantage is the minimal time commitment for incremental budget preparation and the disadvantage is assumption that all existing operations are essential for business.

Indirect Expense (Cost): All of the charges (in dollars) that are part of doing business but are not directly related to the cost of the test being evaluated; also known as *overhead*. Examples include marketing, licenses, and information systems requirements.

Influence Approach: An approach to leadership in which leadership is an influence or social exchange process.

Information Management: The set of processes that ensures the confidentiality and integrity of patient information and test results. This quality system essential includes the activities of using, manipulating, and transferring the patient information, test results, and reports in the laboratory's paper and/or electronic information systems.

Inpatient: A patient receiving care while in the hospital.

Input-Throughput-Output Mechanism: A process that takes a product and/or information (concerning the product) from the environment (input); transforms, converts, and processes it (throughput); and then exports a changed product back into the environment (output).

Insight: A suggested leadership quality that refers to the ability to determine and understand clearly the nature of things, which is often accomplished through intuition.

Instructional/Educational Objectives: Clearly stated directives written in measurable terms for the purposes of achieving goals related to instruction.

Integrity: A suggested leadership quality that is based on the premise that the value individuals place on themselves and others is paramount to being effective.

Interface: Specialized software and hardware connections between different information systems that allow the systems to communicate with each other, even when the systems use different programming languages.

Internal Audit: An internal assessment tool conducted by laboratory staff. An internal audit reviews a specific laboratory process and determines by examination of documents, records, interviews, and observations whether the process meets applicable requirements and follows the laboratory's policies, processes, and procedures.

Internal Failure Costs: Represent costs incurred before delivery of the product or provision of a service; considered "bad" quality costs.

Interview: In-person, oral process that serves as confirmation of a perspective employee's application and to fill in any gaps.

Job: An arrangement through which work is done; products or services are delivered in the mutual interest of a worker and an employer.

Job Analysis: The analysis and documentation of the tasks, conditions, requirements, and authority arrangements of a working situation.

Job Application: A written document requesting work.

Job Description: A written document describing the tasks, expectations, reporting relationships and other information relative to the employment of an individual; also referred to as a position description.

Joint Decision: A group decision-making technique, also known as democratic style, in which the leader shares the problem with the relevant team members as a group. Together alternatives are generated and evaluated. The group strives to reach a consensus that determines the decision made.

Just Cause: A standard by which adverse employment actions may be assessed to determine whether they were appropriately taken and generally includes at least five factors: forewarning, proper investigation, evidence, lack of discrimination, and penalty meets the offense.

Justice: An ethical principle requiring fairness in distribution of burdens and benefits; often expressed in terms of treating persons of similar circumstances or characteristics similarly.

Keirsey Temperament Sorter: A system developed by David Keirsey and adapted from the Myers-Briggs Type Indicator questionnaire for identifying actions and attitudes associated with 16 personality types.

Laboratory Information System (LIS): A class of software used to handle information produced from laboratory testing. As such, all laboratory information systems function within the framework of a computer network.

Leaders: Individuals who influence the opinions and attitudes of others to accomplish a mutually agreed on task while maintaining integrity and moral purpose of all involved. Leaders are central individuals who guide others in achieving a goal.

Leadership: A quality exhibited by individuals; occurs when one individual attempts to influence the behavior of others (a group) to accomplish goals (either personal or organizational).

Leading: See *Directing*.

Lean Data Management: A process management tool for improving efficiency through eliminating wasteful practices.

Learning Outcome: A desired result achieved by a learner after completing an instructional experience.

Lease: In a lease arrangement, monthly payments are determined and spread over a specified period of time, and are based on the purchase price plus interest, taxes, insurance, and maintenance. Typically, the lease option is used when lump sum capital dollars are not available to outright purchase.

Legitimate Power: The type of power derived from a person's position or job in an organization.

Liabilities: The obligations that an organization has to its creditors. These may be short-term, due in one year or less; or long-term, greater than one year.

Liquidity Ratios: Ratios used to determine the organization's ability to meet short-term debt obligations.

Local Area Network (LAN): A computer network that connects computers and devices in a geographically small area.

Mainframe Computer: A high-performance computer that functions as a server or mainframe constructed for durability and high volume storage.

Maleficence: The act of committing harm to ourselves or other people.

Managed Care: A means of providing health care services within a network of health care providers, with the goal of ensuring high quality and cost effective health care to the patients belonging to a managed care plan.

Management: Achieving organizational goals in an effective and efficient manner by working with and through people.

Management Accounting: The analysis of cost and revenue data that provides information on operations and budgeting for managers.

Management Review: The laboratory's management team should carefully review the quality report and set priorities for the problems that need the most immediate attention. Problems can be prioritized by considering all of the issues and the laboratory's situation, importance of the problems will be unique to each laboratory.

Managerial Cost Accounting: A system for providing an analysis of cost information used in decision-making.

Managers: Individuals, usually administrators, who are able to influence decisions and actions.

Market: A web of interactions among those who have commercial relationships or the potential for such relationships with other buyers and sellers of similar commodities.

Market Analysis: A continuous cyclical process of analyzing marketing opportunities, developing a marketing strategy, planning and implementing the plan, and revising the plan by responding to market forces.

Market Demand: The determination of how many current customers in a particular market purchase a product or service.

Market Segmentation: The breaking up of markets into smaller, more manageable pieces.

Marketing: A process by which individuals and groups obtain what they want through creating, offering, and exchanging products or services of value with others.

Marketing Concept: A business philosophy whose central tenet is that the key to achieving the goals of the organization consists of being more effective than the competition in satisfying the needs, wants, and demands of the customer.

Marketing Environment: The surroundings that influence the marketing and business planning of a company including demographics, economic climate, political, legal, and societal structures, available technologies, and natural resources.

Marketing Mix: The set of tools that a firm uses to pursue their marketing objectives. These tools include product, price, place, and promotion.

Marketing Plan: An action plan or a roadmap to guide the company from one place to the next. Aspects of the plan include descriptions of the products or services, as well as their benefits and features, target markets and corresponding buying habits, competing products or services, and the customer problem that the product or service is designed to eliminate.

Marketing Research: A technical and systematic approach to obtain data relevant to a specific market. It is the systematic design, collection, analysis, and reporting of data and findings relevant to a specific marketing situation.

Matrix Organizations: Organizations that take advantage of the skills or functions present; this structure works best when the demands of the environment are changing and uncertainty is the norm; skill diversification, also known as cross-training, is encouraged.

Mechanistic Structure: An organizational model that consists of a highly structured environment with communication from the top down and reliance on authority-obedience relationships; appropriate in environments of slow change and relative stability.

Microcosting: The process of determining the actual cost of performing a billable procedure (cost-per-test).

Mission Statement: A document that states the purpose, attitude, and core competencies of a group, department, or an institution.

Mixed/Semi-Variable Costs: Costs that change in increments based on workload or volume change.

Moderate Complexity Testing: The middle level of laboratory testing determined by the examination of knowledge, training and experience, and calibration, quality control, and proficiency testing materials plus four other criteria.

Myers-Briggs Type Indicator: A method of identifying actions and attitudes associated with 16 predefined personality types. Individuals take a self-assessment and the pattern of their answers correlates with these personality types.

Natural Environment: An aspect of the marketing environment that deals with raw materials and available energy to manufacture a company's products.

Net Income: The amount of net revenue minus operating expenses for a given period. Net income is presented as the bottom line of the income statement.

Net Present Value: A calculation used to indicate the current value of income generated in the future discounted at an estimated percentage equal to the inflation rate over the years of income generation. This demonstrates the concept that the value of a dollar today is more than the value of a dollar in the future.

Network Structures: Structures consisting of specialized units, either internal or external to the organization, that are linked together by informal or formal agreements.

Networking: Utilizing the relationships in your organization, profession, or industry. Capitalizing on the knowledge and expertise of colleagues and peers; extracting information, encouraging, and partaking in collaborative efforts.

Niching: A marketing strategy consisting of a company focusing on a specific subsection of a market.

Non-Billable Procedure: A laboratory procedure that contributes to the generation of a billable test result, but that is not directly reimbursable; examples include standards, quality control specimens, and repeat testing of samples.

Nonconformance: Processes that detect, report, evaluate, and correct events in laboratory operations that do not meet the laboratory's requirements.

Nonmaleficence: Do not inflict unjustified harm to ourselves or other people.

Nonwaived Testing: For quality control and quality assessment CLIA requirements, moderate and high complexity are grouped and referred to as nonwaived testing.

Not-for-Profit Entity: An organization (such as a community-based hospital) in which the profits made are not taxed, and are held by the organization to further its cause. Such organizations exist to provide a service such as health care.

Objectives: Directives developed to accomplish established goals.

Occupational Safety and Health Administration (OSHA): A federal organization that is responsible for regulations relating to the general workplace safety and protecting the health of U.S. workers.

Open System: A system that is in active exchange with its environment.

Operating Budget: An overall plan that identifies the expected resources and expenditures of an entity for a given future period of time, usually one year.

Operating Margin: Refers to the profits that are generated from the excess of revenues received for providing a service.

Opportunities for Improvement: A step in the Plan-Do-Check-Act (PDCA) cycle, a quality improvement process.

Organic Structure: An organizational model consisting of an environment that features decentralized decision-making and encourages adaptability and flexibility; appropriate in environments of change.

Organizational Structure: The way in which an organization divides its tasks and coordinates them for overall goal achievement. Commonly represented visually as an organization chart.

Organizing: The process of determining the steps needed to implement a successful plan.

OSHA's Standard Precautions: Standards set by the Occupational Safety and Health Administration (OSHA) for the handling of biological specimens, formerly known as Universal Precautions. These standards mandate that all blood, body fluids, tissue, and other potentially infectious materials be treated as equally hazardous.

Outcomes Assessment: The final quantitative and qualitative evaluation of the effectiveness of the plan used to obtain an organizational goal.

Outpatient: An ambulatory patient who visits the hospital for services but is not admitted to the hospital.

Overconfidence Trap: A decision-making trap in which the manager believes that they are better at making forecasts or estimates than they actually are; such individuals are overly confident about their ability to predict leading to a narrow range of possibilities.

Overhead: See *Indirect Expense (Cost).*

Owner's Equity: The book value of the organization.

Pareto Chart: A graphic technique designed to help identify major factors and distinguish between the "vital few" causes and the potentially less significant ones of a given problem. It is based on the Pareto principle, which states that approximately 80% of the problems can be attributed to 20% of the causes (also known as the 80/20 rule).

Passion: A suggested leadership quality that refers to the excitement and enthusiasm a leader possesses about the leadership role and all of its components.

Path of Workflow: A sequence of processes in the laboratory that begins with the input of the clinician's ordering of a test through the activities of sample collection, sample transport, sample receiving and accessioning, testing, review, report preparation, and report delivery and ends with the output of accurate test results and interpretations back to the clinician.

Patient Test Management: The aspect of laboratory testing concerned with maintaining sample integrity and positive patient identification throughout the testing process. Defined policies and procedures must be in place to ensure proper patient preparation, sample integrity, and identification from sample collection through test result reporting.

Payback Analysis: A calculation that identifies the length of time it will take to recover the initial expenditure for a project or providing a service. The calculation used is P/I where P = the purchase or investment cost and I = the annual income or revenue generated by the service.

Payback Period: The time it will take to generate the incoming revenue that compensates for the money paid out for an item such as a piece of equipment; a ratio that identifies the time it will take for revenue or other positive cash flows to cover the initial outlay related to an investment project.

Payer: The individual, government agency, or insurance group that pays for the care of a patient.

Per Case: A type of reimbursement payment methodology whereby a provider and insurer agree on a per case reimbursement rate. This rate is based on the premise that certain diagnoses and procedures have a relatively similar treatment protocol.

Per Diem: A type of payment methodology whereby a set amount of reimbursement is agreed upon based on a per day rate that a patient is in the hospital.

Performance Development: An actively ongoing two-way process between employee and supervisor for communicating about the employee's job performance designed to help them achieve excellence in their position and create job satisfaction. Processes involved include goal setting, feedback, guidance, motivation, evaluation, and development planning.

Performance Evaluation: The periodic comparison of measured actual performance to the requirements stated in the job description.

Performance Objectives: Specific directives developed for the accomplishing of established goals that deal with job performance.

Personnel Budget: The portion of the expense budget that includes all expenses related to personnel such as salaries, fringe benefits, vacation, holidays, and shift differentials.

Personnel Development: A function of management that refers to encouraging and providing opportunities to staff employees to gain additional knowledge for personal and professional growth. In-services and continuing education lectures are examples of such opportunities.

Place: A marketing mix tool that refers to the "how and where" a product or service is offered to the buying public.

Planning: The management function that clarifies the process of attaining organizational goals. It includes activities such as data gathering, assessment, risk calculation, and determination of strategy.

Plus/Minus/Interesting (PMI): A tool developed to evaluate the pros and cons of decision-making options. It consists of a table with space for writing in the information that matches these three columns: plus (positive points of taking the action), minus (negative points of taking the action), and interesting (extended implications of taking the action, both positive and negative in nature).

POCT: Point-of-Care Testing.

Political and Legal Environment: An aspect of the marketing environment that consists of pertinent political and legal issues related to federal government agencies, legislation, and lawsuits.

Position Description: A listing of all of the essential and nonessential functions of a job, including requirements related to education and experience; also referred to as a job description.

Positive Attitude: Optimism, and the vitality it generates, independent of changing circumstances, that are essential for personal and professional advancement and achievement.

Positive Self-Esteem: A suggested leadership quality that refers to the ability of leaders to believe in themselves by working selflessly to support others working toward the common good of the organization.

Postanalytical Phase: The phase of workflow that consists of finalizing and reporting test results.

Power: The capacity to influence others' behavior.

Preanalytical Phase: The phase of workflow that consists of the steps taken before actual testing.

Premiums: The dollar amount charged by the insurer to individuals to insure against specific risks.

Prevention Costs: Represent the costs of laboratory activities specifically designed to prevent poor quality in laboratory services. Prevention costs are considered "good" quality costs because the related activities prevent errors or problems altogether.

Price: A marketing mix tool that refers to the amount of money a customer pays for a product or service.

Private Accounting: The activities performed by an entity for its own managerial activities.

Private Payers: Refers to commercial insurers (such as Anthem Blue Cross) that pay for the care of a patient.

Problem Solving: The process of identifying and defining a problem, determining what happened to cause it, and what steps or possible solutions will be necessary to solve it.

Procedure: Procedures provide instructions for each activity in the larger process.

Process: A set of interrelated resources and activities that transforms inputs into outputs.

Process-Based Structures: Emphasize the lateral relationships in an organization and allow the organization to use resources for customer satisfaction. The process-based structure focuses around the process driving the structure and the customer defining the performance.

Process Control: A set of activities that ensures that a given work process will keep operating in a state that is continuously able to meet process goals without compromising the process itself.

Process Designs: Broad overall plans used to develop and design a process or way of completing work or doing a task. Once the process design is developed, workflow can be analyzed.

Process Management: A systematic data based approach to improving performance by continuously monitoring the performance of processes and identifying opportunities for improvement using proven problem-solving methods without sacrificing quality.

Process Management Tools: Standardized process improvement methodologies used in process management (i.e., FOCUS-PDSA, Six Sigma, etc.).

Product: A marketing mix tool that refers to what a firm offers to the public for sale.

Production Concept: A business philosophy that suggests that customers will buy goods in adequate volume at a low enough price.

Professional: One who adheres to the technical or ethical standards of a profession.

Proficiency Testing (PT): A mechanism to assess the internal quality for CLIA regulated analytes in testing sites performing moderate and/or high complexity testing. Laboratories enroll in a program whereby they periodically receive "unknown" specimens and are required to test them just like the patient samples. Results are sent to the program administrator for grading. Corrective actions are in place for laboratories that do not meet the criteria established by the administrator.

Profitability Ratios: Ratios that demonstrates the organization's efficiency of operations.

Program Budget: A type of budget created based on a specific program matrix that includes all proposed services and the resources required.

Promotion: A marketing mix tool that refers to the means by which a company communicates and promotes its products to its target market.

Prospective Payment System (PPS): A payment system in which hospitals receive a set amount of reimbursement per patient discharge. This system incorporates the Diagnostic Related Group (DRG)-based reimbursement system for all Medicare inpatients.

Provider: Refers to the hospital, the outpatient department, the physician, or other health care professional who furnishes care to the patient.

Provider-Performed Microscopy Procedures (PPMP): A CLIA certificate issued to a laboratory for physicians, midlevel practitioners, or dentists to perform PPMP procedures (a predetermined list of tests, such as a microscopic urine examination), as well as tests on specimens collected during a physical examination. Laboratories with this category CLIA certificate may also perform waived testing.

Prudence Trap: A decision-making trap that managers fall into when faced with a high-stakes decision. These individuals tend to adjust their estimates or forecasts "just to be on the safe side."

Psychomotor Domain: A category of learning that involves the actual performing of identified tasks, such as performing laboratory tests, or skills.

Public Accounting: The making available of financial activities to regulatory, government, and private accounting firms for both informational purposes and to meet regulatory requirements.

Quality: The degree to which a product or service meets requirements.

Quality Assurance (QA): Ensuring the overall quality of the testing process accomplished by the development of a written plan that includes a mechanism to evaluate the effectiveness of the laboratory's policies and procedures, identify and correct problems, ensure reliable and prompt reporting of results, and testing performed by competent individuals. QA is a set of planned actions to measure and provide confidence that the performance of laboratory processes that influence the quality of the laboratory's results and reports (other than testing), are working as expected, individually, and collectively.

Quality Control (QC): Provides control only of test methods by testing and documenting prepared samples with known expected results before or in conjunction with unknown patient samples. Includes having written procedures in place for the monitoring of and evaluating the quality of the analytic testing of each test performed to ensure accuracy and reliability of patient results and reports.

Quality Costs: The costs of preventing quality problems, measuring quality levels, controlling and/or inspecting quality levels, and failing to accomplish the desired quality levels.

Quality Indicators: The quality indicators monitored in the laboratory's QA program are also helpful but do not usually cover all important aspects of the laboratory's path of workflow. Can be used to determine measurable failure costs.

Quality Management (QM): Actively and continuously validating that processes work as intended before implementation; monitoring process performance; knowing where the problems are; continuously determining root causes of problems and removing them; and documenting the actions taken. In QM organizations, quality is everyone's job all the time—to make their best professional contributions to patient care and safety.

Quality Management System (QMS): A quality management system (QMS) is the means to organize all the management activities that support the laboratory's preanalytic, analytic, and postanalytic processes in a way that meets applicable requirements. QMS provides a framework for building quality principles and practices into *all* laboratory operations, starting with test ordering and proceeding through delivery of test reports.

Quality System Essentials (QSEs): A model for a generic quality management system that meets all the requirements of U.S. laboratory regulatory and accreditation organizations has been published by the Clinical and Laboratory Standards Institute (CLSI) in a guideline that describes how to use 12 Quality Systems Essentials (QSEs) as a means to organize all the policies, processes, and procedures that any laboratory needs to meet those requirements.

Random Access Memory (RAM): A type of computer data storage, which has a very fast transfer rate, allowing rapid access to stored data that is processed, or is waiting to be processed by the CPU.

Rate of Return: The ratio of the annual revenue to the price of the project calculated as follows: I/P where I = the annual income or revenue generated and P = the cost of providing the service or original investment in the project.

Ratio Analysis: The use of ratios to compare an aspect of one organization to that of another; a specific example is comparing laboratory operations of one institution to those of another.

Reagent Rental: An agreement that usually commits the laboratory to a minimum volume of reagent purchased over a specified period at a set price. The cost of the instrument is included in the reagent cost.

Reasonable Accommodation: A duty incumbent on employers under the Americans with Disabilities Act (ADA) to provide qualified employees and candidates with remedial measures or devices, absent an undue burden on the organization.

Recallability Trap: A decision-making trap associated with bias in terms of "it worked before." Managers in this trap get caught in using past experiences to forecast the future and are thus overly influenced by those past events that left a strong impression on them.

Reciprocal Approach: An approach to leadership in which a relational and shared process includes a strong emphasis on followership.

Records: Records capture the results or outcomes of performing procedures and testing in written forms or electronic media such as manual worksheets, instrument printouts, tags, or labels.

Redundancy: The utilization or setting up of backup systems such as hard drives, to maintain proper equipment functionality, if their equivalents were to fail.

Referent Power: Exists when the power-holder is liked, respected, or admired by others. Referent power represents a more profound base of power than those based on incentives or threats.

Registration Certificate: A CLIA certificate issued to enable laboratories to conduct waived, moderate, and/or high complexity laboratory testing.

Regulatory Requirements: Standards that are required by federal law.

Relational Database: A structured set of data organized into tables that link records together through common data elements in the tables. Records are retrieved from multiple tables by matching the common data elements in those tables.

Remedial Action: The immediate action taken by the person discovering the nonconformance is known as remedial action and is the initial quick-fix solution. Remedial actions most often do not address the real cause of the problem, which can be determined only through investigation.

Request for Proposal (RFP): A document used by laboratories to solicit bids from various vendors. It includes specific requirements and questions concerning each vendor's product capabilities. Vendors may include in their bids proposed solutions to certain problems outlined in the RFP.

Resource Allocation: The distribution of resources.

Resource Based Relative Value Scale (RBRVS): The payment system used for reimbursing physicians for services rendered. A payment rate is calculated based on geographic region, service performed, malpractice costs, and practice overhead.

Resource Management: The justification and accountability of resources.

Respect for Persons: A principle stating that (1) individuals should be treated as autonomous agents, and (2) persons with diminished autonomy are entitled to protection.

Responsibility: Assignment for accomplishing a goal.

Resume: A short document that lists only the most relevant experiences, qualifications, skills, certifications, and other information relevant to the job. It is typically one or two pages in length, depending on your experience, or the position you are applying for (employers may have their own requirements).

It is meant to be persuasive and should highlight your strengths, and provide proof of how your potential employer will benefit from hiring you.

Retained Earnings: In a for-profit organization, represent the company's earnings over time less any dividends distributed.

Return on Investment (ROI): A profitability ratio used to demonstrate the organization's efficiency of operations. A dollar amount that is used when evaluating the cost versus rent or lease option; calculated by taking the profit margin and multiplying it by asset turnover. The goal is to at least breakeven on the return.

Revenue Budget: A document that identifies each of the different types of revenue to be earned, according to the period in which it will be earned.

Revenues: Monies that the laboratory receives or is entitled to receive (i.e., income) for the services and testing it has provided.

Reward Power: The capacity to influence others by providing positive rewards. Positive rewards may include raises, promotions, assignment of preferred tasks, recognition, etc.

Rolling Budget: A continuous budget that is updated periodically in preparation for the next budget cycle; a rolling budget for a 12-month period is typically reviewed and revised every quarter.

Router: A device that connects area networks to national networks that make up the Internet, or World Wide Web.

Sales Concept: A business philosophy that promotes factory products sold by aggressive selling.

Scatter Diagram: A plot of one variable versus another to see if there is any relationship between the two variables.

Scheduling: Assigning a worker to a specific task or work area.

Self-Contained Unit Structure: An organizational model that centers around a common basis such as a discipline, location, customer group, or technology; in this model, the components that make up the common basis function using their own expertise and supervision, hence the term self-contained.

Self-Esteem: A suggested leadership quality that includes selflessly supporting people toward the common good of the organization.

Self-Payers: Those individuals who do not have any other type of insurance and must pay for their own health care.

Self-Scheduling: A scheduling program that allows employees to have more control over their schedules and gives them more flexibility.

Semivariable Costs: Expenses incurred in the laboratory that will vary but only incrementally based on workload volume change. An example of such a cost is a technologist's salary.

Sense of Humor: A suggested leadership quality that refers to the ability of leaders to incorporate laughter (humor) at appropriate times, especially during highly stressful instances.

Shewhart Cycle: A problem-solving approach that incorporates scientific principles of analysis. It is a continuous circular process that includes four steps: Plan, Do, Check, and Act (PDCA).

Situational Contingency Approach: Since the 1960s, situational contingency approach has emerged, focusing on the importance of the context of the situation in explaining leader effectiveness. The central point of the contingency approach is that the leadership style needed would change with the situation.

Six Sigma: A process management methodology that focuses on improving quality and eliminating errors. The underlying assumption of the Sigma methodology is that the cause of a defect or failure is variation.

Spaghetti Diagram: Also known as a Standard Work Chart; is tracking on paper the path of the person or persons performing the process tasks. Called a Spaghetti Diagram because of the lines drawn to trace the operation sequence, this step-by-step documentation is a visual creation of the flow and describes the actual activities, distance from the last step, estimated task time, observations, and return rate.

Staffing: The hiring, training, scheduling, and retaining of the employee who will be doing the work or task.

Standard Operating Procedures (SOPs): Comprehensive written instructions for processes that are completed on a regular basis.

Subspecialties: A subordinate field of specialization.

Supervisory: The lower levels of management.

Surcharge/Cost Plus Method: Using the surcharge/cost plus method, the actual cost of performing the test is determined using the microcosting method. The total cost is then multiplied by a factor (e.g., 1.5 times cost) or a dollar amount is added to the cost (surcharge) to arrive at the final price.

SWOT Analysis: An analysis to determine the Strengths, Weaknesses, Opportunities, and Threats facing the organization; may give a different view from that presented in the budget process.

System: A collection of interdependent, interconnected elements that constitute an identifiable whole.

Systems: Made up of individuals who share a common purpose and perform tasks in service of that purpose.

Task/Production Management: Individual activities based on the manager's needs and that of the organization, not on the individual. This creates a submissive, passive, and dependent feeling in the individual. Individual frustration, resentment, and underproduction often result.

Tasks: The routine duties for which a laboratory manager is held responsible and accountable.

Taxonomy Levels: Levels/categories of learning designed to aid an instructor in defining appropriate learning outcomes.

Technological Environment: An aspect of the market environment that deals with advancements in technology such as the advent of cellular phones, satellite television, DNA technology, and numerous new medications.

Telehealth: The delivery of health-related services and information with telecommunications technologies.

Telemedicine: Practicing medicine from a distance, usually using video conferencing, e-mails, or telecommunications.

The Joint Commission (TJC): A voluntary organization that accredits more than 80% of the U.S. health care organizations. Formerly known as Joint Commission on Accreditation of Health care Organizations.

The Laboratory Accreditation Program of the College of American Pathologists (LAP-CAP): Accredits only laboratory testing sites and not the entire health care organization. Similar to TJC, emphasizes an overall total quality management approach and continuous quality improvement for the entire analytical process, including management of pre-analytical, analytical and postanalytical errors.

Theory X-Theory Y: A model designed for managers to operate by that is based on the premise that two sets of expectations (known as X and Y) about employees' attitudes and abilities ultimately influence their work performance. The Theory X manager is likely to compensate for the shortcomings of the workers and tends to be dictatorial and autocratic. The Theory Y manager possesses a more optimistic set of expectations, suggesting that workers are highly motivated, self-disciplined, and creative problem-solvers, thus capitalizing on worker strengths.

Theory Z: A theory based on McGregor's Theory Y. The Z-philosophy implies that changing societal goals must be included in the workplace and that productivity and rewards are not the only objectives of workers, but other issues such as quality of their work lives have a significant impact on their performance.

Title VII of the Civil Rights Act of 1964: A federal law that prohibits discrimination based on race, color, creed, religion, national origin, and sex.

Total Quality Costs: Is a measure of both "good" and "bad" quality costs.

Trait Approach: A historical approach to leadership that resulted in the generation of lists of personal traits that supposedly guaranteed successful leadership to those individuals possessing them; such traits include height, charisma, and intelligence.

Training: Teaching a worker the department policies and procedures.

Trend Analysis: A management tool that examines an organization's performance over a given period.

Unlawful Harassment: Occurs as the result of an individual exhibiting inappropriate behaviors based on sex (whether or not of a sexual nature), color, race, national origin, religion, protected activity, disability, or age.

Unit Costs: See *Cost-per-Test.*

USDHHS: United States Department of Health and Human Services; also referred to as HHS (Health and Human Services).

Validation: Documented evidence that provides a high degree of assurance that a system or process will function consistently as expected; the managed process of determining that something accomplishes what it is intended to accomplish. Validation challenges all activities in a new process to provide a high degree of assurance that the process will work as intended in the live environment.

Value: The worth of a product or service in money or goods.

Value Chain: The process of creating customer value, described by Michael Porter as a chain, which includes the support activities and primary activities. The value chain has four levels of support activity represented by the vertical links in the chain, and five primary activities of a firm, represented by the horizontal links of the chain. The support activities include: firm infrastructure, human resource function, technology, and materials management. Primary activities include inbound and, outbound logistics, operations, marketing/sales, and customer service. Both vertical and horizontal links in the chain lead to increasing profit margin. Laboratory inbound logistics include all the steps of getting the specimen into the laboratory.

Variable Costs: Expenses that vary based on workload volume and change in direct relationship to that volume. Examples include reagents and supplies.

Variance Analysis: The process of analyzing and evaluating differences between actual and budgeted performance.

Variation: Disparity or difference in the act, state, result, or process.

Vision: A suggested leadership quality that refers to the ability to "see the big picture" to determine strategic/future directions of a department and/or organization. It also refers to the ability to effectively communicate such directions to others.

Waived Tests (WT):   Laboratory tests considered simple and foolproof (such as glucose monitoring via devices cleared by the FDA for home use). Tests in this category are determined by examining seven specific criteria including reagents and materials preparation and characteristics of the operation steps.

Waiver: A CLIA certificate that permits a site to perform only those test methods identified as waived.

Wide Area Network (WAN):   A computer network that connects computers and devices in a large geographic area.

Workflow: The process of work through a workstation or department from the beginning to the final product/end of the task.

Work Group: A group of employees working together in various capacities with the goal of accomplishing work-related tasks.

Zero-Based Budget: A budgeting method by which the appropriate manager must annually reevaluate all activities to decide whether they should be eliminated or funded; projects are approved based on funds availability and funding levels are determined by priorities. Each year every department manager is required to justify the entire unit budget as though it were totally new.

Index